Pain Management

Ahura Bassimtabar

Pain Management

A Scientific Compendium for physiotherapists

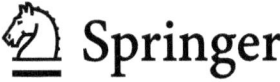 Springer

Ahura Bassimtabar
Deutsche Sporthochschule Köln
Köln, Germany

ISBN 978-3-662-71561-1   ISBN 978-3-662-71562-8 (eBook)
https://doi.org/10.1007/978-3-662-71562-8

© The Editor(s) (if applicable) and The Author(s), under exclusive license to Springer-Verlag GmbH, DE, part of Springer Nature 2025

This work is subject to copyright. All rights are solely and exclusively licensed by the Publisher, whether the whole or part of the material is concerned, specifically the rights of translation, reprinting, reuse of illustrations, recitation, broadcasting, reproduction on microfilms or in any other physical way, and transmission or information storage and retrieval, electronic adaptation, computer software, or by similar or dissimilar methodology now known or hereafter developed.
The use of general descriptive names, registered names, trademarks, service marks, etc. in this publication does not imply, even in the absence of a specific statement, that such names are exempt from the relevant protective laws and regulations and therefore free for general use.
The publisher, the authors and the editors are safe to assume that the advice and information in this book are believed to be true and accurate at the date of publication. Neither the publisher nor the authors or the editors give a warranty, expressed or implied, with respect to the material contained herein or for any errors or omissions that may have been made. The publisher remains neutral with regard to jurisdictional claims in published maps and institutional affiliations.

This Springer imprint is published by the registered company Springer-Verlag GmbH, DE, part of Springer Nature.
The registered company address is: Heidelberger Platz 3, 14197 Berlin, Germany

If disposing of this product, please recycle the paper.

Gender Disclaimer

For the purpose of better readability, gender-specific writing is omitted. The generic masculine is used, whereby all genders (masculine, feminine, diverse) are equally meant.

Preface

Receiving the opportunity from the renowned Springer Publishing House to write a textbook on pain fills me with deep gratitude and at the same time with the awareness of a great responsibility. Even during my time being a physiotherapy trainee, I found the abstract treatment of the topic 'pain' unsatisfactory—there was a large discrepancy between the limited understanding of the underlying mechanisms and the abundance of therapy approaches for pain relief that were taught to us.

In therapeutic practice, a kaleidoscope of different approaches and explanatory models is revealed, with the market seemingly living off the constant introduction of new, preferably complex-seeming theories. This is extremely unsatisfying, both for me as a therapist and for the patients, who must be completely confused when they present the same problem to three different therapists and receive three different explanations. The reasons for this, in my opinion, are manifold: There is a lack of a uniform, nation-/worldwide curriculum, the existing curricula are only inadequately oriented towards evidence-based guidelines, and the basic knowledge about the symptom of pain is still very, let's say, expandable. In addition, a large number of professional groups in the context of pain therapy feel compelled to market their own approaches in order to underpin their right to exist.

I do not have a patent solution to remedy these shortcomings at hand. However, a start can be made in knowledge transfer. While experts and politicians argue about the academization of physiotherapy, the setting in which high-quality knowledge combined with clinical expertise is taught and learned is irrelevant in my eyes. The content must be correct. Why not through a book that addresses fundamental questions: What is pain? How and why does it occur? Which factors lead to chronification? And how can it be alleviated? This book not only competes with existing practice and teaching, it hopefully enhances them and becomes an indispensable part of pain education. Not because I am a particularly great author, but because I fill existing and proven gaps with the contents of this book; through insights that already exist. As my first work in the field of specialist literature, this vision may seem daring. Premieres carry both risks and opportunities: They can fail, like the Wright brothers' first attempt to get a motorized airplane off the ground, or triumph, like Walt Disney's first animated film "Snow White and the Seven Dwarfs". Whether I succeed in setting a milestone in pain literature with this textbook remains to be seen. But just as Disney was not primarily after fame, but innovation in the animation field, so my main goal is to make a substantial contribution to the understanding and treatment of pain, regardless of commercial success. I eagerly await whether I will succeed in this.

Ahura Bassimtabar

Acknowledgment

I'll make it brief. Everything in my life I owe to my father. His actions have shaped me so deeply that I can hardly find words to express my gratitude. A big thanks also goes to my little, or rather younger, brother, who always stands by my side, everywhere and at all times. Moreover, successful professional careers are never just the product of one's own performance, but also of situational promotion, support, and appreciation by colleagues and mentors. To all friends and colleagues, whether in sports physiotherapy, university, teaching, research, or professional politics, I would like to express my heartfelt thanks at this point.

Contents

1 **Pain—The History** 1
   1.1 Spirituality and Religions 2
   1.2 Medicalization 6
   1.3 Neuroscience and Cognition 10
   References... 16

2 **The Neurobiology of Nociception** 19
   2.1 Transduction 24
   2.2 Transmission 27
   2.3 Modulation... 33
   2.4 Perception 39
   2.5 Forms of Pain... 41
   References... 45

3 **The Neurobiology of Pain**.................................... 49
   3.1 Pain-Relevant Brain Areas............................... 53
   3.2 Acute Pain Interpretation 57
   3.3 Chronic Pain Perception 64
   3.4 Neuroplasticity.. 72
   3.5 Sensitization.. 74
   3.6 The Bio-psycho-social Model as a Solution? 80
   References... 81

4 **The Postural-Structural-Biomechanical (PSB) Model** 93
   4.1 Postural Deficitsglenohumeral Internal Rotation Deficit......... 95
   4.2 Movement Deficits..................................... 101
   4.3 Structural Deficits 110
   4.4 PSB Therapies 112
   References... 118

5 **Examination and Treatment of Pain** 131
   5.1 Pain Education.. 132
   5.2 Investigation.. 137
      5.2.1 Medical History 137
      5.2.2 Clinical Tests 138

		5.2.3	Questionnaires	142
		5.2.4	Documentation and Illustration	146
	5.3	Therapy		149
		5.3.1	General Recommendations for Pain Therapy	150
		5.3.2	Specific Recommendations for Pain Therapy	152
		5.3.3	Change Management	162
	References			165
6	**Exercise Planning in Pain Therapy**			179
	6.1	A Progressive Approach		179
		6.1.1	Movement Modification	180
		6.1.2	Are Pains Allowed During Exercises?	183
	6.2	Specific Exercise Recommendations		185
		6.2.1	Chronic Lower Back Pain	186
		6.2.2	Chronic high cervical pain	196
		6.2.3	Chronic Neck Pain	206
		6.2.4	Chronic Shoulder Pain	212
		6.2.5	Chronic Knee Pain	216
	References			231

Glossary of Abbreviations

ACC	anterior cingulate cortex
ACT	Acceptance and Commitment Therapy
ADL	activities of daily living
AH	Anterior horn
AMPA	α-Amino-3-hydroxy-5-methyl-4-isoxazole-propionic acid
ATP	Adenosine triphosphate
BDNF	brain derived neurotrophic factor
BL	Prone position
BMS	basic motor skill
BPSM	bio-psycho-social model
BWS	Thoracic spine
C	Celsius
CBT	cognitive-behavioral therapy
CFT	Cognitive Functional Therapy
CGRP	Calcitonin Gene-related Peptide
CIPA	congenital insensitivity to pain with anhidrosis
CM-PF	Centrum medianum and Ncl. parafascicularis of the thalamus
cm	Centimeter
CMS	Constant-Murley Score
Comp.	Comparison
CNS	central nervous system
COX	Cyclooxygenase
CPM	conditioned pain modulation
CRPS	complex regional pain syndrome
CSI	Central Sensitization Inventory
CWP	Chronic Widespread Pain
DASH	Disabilities of arm, shoulder, hand
DLPFC	dorsolateral prefrontal cortex
DMN	Default Mode Network
DNIC	diffuse noxious inhibitory control by painful stimuli
EAA	excitatory amino acid
e.g.	for example
EKPQ	Essential Knowledge of Pain Questionnaire

ESAS	Elbow Self-Assessment Score
FAB-Q	Fear Avoidance Belief Questionnaire
FAOS	Foot and Ankle Outcome Score
Fig.	Figure
FT	Fiber thickness
FHP	forward head posture
fMRI	functional magnetic resonance imaging
GA	Graded Activity
GABA	Gamma-Aminobutyric Acid
GAP	growth associated protein
GCT	Gate Control Theory
GE	Graded Exposure
GIRD	glenohumeral internal rotation deficit
GMD	grey matter density
GMI	Graded Motor Imagery
HH	Posterior horn
HIT-6	Headache Impact Test-6
HOOS	Hip Disability and Osteoarthritis Outcome Score
IASP	International Association for the Study of Pain
ICF	International Classification of Functioning, Disability and Health
IL-N	intralaminar nuclei
kg	Kilogram
KOOS	Knee Injury and Osteoarthritis Outcome Score
KTW	Knee to Wall
lOFC	lateral orbitofrontal cortex
LT	Lissauer's Tract
LTP	long-term depression
MBSR	mindfulness-based stress reduction
MCC	middle singular cortex
mg	Milligram
MHQ	Michigan Hand Outcomes Questionnaire
mm	Millimeter
mPFC	medial prefrontal cortex
MRI	Magnetic Resonance Imaging
MT	Manual Therapy
Myel.	Myelination
N	Newton
N.	Nerve
NAA	N-Acetylaspartate
Ncl.	Nucleus
ND	navicular drop
NDI	Neck Disability Index
NGF	nerve growth factor
NK-1	Neurokinin-1
NLG	Nerve conduction velocity

NMDA	N-Methyl-D-Aspartate
NPQ	Neurophysiology of Pain Questionnaire
NRPS	Numeric Rating Pain Scale
NSLBP	nonspecific low back pain
ODI	Oswestry Disability Index
OFC	orbitofrontal cortex
PA	physical activity
PAG	periaqueductal gray
PCS	Pain Catastrophizing Scale
PDI	Pain Disability Index
PFC	prefrontal cortex
PNE	Pain Neuroscience Education
PRMD	Pain-Related Movement Dysfunction
PSB	postural-structural-biomechanical
rACC	rostral anterior cingulate cortex
RMDQ	Roland Morris Disability Questionnaire
rNPQ	revised Neurophysiology of Pain Questionnaire
ROM	Range Of Motion
RVM	rostral ventromedial medulla
S1	primary somatosensory cortex
S2	secondary somatosensory cortex
SDT	sensory discrimination training
SIA	stress-induced analgesia
SIAS	anterior superior iliac spine
SIJ	Sacroiliac joint
SIPS	superior posterior iliac spine
S-LANSS	selfreported Leeds Assessment of Neuropathic Symptoms and Signs
TENS	transcutaneous electrical nerve stimulation
TNF-α	Tumor necrosis factor alpha
TP	Time point
TrkA	Tyrosine Kinase-A
TRP	transient receptor potential channels
TSK-11	Tampa Scale of Kinesiophobia-11
VAS	visual analogue scale
Vgl.	Comp.
VPI	ventroposteroinferior
VPL	ventroposterolateral
VPM	ventroposteromedial
vlPFC	ventrolateral prefrontal cortex
W	Work
WDR	wide dynamic range
WHO	World Health Organization
YLD	years lived with disability

List of Figures

Fig. 2.1	Fiber type-dependent pain response, own production	23
Fig. 2.2	Temperature-specific TRP types, own production.	25
Fig. 2.3	Descartes pain pathway. (from the book "Traite de l'homme" 1664, public domain). https://upload.wikimedia.org/wikipedia/commons/8/8a/Descartes-reflex.JPG	27
Fig. 2.4	Nociceptive transmission. primary neuron (yellow), secondary neuron (orange) and tertiary neuron (red)	28
Fig. 2.5	Pathways of the spinal cord (by Polarlys, 05.06.2006, unchanged).	29
Fig. 2.6	Lissauer's tract (LT), own production. PH = posterior horn, AH = anterior horn	30
Fig. 2.7	Laminae of the spinal cord, own production	31
Fig. 2.8	Transmission path of nociceptive signals, own production.	32
Fig. 2.9	Nociceptive inhibition, own production 1.1 = Nociceptive influx through a noxious stimulus, 2.1 = New stronger nociceptive influx through a larger noxious stimulus in another area, 1.2 = Attenuation of the weaker nociceptive influx, 2.2 = Constant, but in relation stronger, nociceptive influx of the second stimulus..	38
Fig. 2.10	Pain dimensions 1, own illustration.	41
Fig. 2.11	Pain dimensions 2, own illustration.	41
Fig. 3.1	Perception formation	50
Fig. 3.2	Aspects of pain perception (graphically).	52
Fig. 3.3	Aspects of pain perception (anatomically). The arrows for point 3. (Modulation) represent the influences by the interneurons and descending pathways	52
Fig. 3.4	Cold application with different colors, own production	60
Fig. 3.5	Man at his PC, own creation	76
Fig. 3.6	Woman opening the door, own production	77
Fig. 3.7	Angry man, own production	77
Fig. 3.8	Allodynia and hyperalgesia, own production	78
Fig. 4.1	Anterior position of the head, own illustration	97
Fig. 4.2	Lumbar curvature, own production	98

Fig. 4.3	Pelvic obliquity, own production	100
Fig. 4.4	Right knee valgus, own production	103
Fig. 4.5	Navicular Drop. Distance between the ground and the tuberosity of the navicular bone, own production	105
Fig. 4.6	Right scapular dyskinesis, own production	106
Fig. 4.7	Lifting with a rounded back, own production	108
Fig. 4.8	Angle of pressure	114
Fig. 4.9	Course of pressure	114
Fig. 4.10	Strength of pressure	114
Fig. 4.11	Amplitude of pressure	114
Fig. 4.12	Speed of pressure	115
Fig. 4.13	Frequency of pressure	115
Fig. 4.14	Area of pressure	115
Fig. 5.1	Protectometer, own production	134
Fig. 5.2	ICF, own creation	137
Fig. 5.3	Graph with clinical pain reports. (Own creation)	147
Fig. 5.4	Correction to the middle, own creation	165
Fig. 6.1	Comfort and discomfort zone, own production	181
Fig. 6.2	Pain monitoring, own production. Action plan for 1. Pain intensity, 2. -increase and 3. -duration	185
Fig. 6.3	painful deadlift	187
Fig. 6.4	painful bending	187
Fig. 6.5	Knees to chest bilaterally. Continuing lumbar spine flexion over maximum hip flexion with emphasis through a towel	188
Fig. 6.6	Knee to chest unilaterally. Regression to 6.5, less continuing lumbar spine flexion due to contralateral hip extension	188
Fig. 6.7	Knees to chest bilaterally with head elevation. Progression to 6.5. More flexion pre-setting from cranial and more continuing lumbar spine flexion	188
Fig. 6.8	Lumbar spine flexion from standing position. Closer to the problematic movements than a flexion from the supine position	189
Fig. 6.9	Lumbar spine flexion from standing position with band. Progression of intensity compared to 6.8.	189
Fig. 6.10	Lumbar spine flexion from standing position with elbow support. Progression of kinematics compared to 6.8. The elbow support provides more upper body inclination and more hip flexion, thus more deep lumbar spine flexion	189
Fig. 6.11	Lumbar spine flexion from sitting position	190
Fig. 6.12	Lumbar spine flexion with upper body inclination from sitting position	190
Fig. 6.13	Lumbar spine flexion from assisted standing position	191

Fig. 6.14	Lumbar spine flexion from standing position with support. By transferring weight through the hands, the patient can be given a sense of security and the load can be reduced. In addition, the upper body inclination is initiated with a neutral lumbar spine and the lumbar spine flexion is added later. From a cognitive perspective, this is not the bending movement that the patient has stored as painful...................	191
Fig. 6.15	Relieving bending movement with band. Grasp a sufficiently firm band with the palms of your hands, which takes some body weight. This allows a more relaxed position for the patient and possibly less protective tension of the posterior muscle chain..	192
Fig. 6.16	Bending with antagonistic resistance. By working the anterior muscle chain against the band, the focus may be shifted away from the painful work of the posterior muscle chain......	192
Fig. 6.17	Indirect lumbar spine flexion on the cable pull. This exercise can indirectly train the lumbar spine. The hip flexion makes the posterior muscle chain and the lumbar spine biomechanically more resilient to flexion, however, this exercise does not imply lumbar spine flexion and the patient may see less risk in this than in direct bending movements. By reversing the Punctum Fixum and Punctum Mobile, a detour is often possible for movements coded as painful...................	193
Fig. 6.18	Jefferson Curl hip and lumbar spine dominant..............	194
Fig. 6.19	Jefferson Curl thoracic spine dominant. Regression to 6.18 through less leverage (biomechanically) and less similar movement to the patient's problematic movement (cognitively), which is hip and lumbar spine dominant. Sometimes it is worth educating the patient to clarify that performing a new movement, such as this one, is a movement modification and not the same movement that usually causes problems. This may make the patient more likely to engage.........	194
Fig. 6.20	Jefferson Curl from assisted standing. Regression to 6.18	195
Fig. 6.21	Lumbar spine flexion with ball from assisted standing. Biomechanical regression to 6.20 through closer weight guidance and less leverage................................	195
Fig. 6.22	Jefferson Curl from sitting. Regression to 6.20 through a more distant position to the patient's problematic bending movement from standing (cognitively), possibly however kinematically seen a progression due to the stronger hip and thus lumbar spine flexion	196
Fig. 6.23	tense cervical spine	197
Fig. 6.24	painful cervical spine rotation	198

Fig. 6.25	Cervical spine rotation from supine position. The weight transfer to the ground usually allows for a safer execution and greater range of motion for the patient	199
Fig. 6.26	Cervical spine rotation from elevated supine position. Progression to 6.25.	199
Fig. 6.27	Thoracic spine-dominant rotation. Through the visual fixation of the moving palms and the rotation of the upper body with horizontal shoulder adduction, the cervical spine is biomechanically rotated further, but the movement is not an implicit cervical spine rotation exercise and may serve as a cognitive opener.	200
Fig. 6.28	Thoracic spine rotation without head rotation. Through the visual fixation of a point and a thoracic spine rotation without head rotation, an indirect counter-rotating cervical spine rotation is created. In the following example, there is a reversal of Punctum Fixum and Mobile, with the thoracic spine rotating to the left and the cervical spine indirectly rotating to the right.	200
Fig. 6.29	Chin-in from supine position. Isometric activation of the high cervical flexors and deep cervical extensors	201
Fig. 6.30	Isometric cervical extension	201
Fig. 6.31	Isometric cervical flexion.	202
Fig. 6.32	Isometric cervical lateral flexion to the left	202
Fig. 6.33	Isometric cervical rotation to the left. It is difficult to create a torque into the rotation with a band. It helps to sit further forward so that the pull goes dorsolaterally.	203
Fig. 6.34	Isometric cervical rotation to the left with the hand. With the hand, a better anti-rotation activity can be triggered by a pressure on the lateral forehead towards the medial	203
Fig. 6.35	Deep cervical mobilization. The nose always points towards the ground. This achieves movement of deep cervical and high thoracic segments.	204
Fig. 6.36	High cervical mobilization. Nose and head swing along, look forward and down at the back. Progression to 6.35 in individual patient cases, who particularly have problems in high cervical regions	204
Fig. 6.37	Dynamic strengthening of cervical flexion. Example for cervical flexion. Extension from prone position	204
Fig. 6.38	Dynamic strengthening of cervical flexion from overhang. Progression to 6.37 due to larger range of motion.	205
Fig. 6.39	Dynamic strengthening of cervical flexion with band.	205
Fig. 6.40	Dynamic strengthening of cervical rotation with band	205
Fig. 6.41	painful neck	206
Fig. 6.42	painful shoulder abduction.	207

Fig. 6.43	Passive shoulder abduction with fulcrum. By swapping Punctum Fixum and Mobile, the abducting muscles are less activated and indirectly a greater abduction is achieved than would be the case actively against gravity.	208
Fig. 6.44	Assistive shoulder abduction with rod. Progression to 6.43 through more active work of the abducting muscles. The push of the right hand relieves the left shoulder compared to abduction without a rod	208
Fig. 6.45	Shoulder abduction with antagonistic resistance. The adducting muscles are eccentrically active during abduction and can relieve the abducting muscles and facilitate abduction. The movement task is an adduction, which can also be a cognitive approach to the abduction coded as painful.	209
Fig. 6.46	Shoulder abduction with resistance	209
Fig. 6.47	Shoulder flexion with resistance	210
Fig. 6.48	Shrugs with resistance	210
Fig. 6.49	Unilateral shrugs. Progression to 6.48 through ipsilateral cervical spine lateral flexion in the concentric phase and contralateral cervical spine lateral flexion in the eccentric phase.	211
Fig. 6.50	Upright Rowing	211
Fig. 6.51	Painful shoulder flexion	212
Fig. 6.52	Painful overhead press	213
Fig. 6.53	Assistive shoulder flexion with rod	214
Fig. 6.54	Shoulder flexion with abutment on the wall	214
Fig. 6.55	Incline Dumbbell Bench Press	215
Fig. 6.56	Adjusted Overhead Press. Another possible regression is the Overhead Press in the closed chain with a barbell or in a guided device	215
Fig. 6.57	Front Raise	216
Fig. 6.58	painful squat	217
Fig. 6.59	painful lunge	218
Fig. 6.60	stiff deep squat	218
Fig. 6.61	B-Stance Squat	219
Fig. 6.62	Hip-dominant squat. Similar to deadlift.	220
Fig. 6.63	Bilateral wall sit	220
Fig. 6.64	Unilateral wall sit. Progression to 6.63	221
Fig. 6.65	Isometric flexed single-leg stand. Regression to 6.63, due to the upper body tilt more involvement of posterior muscle groups	221
Fig. 6.66	Step-Down foot lateral down	222
Fig. 6.67	Stepdown foot ventral down. Regression to 6.66 due to the upper body tilt more knee flexion	222

Fig. 6.68	Bilateral landing from a standstill. This movement is not a jump. (Only a fall occurs from the toe stand, without jumping upwards).	223
Fig. 6.69	Bilateral landing from an elevation	223
Fig. 6.70	Shifted landing from a standstill. Preparation for unilateral landings. The right foot here serves as a light support for weight reduction and for more stability	224
Fig. 6.71	Unilateral landing from a standstill. Progression to 6.70.	224
Fig. 6.72	Shifted landing from an elevation. Preparation for unilateral landing from an elevation. The right foot here serves as a light support for weight reduction and for more stability	225
Fig. 6.73	Unilateral landing from an elevation	226
Fig. 6.74	Deep squat with holding	227
Fig. 6.75	Heel sit variant 1. The near-knee support position allows for better dosing of tolerable pressure on the knee joint	227
Fig. 6.76	Heel-sit Variant 2.	228
Fig. 6.77	Unilateral Knee Mobilization on an Elevation	228

List of Tables

Tab. 2.1 Nerve fiber classification according to Erlanger & Gasser and Loyd & Hunt, own creation 22
Tab. 5.1 Paraphrasing of nocebos, own creation..................... 136
Tab. 5.2 Table with clinical examination results, own production 146

About the Author

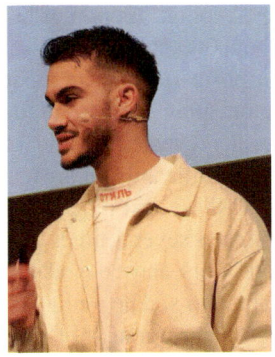

Ahura Bassimtabar (info@edupain.de) Even during his school years, Ahura Bassimtabar felt the desire to pursue a profession that combined his passion for sports and health. This desire led him to physiotherapy, which offered him exactly this connection. After a dual study program, which he completed with the state examination and a successful bachelor's thesis, he continued his education with a part-time master's program in sports physiotherapy at the German Sport University Cologne. There, he graduated as the best in his class.

Bassimtabar began his professional career after his state examination in a physiotherapy practice in Düsseldorf, where he worked with both sports trauma patients and chronic pain patients. His expertise then led him through the youth departments of Fortuna Düsseldorf and Bayer 04 Leverkusen, where he held the position of head of the physiotherapy department, among other things, and into the professional team of Bayer 04 Leverkusen. Today, he looks after the players of the Werkself as a physio and rehab coach. In addition to his work as a sports physiotherapist, Ahura Bassimtabar has also been working as a lecturer since 2018. He began his teaching career at vocational schools, where he taught the subjects of sports medicine and medical training therapy. Over time, his focus shifted to university teaching, where he lectured at the Niederrhein University of Applied Sciences and the Fresenius University of Applied Sciences, among others. Today, his focus is on teaching in the master's program of sports physiotherapy at the German Sport University Cologne. There, he teaches the master's students sports physiotherapy screening methods as well as his self-developed and newly introduced subject **Modern Pain Science**, which deals intensively with modern approaches to pain research and treatment. In addition to his passion for sports physiotherapy, Bassimtabar developed a deep fascination for Pain Science and pain neuroscience. He was disturbed by the fact that he did not know the exact mechanisms of pain onset, chronification, and relief well enough, even though he was taught numerous pain-relieving techniques. Since then, he has been self-taught in current pain research, which he felt was inadequately taught in his training. He dedicated his bachelor's thesis to the variability of individual pain perception. As part of his master's thesis, he surveyed about 300 physiotherapists nationwide shortly before their professional start about their knowledge of the symptom pain and the influence of pain education. The results revealed significant knowledge gaps that could be significantly improved by pain education. He published these and other findings from other studies he designed several times and presented them at various trade fairs and congresses, where he advocates for the adaptation and upgrading of physiotherapy curricula through the integration of pain neuroscience findings. These experiences motivate him to anchor the topic of **Modern Pain Science** in teaching. Today, he teaches this essential topic from his point of view at various universities and has written this textbook out of this motivation to reach as many therapists as possible. In addition, he has launched the education campaign **EDUPAIN** to advance the transfer of current pain neuroscience findings into practice. In addition, he is doing his doctorate part-time at the DSHS at the Institute for Circulatory Research and Sports Medicine in the Department of Molecular and Cellular Sports Medicine and conducts prospective studies, including biomarker reactions after muscle injuries.

Pain—The History

Abstract

The understanding of pain has evolved from early mystical-religious interpretations to complex scientific theories. Ancient philosophers and physicians began to view pain from a medical perspective. In the 17th–19th centuries, medical advancements led to new analgesics and anesthetics. Various theories emerged: from Descartes' linear model, through the specificity and intensity theory, to the groundbreaking gate-control theory by Melzack and Wall in 1965. This was the first to integrate psychological factors into pain processing. Later approaches, such as the neuromatrix theory and the bio-psycho-social model, emphasized the multidimensionality of pain. Behavioral therapeutic and cognitive methods gained importance. Today, pain is understood as a complex interplay of physical, emotional, and social factors. The integration of this holistic view into research and practice remains a central challenge for future pain therapies.

What is pain? Describe it in one word.—This would be a question, the answer to which could quickly lead to the nature of pain. Descriptions such as *unpleasant, burdensome* or *suffering* would apply. The official definition of the International Association for the Study of Pain (IASP) is: "Pain is an unpleasant sensory and emotional experience associated with actual or potential tissue damage, or described in terms of such damage." (Raja et al., 2020). We can agree that pain—fundamentally—is unpleasant. We associate pain with an experience of suffering. What lies behind it has undergone a significant change over time.

1.1 Spirituality and Religions

Medicine and healing methods have probably existed as long as pain has. And pain has probably existed as long as humans have. This assumption is based on the evolutionary development of humans and the function of pain as a vital protective mechanism. Pain warns of dangers and motivates behavioral changes that ensure survival (Nesse & Schulkin, 2019). Thus, pain and the need for pain relief are among the primal phenomena of human history. However, the significance of pain has undergone a change over time, this change being closely linked with cultural and religious beliefs. Pain did not always seem to be a medical problem, but was often placed in a spiritual or moral context. Thousands of years ago, pain was considered a **punishment from the gods,** a belief that was widespread in many early cultures. This interpretation of pain as divine intervention reflected the worldview of the time and significantly influenced the handling of pain. People with headaches were thought to be possessed by demons—an explanation that reduced the complexity of the human nervous system and the variety of possible causes of pain to a simple, albeit terrifying formula. This belief led to specific therapeutic approaches, which often had a ritualistic character. There existed in almost all civilizations countless rituals to exorcise evil spirits to alleviate pain. These rituals varied greatly between different cultures, but often had in common that they tried to establish a connection between the physical and the spiritual world. A particularly drastic example of early pain therapies are found corpses whose skull bones have holes. These archaeological finds suggest that holes were drilled into the skull bones to let evil spirits escape (Heidecker, 2009). This practice, known as *trepanation,* is one of the oldest known surgical procedures and was developed independently in various parts of the world. Surprisingly, there is evidence that some patients survived this procedure, which suggests a certain degree of surgical skill and knowledge of hygiene. These early approaches to pain therapy, as alien as they may seem to us today, testify to the deeply rooted human need to understand and alleviate pain. They mark the starting point for a long development of pain therapy that continues into the present and will probably remain a central challenge of medicine in the future.

The pain history of the **ancient world** is a special chapter in the development of medical thinking. In this era, which spanned several centuries, scholars and healers began to view pain not just as divine punishment or demonic possession, but as a phenomenon that could be rationally explained and treated. In early antiquity, the concept of pain was still heavily influenced by mythological and religious beliefs. However, with the development of the healing arts, a new era of thinking about pain began. In particular, the natural philosophers began to seek natural explanations for physical phenomena, which also influenced thinking about pain. These early approaches paved the way for more profound philosophical and medical considerations of pain. One of the first comprehensive philosophical engagements with the topic of pain can be found in Plato, one of the most influential thinkers of antiquity.

Plato distinguished between mental and physical pain, with pain, regardless of its cause, always being the end of pleasure, and pleasure the end of pain (Jungnitz, 2017). This distinction reveals a fundamental philosophical insight: pain, whether physical or psychological in nature, is perceived as an undesirable state. This early philosophical perspective reveals the deep-rootedness of the concept of pain in human experience and collective thinking. Plato conveys that pain and pleasure are opposing states that exclude each other and significantly shape human existence in their interaction. It becomes clear that the pursuit of pleasure and the avoidance of pain are central drivers of human action and thinking; a principle that is still reflected in many scientific and philosophical considerations today.

Aristotle defined the 5 senses as touch, sight, smell, hearing, and taste. In doing so, he assigned pain to the sense of touch, thereby indirectly excluding the possibility of pain perception without a sensory basis (Hicks, 1907). This classification of pain as part of the sense of touch had a profound influence on pain research for centuries. It illustrates the challenges of understanding pain as an independent phenomenon. Aristotle's perspective highlights the historical challenge of recognizing the complexity and multi-dimensionality of pain beyond pure sensory perception. This early conceptual anchoring and possibly incorrect orientation significantly influenced the scientific understanding of pain and shaped the methods and approaches of pain research into modern times.

Hippocrates was the first physician who attempted to systematically medicalize pain. He did not interpret pain as an independent disease, but as a symptom of an underlying pathology. He attributed this pathology to an imbalance of the four so-called *bodily fluids:* blood, phlegm, yellow bile, and black bile. The humoral pathology, as this model is called, formed the foundation for Hippocrates' entire understanding of health and disease. Within this framework, pain was considered an indication of an imbalance in the body. This humoral pathological view led Hippocrates to see pain as an expression of a systemic problem. His therapeutic methods therefore aimed to correct the supposed imbalance of bodily fluids. He achieved this through measures such as a tailored diet, lifestyle changes, and specific medical interventions, including bloodletting. By medicalizing pain in this way, albeit with theories that are unprovable or refuted from today's perspective, Hippocrates laid the foundation for a holistic understanding of pain that takes into account both the physical and systemic aspects of human health.

Galen expanded on Hippocrates' thoughts and saw tissue damage as the sole cause of physical pain. Galen's contribution to pain research was significant as he attempted to trace pain back to concrete physical changes in the body. He developed a detailed theory about the origin and transmission of pain based on his conception of the nervous system. Galen believed that pain was caused by a disruption of the normal function of nerves, which he viewed as hollow tubes through which the *Spiritus animalis* flowed (Rocca, 2003). In his opinion, pain arose when these *souls* were blocked or disturbed by tissue damage. Although this theory is incorrect from today's perspective, it was an important step towards a physiological understanding of pain.

Avicenna, also known as Ibn Sina, developed in his work *Canon of Medicine* a comprehensive theory of pain that significantly differed from previous philosophical and medical ideas. Avicenna assumed that pain was caused by a disruption of the normal function of tissues and organs, which included a wide range of possible causes of pain. Avicenna saw a change in the state of tissues and organs as the cause of pain, not just or only damage (Tashani & Johnson, 2010), and postulated pain as an independent sensory perception, unlike Aristotle (Naderi et al., 2003). Avicenna's contribution to pain research was revolutionary for his time. He recognized that pain is not only caused by obvious injuries or damage, but can also arise from subtler changes in the body. This allowed for a more nuanced understanding of pain causes and mechanisms. Furthermore, Avicenna's conception of pain as an independent sense was a significant advancement. He argued that pain is a unique sensory experience that differs from other sensory perceptions. He also recognized the psychological aspects of pain and emphasized the importance of the patient's emotional and mental state in pain perception and management. This was a significant step towards a holistic understanding of pain that takes into account both physical and psychological components. In addition to traditional methods, such as the application of herbal remedies and surgical interventions, Avicenna emphasized the importance of careful diagnosis and individual adaptation of therapy. He recommended specific measures to restore balance in the body, such as dietary adjustments, physical exercises, and psychological support, which represents an early form of multimodal pain therapy. Avicenna's comprehensive and differentiated view of pain had a lasting impact on medical practice and the theoretical engagement with pain. His ideas laid the groundwork for later developments in pain research and therapy and mark a decisive turning point in the history of pain medicine.

Despite these explanatory attempts by many different philosophers and natural scientists, pain was not always and universally recognized as a medical problem. The theories of Hippocrates, Galen, and Avicenna often coexisted and were interpreted and applied differently depending on the cultural and historical context. The recognition of pain as an independent medical problem was a lengthy process that spanned centuries and was influenced by various philosophical, religious, and scientific currents. It was not until the advent of modern medicine and particularly neurobiology in the 19th and 20th centuries that a comprehensive scientific understanding of pain began to develop, building on the insights of these early thinkers.

Religiously, in Judaism and Christianity, pain was considered a **test of faith,** which is evident in the story of Job: Although the devil did terrible things to Job, a rich and pious man, causing him to suddenly suffer poverty and severe pain in an attempt to turn him away from God, he never lost his faith in God. Although he complained frustratedly about his situation, he never questioned the existence of God and continued to submit to him. God eventually rewards Job's loyalty. Because he remained faithful to his God in all his suffering, poverty, and sorrow, God frees him from the disease and blesses his further long life. In this case, the pain was a test from God and its alleviation came after acceptance and endurance of the situation through God's redemption. The crucifixion of Jesus Christ is also a topic of pain. He accepted the agonizing death, which is believed to have brought salvation and blessing to the believers. Pain is a suffering and healing phenomenon at the same time. A feeling without which there would be no life. Or a feeling that makes life more enjoyable in its absence. Because one appreciates being pain-free when one experiences pain. Just like youth, which one only appreciates when it is over. The perceived connection between advanced age (with the accompanying loss of youth) and chronic pain syndromes (characterized by reduced pain freedom) has also developed into a recurring narrative in societal perception. Statements like "My aged musculoskeletal system can no longer withstand these stresses and constantly hurts" raise the question of whether the described pain conditions are primarily due to the biological aging process.

In Islam too, pain is closely associated with suffering. The believer is admonished to perform good deeds in this world, otherwise, the fires of hell threaten in the hereafter—a state of extreme torment and pain. Pains in this world are considered a test from God, through which the believer should practice patience and perseverance, without losing trust in God or questioning his fate. This theological perspective suggests that pain is seen as a way to promote spiritual growth and character strength. Whether religious people perceive pain differently or deal with it differently because they see it as divine punishment or a test is a question that science cannot definitively answer. However, studies from psychology and pain research have shown that individual coping with pain is strongly influenced by cultural, social, and personal beliefs (Lasch, 2000; Peacock & Patel, 2008). However, there is a lack of systematic studies that isolate and analyze the specific influence of religious beliefs on pain management. It is nevertheless clear that pain—even in religious contexts—is not seen as joyful states. In religious teachings, pain is considered a means to purify oneself spiritually and to grow internally. This view can help those affected to develop a positive attitude towards their suffering and to find a deeper meaning in their painful experiences. Nevertheless, pain remains a negative sensation that is physically and emotionally burdensome.

In the Middle Ages, pain was also seen as a way to purify the soul through suffering. This idea was deeply rooted in Christian theology and medieval worldview. Pain and suffering were not only seen as inevitable aspects of human existence but also as a path to spiritual perfection and as a means to repent and atone for sins. This interpretation of pain as a spiritual tool led to a complex relationship between physical suffering and religious experience. **Self-flagellation**—a ritual in which one inflicted pain on oneself and imitated the suffering of Jesus Christ— was practiced to get closer to God and heaven. This practice, which appeared in various forms, ranged from fasting rituals to wearing rough penitential garments to more extreme forms of physical punishment. Flagellants, groups of penitents who publicly flogged themselves, were a particularly visible example of this tradition of self-flagellation. The imitation of Christ's suffering, known as *imitatio Christi,* was understood as a path to spiritual purification and as an expression of deep piety (Mowbray, 2009).

In contrast, the 18th century saw a fundamental shift in the philosophy of pain and well-being. With the advent of **hedonistic utilitarianism,** significantly shaped by philosophers such as Jeremy Bentham and John Stuart Mill, the understanding of pain underwent a significant realignment. In hedonistic utilitarianism, human well-being is primarily defined by the sensation of pleasure and joy, as well as by the absence of suffering and pain. This perspective represents a sharp deviation from the medieval view, in which pain was often seen as a necessary means for moral or spiritual purification. In hedonistic philosophy, the pursuit of maximum pleasure and the avoidance of suffering are central. The basic assumption is that human well-being is highest when pleasure is maximized and suffering is minimized. This view leads to pain being seen not only as an unpleasant state, but also as a serious threat to general well-being. In this era, pain is no longer mitigated by religious or spiritual interpretations, but is seen as something to be avoided in order to achieve the highest possible level of quality of life and personal happiness. This philosophy influences medical practice, as the focus increasingly lies on the alleviation of pain to promote individual well-being. The spread of hedonistic ideas favors developments such as the introduction of anesthetics and the establishment of pain management strategies aimed at minimizing suffering and maximizing well-being. In contrast to the medieval notion that pain has a spiritual significance or serves as a test, hedonistic utilitarianism views pain as a purely negative experience that should be avoided to ensure an optimal life. This philosophy represents a paradigm shift that forms the basis for modern approaches in pain therapy. While the Middle Ages interpreted pain as a test of faith, the 18th century primarily saw pain as an obstacle to personal happiness and well-being that needs to be overcome.

1.2 Medicalization

Previously, many doctors began in the 16th century to increasingly view pain as a **medical problem** and to search for physical causes of pain. The use of medication against pain became popular. Many European doctors began to use opium for pain relief. By 1800, ether and chloroform were introduced as anesthetics for childbirth and later for surgery. However, this medical revolution was not welcomed by all. On the one hand, there were ethical debates about operations on an unconscious person, on the other hand, religious protests: anesthetics would disregard God's laws and, for example, take away the chance for the birthing mother to strengthen her faith through pain and to sacrifice her own well-being for her child (Meldrum, 2003). Here, the discrepancies in the views and definitions of pain became clear again. Ultimately, anesthesia prevailed due to the numerous advantages of medical interventions. In the 1900s, morphine and heroin were used as painkillers. A simple and effective way to relieve acute pain. At the latest then, doctors found themselves in a dilemma, prescribing morphine and heroin as painkillers to improve the quality of life of their patients, but at the same time fearing that these therapies could lead to dependence and addiction (Collier, 2018). However, chronic pain patients were caught in a dilemma: neither did the opiates help in the long term, nor was there a good explanation for their pain, as doctors found no obvious pathology in many pain patients. The importance of chronic pain, which persisted despite the administration of opiates, increased. Today we know that pain that is not explainable musculoskeletally or neurally is not synonymous with psychological problems (Gagliese & Katz, 2000). Back then it was different. Patients whose chronic pain seemed inexplicable were often condemned as malingerers or referred to a psychiatrist due to supposed psychological problems. This opened up a new field of pain research at the neurobiological level, where neurosurgical and psychoanalytic disciplines came together and tested new therapeutic approaches. Due to strong regulation of opiates by law, chronic pain patients had few therapy options: psychotherapy or neurosurgery. Here, new approaches were developed to alleviate pain. Neurosurgically, attempts were made to stop the nociceptive influx into the central nervous system (CNS), for example by crushing or resecting local nerves, which logically had more disadvantages than advantages. The French doctor René Leriche was the first doctor to use procaine (a local anesthetic synthesized by Alfred Einhorn in 1905) as a standard and in large quantities for the therapy of patients with nerve pain, in order to stop all afferent sensory transmissions. If this method did not lead to the desired success, the ligation—a kind of tying off—of the sympathetic nerve fibers/ganglia, which supplied the affected extremity, followed. Here, the idea was pursued that patients would no longer feel pain if no afferent nociceptive signals reached the brain anymore.

During the **Second World War,** Henry K. Beecher, a renowned anesthetist from Harvard and military doctor of the USA, made a startling discovery for the time, which fundamentally questioned the established understanding of pain. He observed that soldiers who had been severely wounded on the battlefield often complained of less pain than patients at home who had only suffered minor injuries (Beecher, 1946). These observations posed a radical challenge to the hitherto generally accepted notion that the intensity of pain was directly proportional to the degree of tissue damage. Previously, it was largely taken for granted that the condition of the tissue had a linear relationship to the intensity of pain—the more severe the injury, the more intense the pain. The idea that pain and tissue damage had a clear, predictable connection was considered a fundamental principle by the medical community. However, Beecher found that this assumption did not always hold true and discovered that the degree of tissue damage did not necessarily correlate with the severity of the pain experienced. This insight was groundbreaking as it opened up new perspectives on the complex nature of pain. The soldiers, who were in a war scenario, might have experienced altered pain perception due to various factors such as adrenaline, group cohesion, or the direct threat of death. In contrast, civilian patients, although they had less severe injuries, might have suffered more from pain due to other stressors such as emotional burdens, worries about the healing process, or the lack of immediate support. Beecher's observations led to a radical rethink in pain research. Instead of viewing pain solely as a direct result of tissue damage, it was increasingly recognized as a multifactorial phenomenon that encompasses both physiological and psychological dimensions. This insight ushered in a new era in pain research and therapy, calling for an integrative approach to consider the diverse factors that can influence the pain experience.

In 1965, Ronald Melzack, a Canadian psychologist, and Patrick Wall, a British neurophysiologist, laid the foundation for modern pain science, which allowed entirely new perspectives on pain onset and processing: The Gate-Control Theory (GCT), which was complementary and also partly contrary to Descartes' theory of pain. A brief look back: In the 17th century, **Descartes** assumed that when peripheral tissue is injured, sensory channels (today: nociceptors) are activated and pain signals reach the brain directly and linearly, where the pain is perceived. This, in turn, activates motor channels to avoid the sensory stimulus—a protective function. He also suspected that the stronger this peripheral sensory channel is stimulated, the more clearly the pain would be perceived in the brain (Descartes, 1664). The onset of pain is thus based on a peripheral, mechanistic, and purely body-based phenomenon, which is merely relayed to the brain, perceived there, and reacted to motorically. In 1856, before Beecher's discoveries and the GCT, the physiologist Moritz Schiff expanded these considerations and established the **Specificity Theory,** which was later particularly strongly represented by the physiologist Max von Frey. This Specificity Theory describes that each somatosensory modality has a specific receptor and an associated afferent nerve fiber, which reacts to a specific stimulus. The pain receptors would transmit the pain information directly to the brain. The Specificity Theory postulates that there are special nerve endings that are solely responsible for the perception of pain. These react selectively to painful stimuli and transmit this information via specific nerve fibers to the spinal cord and further to the brain. According to this theory, there is a direct, linear relationship between the painful stimulus, the activation of the nociceptors, and the pain sensation. According to this theory, accompanying emotions are understood as reactions to the initial pain information, but they do not directly influence the pain itself. Some medical treatments, including neurosurgery and nerve blocks, rely on this approach. The Specificity Theory separates biological and psychological aspects of pain experience from each other. This separation implies that the pain sensation is purely physical-damaging (noxious) in nature and has no psychological influences. Therefore, the theory is not able to adequately explain chronic pain syndromes, especially when there is no organic basis for the pain. Another problem with this theory is that it does not provide an explanation for why pain can persist after the underlying injury has healed. According to this theory, pain should no longer exist once the tissue damage has been eliminated.

At that time, pain was still considered, alongside for example the sense of smell or touch, as one of these somatosensory modalities (Moayedi & Davis, 2013). This model suggests that the sensation of pain has a specific receptor with a corresponding specific pathway to the brain. Whether pain can thus be interpreted as a sense remained open. Some argued that pain differs from other senses because it

1.2 Medicalization

is inherently unpleasant (Boring, 1942). In the writings of Plato, pain was always described as an emotion (Schmitter, 2021).

From 1874, a counter-movement to the specificity theory formed, which advocated for the **intensity theory,** also known as the summation theory. This was developed by the neurologist Wilhelm Erb based on the considerations of Erasmus Darwin and states that any sensory stimulus can be perceived as painful if it is intense enough. Pain does not represent an independent sensory modality (Dallenbach, 1939). Rather, it is about an unusual change in state (recalling Avicenna), which can be interpreted as a danger and thus perceived as painful. In contrast to the specificity theory, which assumed specific pain receptors, the intensity theory postulated that all sensory nerve fibers can potentially transmit pain signals. This theory explained why sometimes even non-painful stimuli can be perceived as painful if they exceed a certain intensity. For example, a light pressure on the skin can be perceived as pleasant, while strong pressure causes pain. The intensity theory also provided an explanation for phenomena such as hyperalgesia, where normally non-painful stimuli are perceived as painful.

In 1906, the British neurophysiologist Charles Sherrington coined the term **nociceptor**—a receptor that specifically responds to noxious stimuli and triggers protective reflexes and pain (Sherrington, 1906). The introduction of the term nociceptor bridged the gap between the intensity and specificity theories. A specific receptor that reacts when the danger becomes large enough and noxious. Sherrington acknowledged the existence of specialized receptors as proposed by the specificity theory, but also took into account the importance of stimulus intensity as emphasized by the intensity theory. Nociceptors respond selectively to potentially tissue-damaging stimuli, regardless of whether they are mechanical, thermal, or chemical in nature.

Returning to the observations of the severely wounded soldiers of Beecher, who were not really suffering from severe pain, or conversely to the patients suffering from tormenting chronic back pain, without any detectable medical lesion, all prevailing theories seemed unable to unite the diversity of pain perception. These theories fall in line with observations where patients suffer from pain without any detectable pathology or lesion, while others have little to no pain despite larger lesions. One must praise Descartes for his theories set up in the 17th century without advanced diagnostic technologies. He defined the brain as the perception center of pain (even though we know today that the brain is more than just a perception center in the receiver role). And as a natural scientist, he unsurprisingly contradicted with his theory against the mystical/religious view, according to which pain was seen as God's punishment or atonement for guilt. Pain increasingly evolved from a philosophical-religious topic to a pathological-medical topic—to a physical warning signal.

During the pain research of the 20th century, scientists faced fundamental questions, the answers to which were not fully possible with the existing theories. These questions reflect the complexity and multifaceted nature of the pain experience and show that the existing models could not explain all facets of pain perception. The most important open questions that remained unanswered at this time include:

- Why do the degree of damage and the intensity of pain not correlate with each other?
- Why do some people feel little to no pain after severe injury?
- Why do seemingly harmless stimuli cause severe pain in other people?
- Why does the area or quality of pain change over time?
- Why does pain persist despite the apparent healing of the injury?
- Why are there chronic back pain patients, without finding a biological/medical lesion in them?

1.3 Neuroscience and Cognition

The difficulties in finding a consistent answer to these questions led researchers like Melzack and Wall to intensively search for new explanatory approaches. The **Gate-Control Theory** (GCT) attempted to achieve something that other theories never included: to make the variability and diversity of pain perception explainable. In other words: to specify the apparent unspecificity of pain manifestation. For this, the solution was sought not in the pain area, but in the processing area: in the CNS.

The GCT, developed in 1965, marked a turning point in pain research and revolutionized the understanding of pain perception and processing. For the first time, a theory seemed to allow for the diversity and complexity of pain experience and integrated physiological, psychological, and cognitive aspects into a coherent model. The GCT postulates that there are special fibers for nociception, namely the thin C- and Aδ-fibers, which differ from the fibers for the sense of touch, the thicker Aβ-fibers. These different fiber types converge in the dorsal horn of the spinal cord and meet there. The dorsal horn acts in this model as a kind of neural switchboard that regulates the flow of information and decides which signals are forwarded, which are blocked, and which additional modulations take place. Melzack and Wall suspected that the substantia gelatinosa in the dorsal horn acts like a *Gate* or gate, which establishes and modulates the transmission of the incoming sensory information from the primary afferent neurons to the interneurons in the spinal cord. These interneurons play a key role in forwarding the signals to the secondary dorsal horn neuron by further regulating and filtering the flow of information. The gating mechanism is controlled by the activity level in the thick and thin fibers. The thicker Aβ-fibers have an inhibitory effect and tend to close or inhibit the gate. In contrast, the narrower C- and Aδ-fibers have an excitatory effect and tend to open or excite the gate. This interplay explains why, with an incoming nociceptive stimulus, which is conducted via C-fibers, for example, the nociceptive signal triggered by the noxious stimulus can be inhibited and the pain alleviated by simultaneous activation of the thicker Aβ-fibers—for example by light, non-noxious rubbing at the injury site. A particularly innovative aspect of the GCT is the consideration of descending fibers, which originate in supraspinal regions of the brain and project to the dorsal horn. These descending pathways can also influence the gating mechanism and modulate signal processing at the spinal cord level. This opened up for the first time a scientific explanation for the influence of cognitive and emotional factors on pain perception. The fact that descending pathways can influence impulses at the spinal cord level can explain why pain is perceived differently depending on the situation or state of mind, as the gate can be opened more easily in certain situations, allowing more nociceptive signals to reach the brain when the individual is in a negative mood. Conversely, when experiencing joy and positive moods, serotonin and endorphin are released, which can inhibit the transmission of nociceptive signals from the primary to the secondary dorsal horn neuron. This cognitive influence on the gate at the spinal cord level is one of the possible explanations for why athletes only notice certain injuries after the competition, or why people with depression have a higher prevalence of chronic pain (Bair et al., 2003).

The GCT describes how nociceptive impulses at the spinal cord level are modulated multiple times before they reach the brain. This modulation is carried out by non-noxious signals from the Aβ-fibers and by descending pathways from higher brain regions (Melzack & Wall, 1965). This complex interaction explains why pain perception does not linearly correlate with the intensity of the noxious stimulus, but is influenced by various factors. The GCT has far-reaching implications for the understanding and therapy of pain. It provides an explanation for phenomena such as the analgesic effect of distraction or meditation, the effectiveness of techniques such as TENS (transcutaneous electrical nerve stimulation), and the variability of pain perception between individuals and in different situations. The theory has also highlighted the importance of psycho-social factors in pain therapy. It supported the development of bio-psycho-social models of pain and promoted interdisciplinary approaches in pain therapy. In summary, the GCT has thus united and significantly supplemented the previously dominant theories. On the one hand, it distinguishes between special nociceptors and other sensory receptors, reminiscent of the specificity theory. On the other hand, the GCT states that pain perception occurs when the excitatory signals are greater than the inhibitory ones. This is reminiscent of the intensity theory. Furthermore, it is shown that the nervous system is not a mere conduit as Descartes suspected, but contributes to regulation itself. Furthermore, the GCT added to the complexity and situation-dependency of pain perception, especially through the influence of neurobiological events at the spinal cord level by descending pathways depending on the cognitive, psychological, and emotional status. The brain was added here, not as a passive perception organ, but as an active co-determining organ.

A theory would not be a theory if it did not also have flaws. For example, the GCT presupposed a peripheral noxious stimulus, although this stimulus can be perceived in various ways depending on the situation. However, a peripheral event is not necessary as a prerequisite for pain according to current knowledge. Phantom pains (pains without a peripheral noxious stimulus) could not be explained with the GCT, for example (Melzack, 1996). These limitations led to a paradigm shift in pain research, with the brain moving into the foreground for researchers.

In response to these challenges, Ronald Melzack proposed a new approach: the **Neuromatrix Theory**. This theory postulates that there is neither a specific pain entry point nor a specific perception center in the brain. Instead, the Neuromatrix Theory illustrates that various brain areas from the thalamus to the cortex to the limbic system can interact with each other and in parallel, and can initiate processes even without input (Melzack, 1996; Melzack, 2001). The Neuromatrix Theory does not attempt to diminish the relevance of the sensory input coming from the periphery, but to add the influence of other factors such as emotions, experiences, and expectations and to justify these biologically and neurophysiologically. The term Neuromatrix may seem vague at first, but it is due to the complex nature of the human brain, whose pain-related processes may not be more specifically named in one term. Melzack describes the Neuromatrix as a network of countless neurons and synapses that extends through various parts of the brain. A central concept within this theory is the *Neurosignature*. Repeated patterns of neuronal impulses form this Neurosignature, which is supposed to be individual like fingerprints. This explains why pain perception varies so much between individuals, as each person brings different prerequisites and different Neurosignatures. A crucial aspect of the Neuromatrix Theory is that this Neurosignature exists without needing any input. A sensory and non-noxious input can trigger this Neurosignature, but it is not a prerequisite for pain (Melzack, 2001). This provides an explanation for phenomena such as phantom pains or chronic pains without a recognizable cause. The Neurosignature is the result of the synaptic architecture of the Neuromatrix, which is partly genetically determined and partly modified by sensory experiences. It produces characteristic patterns of nerve impulses that generate pain and other body sensations. The Neurosignature is influenced not only by sensory inputs but also by cognitive processes such as psychological stress and by the influence of the immune system. The Neuromatrix Theory presents pain as a multidimensional experience that is generated by various influences such as cognitive and affective events. It opened up entirely new perspectives for understanding and treating pain. In particular, it provides an explanatory approach for chronic pain syndromes, where often no clear physiological cause can be identified.

The theory has far-reaching implications for clinical practice. It supports multimodal therapy approaches that aim not only to alleviate peripheral noxious stimuli but also to include cognitive, emotional, and behavioral interventions. In addition, the Neuromatrix Theory has inspired the research field of pain imaging. Modern imaging techniques, such as functional magnetic resonance imaging (fMRI), have shown that pain actually activates a complex network of brain regions, supporting the basic assumptions of the theory (Apkarian et al., 2005).

In summary, the Neuromatrix Theory emphasizes the central role of the brain in the experience of pain and provides a comprehensive framework for understanding the diverse and often puzzling aspects of the pain experience. By

1.3 Neuroscience and Cognition

acknowledging the complexity and individuality of pain perception, it has paved the way for personalized and holistic approaches in pain therapy.

Almost simultaneously with the groundbreaking theories of Ronald Melzack and Patrick Wall, the widely used **bio-psycho-social model** (BPSM) was developed in 1977 by George Engel, an American psychologist. Engel aimed to create an integrative understanding of the complex nature of health conditions, including pain, with this model. His model represented a significant advancement in medical and psychological science by challenging the assumption that medical phenomena can be explained exclusively by biological processes. The BPSM postulates that a patient's medical status—particularly in the experience of pain—is determined not only by purely biological or pathological factors but also by psychological and social dimensions. Engel argued that pain should not be considered in isolation. Instead, the interactions between physical health, mental well-being, and social circumstances should be taken into account to get a complete picture of the pain experience. According to Engel, biological factors such as tissue damage or neurological disorders influence the sensation of pain, but they only constitute part of the overall pain experience. Psychological factors, such as stress, anxiety, or depression, can significantly influence perception and pain management. Furthermore, social factors, such as social support, living conditions, or societal expectations, play a crucial role in how pain is experienced and managed.

Contrary to common misinterpretations that view the BPSM as an explanation for the onset of pain due to psychological or social factors, Engel rather describes the possible impacts that pain can have on these areas, as well as the influence these factors exert on the pain experience. The model aims to clarify that pain should not be understood merely as a physical response to an injury or illness. Engel's goal was to expand medical practice and research beyond the purely biological perspective. He aimed for the medical approach to pain relief and therapy to consider both the psychological and social dimensions of pain. The BPSM thus calls for a holistic view of the patient, in which all relevant factors are incorporated into the diagnosis and therapy. In the scientific literature, the BPSM is recognized as a fundamental model for understanding pain and other health conditions, as it emphasizes the need to go beyond traditional medical models and develop a more comprehensive understanding of human well-being (Engel, 1977; Gatchel et al., 2007).

In the late 20th century, further significant approaches emerged in pain research, expanding the understanding of chronic pain and its therapy. **Learning theories,** particularly those of behaviorists like Skinner and Watson, assumed that pain, like other behaviors, was learned from birth and could therefore be unlearned/relearned through targeted interventions (Eysenck, 1976; Cordier & Diers, 2018). This perspective highlighted the importance of psycho-social approaches. The application of learning theory principles in pain therapy led to the development of various behavioral therapeutic techniques. A particularly influential method was operant conditioning, based on the work of Skinner (Gatzounis et al., 2012). This approach assumes that behaviors are reinforced or weakened by their consequences. In pain therapy, this principle was used to promote adaptive behaviors and reduce maladaptive ones. Fordyce et al. (1973) were pioneers in applying this method to chronic pain patients. A concrete example of the application of operant conditioning in pain therapy is the use of reinforcers. Here, patients gained the attention and services of the doctor as positive reinforcement (reward) for being able to manage their pain themselves. This meant adjusting movements and increasing them depending on the pain condition to remain functional. This approach aimed to increase the patients' self-efficacy. From these early approaches, the concept of Graded Activity (GA) developed, which today is considered an important component of many multimodal pain therapy programs. GA is based on the principle of gradual increase of activities. Individual baselines are determined and realistic goals are set, which are gradually increased. This approach aims to reduce fear of movement (kinesiophobia) and improve physical functionality. Recent research, such as that by Macedo et al. (2010), has confirmed the effectiveness of GA in chronic pain patients, especially in combination with cognitive-behavioral therapies (CBT). The development of GA and similar approaches underscores the importance of individualized, active forms of therapy in the treatment of chronic pain. Modification programs like GA and CBT have proven effective for many chronic pain patients (Macedo et al., 2010, Williams et al., 2012; Ehde et al., 2014; Hajihasani et al., 2019; Yang et al., 2022).

Both learning and behavioral therapies respect the multidimensionality of pain and attempt to include and influence perception, emotions, cognition, and beliefs. These approaches are based on the BPSM developed by Engel. Melzack and Wall (1965) also significantly contributed to the understanding of the multidimensional nature of pain by highlighting the role of psychological factors in pain modulation. The patient is encouraged to actively participate in what they think about their problem, what they feel, and what they can control. This approach is based on Bandura's concept of self-efficacy (1977): a person's belief that they can handle a specific task has a significant influence on their actual behavior and performance. In the context of pain therapy, this means that patients who believe they can better control their pain actually achieve better results. The main goal of these therapies is to improve coping—dealing with pain—not pain relief per se. Lazarus and Folkman defined *coping* in 1984 as cognitive and behavioral efforts to manage external and internal demands that are perceived as stressful or exceeding one's resources (Ben-Zur, 2019). In pain therapy, coping encompasses a variety of strategies, including problem-solving, cognitive restructuring, acceptance, and mindfulness. The promotion of adaptive coping strategies aims to improve patients' quality of life, even if the pain cannot be completely eliminated. These therapy approaches showed positive effects on mood, physical function, and also patients' pain levels (Sharp, 2001; Salomons et al., 2004). Of course, pain relief is also one of the goals of these therapies, but the approach differs from other pain therapies: it does not fight against the pain and try to alleviate it (where usually the therapist takes the active role and the patient the passive one), but tries to regulate different dimensions of pain—cognition, emotions, and beliefs—and thereby influence the pain. This approach is in line with the concept of central sensitization, which emphasizes the role of the central nervous system in maintaining chronic pain and underscores the need to address not only peripheral nociceptive sources but also central processing processes (Woolf, 2011). The integration of acceptance- and mindfulness-based approaches into pain therapy, such as Acceptance and Commitment Therapy (ACT), has gained importance in recent years (Hayes et al., 2013). These approaches aim to increase patients' psychological flexibility and promote a non-judgmental attitude towards pain experiences. Studies show that these approaches can achieve comparable or even better results than traditional cognitive-behavioral interventions, especially in terms of long-term improvement in quality of life and functionality (Veehof et al., 2016). Learning and behavioral approaches in pain therapy are based on a comprehensive understanding of the complex nature of pain. They aim to empower patients to actively cope with their pain by addressing cognitive, emotional, and behavioral aspects of the pain experience. This holistic approach has proven effective, not only in terms of pain reduction, but also in improving patients' overall quality of life and functionality.

Critics, however, have objected to these patient-participatory approaches, arguing that the responsibility for the success of the therapy could be completely transferred to the patient and in the event of failure, the patient would be held responsible. Attributing responsibility for a failure to the patient is ethically questionable. On the other hand, the transfer of responsibility in the sense of actively involving the patient in the therapy process and imparting self-management skills is considered important and currently underrepresented. The prevailing paradigm, in which the patient takes a passive role and leaves the intervention entirely to the therapist, is seen as outdated. It is argued that a shift towards a participatory approach in therapy is necessary, in which the patient actively participates in the healing process (Longtin et al., 2010).

Today, pain is considered a multidimensional experience that encompasses physical, emotional, and social aspects. And although, as already mentioned in the introduction, pain is an emotional experience, investigations and therapeutic procedures are traditionally set up and interpreted through the musculoskeletal lens, without including the emotional components (Gilam et al., 2020). Since the BPSM, emotions have come more to the forefront again. The development from a religious-philosophical to a medical view of pain could possibly have effects on the behavior of people with pain experiences. This change in the perception and handling of pain requires further investigation, possibly leading to more caution or even defensive behavior when it comes to a supposedly physical/pathological problem, and not a test of faith. The medicalization of the pain phenomenon has led to a significant expansion of the therapy spectrum. This includes a variety of therapeutic approaches and expertise, which can make the selection of a suitable therapy method complex. The diversity of pain cause interpretations by different disciplines underscores the need for an interdisciplinary approach in pain research and therapy, especially when different experts see different causes for the same pain in the same person. To gain a comprehensive understanding, it is appropriate to investigate the various factors that can contribute to the development of pain. This compendium is intended to serve this purpose.

References

Apkarian, A. V., Bushnell, M. C., Treede, R. D., & Zubieta, J. K. (2005). Human brain mechanisms of pain perception and regulation in health and disease. *European Journal of Pain (London, England), 9*(4), 463–484. https://doi.org/10.1016/j.ejpain.2004.11.001.

Bair, M. J., Robinson, R. L., Katon, W., & Kroenke, K. (2003). Depression and pain comorbidity: A literature review. *Archives of Internal Medicine, 163*(20), 2433–2445. https://doi.org/10.1001/archinte.163.20.2433.

Bandura, A. (1977). Self-efficacy: Toward a unifying theory of behavioral change. *Psychological Review, 84*(2), 191–215. https://doi.org/10.1037/0033-295X.84.2.191.

Beecher, H. K. (1946). Pain in Men Wounded in Battle. *Annals of Surgery, 123*(1), 96–105.

Boring E. G. (1942). Sensation and Perception in the History of Experimental. *Psychology. D. Appleton-Century.* https://ia801507.us.archive.org/12/items/in.ernet.dli.2015.52372/2015.52372.Sensation-And-Perception-In-The-History-Of-Experimental-Psychology_text.pdf. Zugegriffen: 23. Dec. 2023.

Ben-Zur, H. (2019). Transactional Model of Stress and Coping. In V. Zeigler-Hill & T. Shackelford (Eds.), *Encyclopedia of Personality and Individual Differences.* Springer. https://doi.org/10.1007/978-3-319-28099-8_2128-1.

Collier R. (2018). A short history of pain management. *CMAJ: Canadian Medical Association journal = journal de l'Association medicale canadienne, 190*(1), E26–E27. https://doi.org/10.1503/cmaj.109-5523.

Cordier, L., & Diers, M. (2018). Learning and Unlearning of Pain. *Biomedicines, 6*(2), 67. https://doi.org/10.3390/biomedicines6020067.

Dallenbach, K. M. (1939). Pain: History and present status. *The American Journal of Psychology, 52,* 331–347. https://doi.org/10.2307/1416740.

Descartes R. (1664) Treatise on Man. *angepasst von Clerselier C., übersetzt von Sloan P. R.* https://www.coretexts.org/wp-content/uploads/2010/08/DescartesTreatiseMnfin.pdf. Zugegriffen: 10. Dec. 2023.

Ehde, D. M., Dillworth, T. M., & Turner, J. A. (2014). Cognitive-behavioral therapy for individuals with chronic pain: Efficacy, innovations, and directions for research. *The American Psychologist, 69*(2), 153–166. https://doi.org/10.1037/a0035747.

Engel G. L. (1977). The need for a new medical model: A challenge for biomedicine. *Science (New York, N.Y.), 196*(4286), 129–136. https://doi.org/10.1126/science.847460.

Eysenck, H. J. (1976). The learning theory model of neurosis: A new approach. *Behaviour Research and Therapy, 14*(4), 251–267. https://doi.org/10.1016/0005-7967(76)90001.

Fordyce, W. E., Fowler, R. S., Jr, Lehmann, J. F., Delateur, B. J., Sand, P. L., & Trieschmann, R. B. (1973). Operant conditioning in the treatment of chronic pain. *Archives of physical medicine and rehabilitation, 54*(9), 399–408. https://static1.squarespace.com/static/54fe580de4b0e762cd9f4d34/t/5516adbae4b0392be72053d0/1427549626375/Operant+conditioning+in+the+treatment+of+chronic+pain.pdf. Zugegriffen: 03. Jan. 2024.

Gagliese, L., & Katz, J. (2000). Medically unexplained pain is not caused by psychopathology. *Pain Research & Management, 5*(4), 251–257. https://doi.org/10.1155/2000/701397.

Gatchel, R. J., Peng, Y. B., Peters, M. L., Fuchs, P. N., & Turk, D. C. (2007). The biopsychosocial approach to chronic pain: Scientific advances and future directions. *Psychological bulletin, 133*(4), 581–624. https://doi.org/10.1037/0033-2909.133.4.581.

Gatzounis, R., Schrooten, M. G., Crombez, G., & Vlaeyen, J. W. (2012). Operant learning theory in pain and chronic pain rehabilitation. *Current pain and Headache Reports, 16*(2), 117–126. https://doi.org/10.1007/s11916-012-0247-1.

Gilam, G., Gross, J. J., Wager, T. D., Keefe, F. J., & Mackey, S. C. (2020). What Is the Relationship between Pain and Emotion? Bridging Constructs and Communities. *Neuron, 107*(1), 17–21. https://doi.org/10.1016/j.neuron.2020.05.024.

Hajihasani, A., Rouhani, M., Salavati, M., Hedayati, R., & Kahlaee, A. H. (2019). The Influence of Cognitive Behavioral Therapy on Pain, Quality of Life, and Depression in

Patients Receiving Physical Therapy for Chronic Low Back Pain: A Systematic Review. *PM & R: The Journal of Injury, Function, and Rehabilitation, 11*(2), 167–176. https://doi.org/10.1016/j.pmrj.2018.09.029.

Hayes, S. C., Levin, M. E., Plumb-Vilardaga, J., Villatte, J. L., & Pistorello, J. (2013). Acceptance and commitment therapy and contextual behavioral science: Examining the progress of a distinctive model of behavioral and cognitive therapy. *Behavior Therapy, 44*(2), 180–198. https://doi.org/10.1016/j.beth.2009.08.002.

Heidecker, K. (2009). Schädeltrepanationen in der Antike. In C. Brockmann, W. Brunschön, & O. Overwien (Hrsg.), *Antike Medizin im Schnittpunkt von Geistes- und Naturwissenschaften* (S. 259–280). De Gruyter. https://doi.org/10.1515/9783110216493.259.

Hicks, R. D. (1907). Aristotle: De anima; with translation, introduction and notes. *Cambridge: University Press.* https://archive.org/details/aristotledeanima005947mbp/page/n29/mode/2up. Zugegriffen: 12. Jan. 2024.

Jungnitz, S. (2017). *Platon. Sind körperliche Freuden wahre Freuden?* GRIN Verlag. https://www.grin.com/document/387716.

Lasch, K. E. (2000). Culture, pain, and culturally sensitive pain care. *Pain management nursing: Official journal of the American Society of Pain Management Nurses, 1*(3 Suppl 1), 16–22. https://doi.org/10.1053/jpmn.2000.9761.

Longtin, Y., Sax, H., Leape, L. L., Sheridan, S. E., Donaldson, L., & Pittet, D. (2010). Patient participation: Current knowledge and applicability to patient safety. *Mayo Clinic Proceedings, 85*(1), 53–62. https://doi.org/10.4065/mcp.2009.0248.

Macedo, L. G., Smeets, R. J., Maher, C. G., Latimer, J., & McAuley, J. H. (2010). Graded activity and graded exposure for persistent nonspecific low back pain: A systematic review. *Physical Therapy, 90*(6), 860–879. https://doi.org/10.2522/ptj.20090303.

Meldrum, M. L. (2003). A capsule history of pain management. *JAMA, 290*(18), 2470–2475. https://doi.org/10.1001/jama.290.18.2470.

Melzack, R., & Wall, P. D. (1965). Pain mechanisms: A new theory. *Science (New York, N.Y.), 150*(3699), 971–979. https://doi.org/10.1126/science.150.3699.971.

Melzack, R. (1996). Gate control theory: On the evolution of pain concepts. *Pain Forum, 5*(2), 128–138. https://doi.org/10.1016/S1082-3174(96)80050-X.

Melzack, R. (2001). Pain and the neuromatrix in the brain. *Journal of Dental Education, 65*(12), 1378–1382.

Moayedi, M., & Davis, K. D. (2013). Theories of pain: From specificity to gate control. *Journal of Neurophysiology, 109*(1), 5–12. https://doi.org/10.1152/jn.00457.2012.

Mowbray, D. (2009). Pain and Suffering in Medieval Theology: Academic Debates at the University of Paris in the Thirteenth Century. *Boydell and Brewer: Boydell and Brewer.* https://doi.org/10.1515/9781846157516.

Naderi, S., Acar, F., Mertol, T., & Arda, M. N. (2003). Functional anatomy of the spine by Avicenna in his eleventh century treatise Al-Qanun fi al-Tibb (The Canons of Medicine). *Neurosurgery, 52*(6), 1449–1454. https://doi.org/10.1227/01.neu.0000064811.30933.7f.

Nesse, R. M., & Schulkin, J. (2019). An evolutionary medicine perspective on pain and its disorders. *Philosophical transactions of the Royal Society of London. Series B, Biological sciences, 374*(1785), 20190288. https://doi.org/10.1098/rstb.2019.0288.

Peacock, S., & Patel, S. (2008). Cultural Influences on Pain. *Reviews in pain, 1*(2), 6–9. https://doi.org/10.1177/204946370800100203.

Raja, S. N., Carr, D. B., Cohen, M., Finnerup, N. B., Flor, H., Gibson, S., Keefe, F. J., Mogil, J. S., Ringkamp, M., Sluka, K. A., Song, X. J., Stevens, B., Sullivan, M. D., Tutelman, P. R., Ushida, T., & Vader, K. (2020). The revised International Association for the Study of Pain definition of pain: Concepts, challenges, and compromises. *Pain, 161*(9), 1976–1982. https://doi.org/10.1097/j.pain.0000000000001939.

Rocca, J. (2003). Galen on the Brain. Anatomical Knowledge and Physiological Speculation in the Second Century AD. *Studies in Ancient Medicine, 26.* ISBN: 978-90-04-12512-4.

Salomons, T. V., Johnstone, T., Backonja, M. M., & Davidson, R. J. (2004). Perceived controllability modulates the neural response to pain. *The Journal of neuroscience : The official journal of the Society for Neuroscience, 24*(32), 7199–7203. https://doi.org/10.1523/JNEUROSCI.1315-04.2004.

Sharp, T. J. (2001). Chronic pain: A reformulation of the cognitive-behavioural model. *Behaviour Research and Therapy, 39*(7), 787–800. https://doi.org/10.1016/s0005-7967(00)00061-9.

Sherrington, C. S. (1906). Observations on the scratch-reflex in the spinal dog. *The Journal of Physiology, 34*(1–2), 1–50. https://doi.org/10.1113/jphysiol.1906.sp001139.

Schmitter, A. M. (2021). 17th and 18th Century Theories of Emotions. *The Stanford Encyclopedia of Philosophy.* https://plato.stanford.edu/entries/emotions-17th18th/ Zugegriffen: 15. Dec. 2023.

Tashani, O. A., & Johnson, M. I. (2010). Avicenna's concept of pain. *The Libyan Journal of Medicine, 5,*. https://doi.org/10.3402/ljm.v5i0.5253.doi:10.3402/ljm.v5i0.5253.

Veehof, M. M., Trompetter, H. R., Bohlmeijer, E. T., & Schreurs, K. M. (2016). Acceptance- and mindfulness-based interventions for the treatment of chronic pain: A meta-analytic review. *Cognitive Behaviour Therapy, 45*(1), 5–31. https://doi.org/10.1080/16506073.2015.1098724.

Williams, A. C., Eccleston, C., & Morley, S. (2012). Psychological therapies for the management of chronic pain (excluding headache) in adults. *The Cochrane database of systematic reviews, 11*(11), CD007407. https://doi.org/10.1002/14651858.CD007407.pub3.

Woolf, C. J. (2011). Central sensitization: Implications for the diagnosis and treatment of pain. *Pain, 152*(3 Suppl), S2–S15. https://doi.org/10.1016/j.pain.2010.09.030.

Yang, J., Lo, W. L. A., Zheng, F., Cheng, X., Yu, Q., & Wang, C. (2022). Evaluation of Cognitive Behavioral Therapy on Improving Pain, Fear Avoidance, and Self-Efficacy in Patients with Chronic Low Back Pain: A Systematic Review and Meta-Analysis. *Pain research & management, 2022,* 4276175. https://doi.org/10.1155/2022/4276175.

The Neurobiology of Nociception

2

Abstract

Pain is based on complex neurobiological processes. Often, pain is equated with nociception, but nociception is a part of the pain experience. Various nociceptive processes occur from the noxious stimulus to conscious perception. These include transduction, transmission, and modulation. Nociceptors, primarily Aδ and C fibers, respond to various noxious stimuli and transmit signals via the spinal cord to the brain. Transmission occurs via primary, secondary, and tertiary neurons, with important modulation processes taking place in the spinal cord. Facilitative and inhibitory mechanisms influence signal transmission, controlled by neurotransmitters such as glutamate and GABA. Pain perception in the brain is multidimensional and includes not only sensory nociceptive information but also affective and cognitive aspects.

Why is there pain? What does God or evolution think when equipping humans with such an unpleasant feeling? What is the benefit of pain? In the acute case, pain has a protective, almost instructive function. It teaches us not to touch fire, to handle sharp objects carefully, and to protect our bodies in the event of a physical altercation and to avoid attacks. In addition to its protective function, depending on its intensity and duration, it can drastically impair quality of life.

The International Association for the Study of Pain (IASP) was founded in 1973 by John Bonica, an American anesthesiologist who elected himself president.

He tried to build an interdisciplinary pain community. The growing interest in the topic of pain, which followed the Gate-Control article by Wall and Melzack, motivated him to act. In 1973, he invited researchers and clinicians from all over the world to a secluded monastery near Seattle. This was the starting point of the IASP, which today has more than 6700 members from more than 100 countries and 60 specialties and is dedicated to the prevention and therapy of pain. What is pain? An introduction is provided by the current definition of the IASP:

"Pain is an unpleasant sensory and emotional experience associated with actual or potential tissue damage, or described in terms of such damage." (Raja et al., 2020).

From this, four deductions can be made:

1. *unpleasant*—Pain conditions are usually not pleasant and therefore not desirable. This gives rise to the desire to get rid of them.
2. *sensory or emotional experience*—Pain is not just a sense or the result of sensory input. It also has emotional components. No one can describe feelings better than the person who experiences these feelings. The patient's version is the complete reality here. A person's report of a pain experience should be respected. Attempting to confront or contradict the feelings with factual facts could lead to misunderstanding and dissatisfaction.
3. *actual or potential tissue damage*—This underlines that pain does not necessarily have to involve tissue damage or a noxious stimulus.
4. *or described in terms of such damage*—Pain is often described in terms of tissue damage or the risk of damage, even when no damage exists. This is the narrative and language of people who perceive pain—and especially essential for doctors and therapists to pick up on.

Traditionally, pain is described as a result of injury, inflammation, or pathology, which is transmitted to the brain by special pain receptors and perceived there (Goldberg, 2008). However, the term pain receptor is now unpopular and outdated, as pain is an experience generated by the brain, based on many different factors, including nociception, but not exclusively. The term *danger detector* or *warning detector* is now used synonymously with the term nociceptor. Nociceptors (from Latin: nocere = to harm) are nerves that respond to noxious (i.e., harmful or potentially harmful) stimuli. They send signals about the thermal, chemical, or mechanical state of the tissue and thus protect the body from (further) dangers and injuries. They transmit danger or warning information, but not pain to the brain. However, the fact that it hurts as a result is purposeful and functional, otherwise the harmful stimulus would not be avoided. Nociceptors have high activation thresholds and can only be activated by intense and noxious stimuli (Mickle et al., 2015).

Summary
The somatosensory system innervates the skin, muscles, and organs, among other things. The nociceptive system is part of the somatosensory system and connects peripheral tissue to the dorsal horn of the spinal cord (peripheral primary cranial nerves do not end in the spinal cord, but via trigeminal ganglia in the brainstem) through the transport of peripheral sensory-noxious information via the primary neuron, where they are switched contralaterally to the secondary neuron and drawn via the spinothalamic tract to the

lateral thalamus (cranial nerves to the medial thalamus). From the thalamus, the signals reach cortical structures, especially the primary somatosensory cortex, via the tertiary neuron. This is the ascending system. The descending system, in turn, can modulate incoming sensory afferents through synaptic connections between primary and secondary neurons at the spinal cord level. Facilitation is associated with central sensitization, inhibition with analgesia.

Various structures of the peripheral and central nervous system are involved in nociception (conversion of noxious stimuli into electrical signals and their transport to the central nervous system), which will be presented in the following. The term nociceptor refers only to the primary neuron (also called first-order neuron), which begins peripherally in the tissue and ends in the spinal cord. The secondary and tertiary neurons (also called second and third order neurons), which receive and transmit these nociceptive signals, are not nociceptors by definition. In English, they are called nocineurons. However, since the doctrine of nociception traditionally refers not only to the processes of the peripheral primary neuron, but the nociceptor is defined as such, the term nocineuronal system is recommended, which also includes processes beyond the primary neuron (primary, secondary, and tertiary neuron).

Different exteroceptive information from the environment is received by different receptors and nerves and transmitted to the CNS. Somatosensory signals are usually informative, nociceptive signals—as a form of somatosensory signals—are also protective. Pain differs from the classic senses (hearing, smelling, tasting, touching, and seeing) in that it contains both an informative-discriminative component (stimulus intensity, location, and quality) and an emotional component associated with actual or potential tissue damage.

Nociceptors have **free nerve endings,** which can be found in the skin, muscles, bones, joints, and organs. Microscopically, they do not show any specific receptive structure and thus also no structural difference to non-nociceptive free nerve endings (e.g., mechanoreceptors and thermoreceptors). Functionally, it is assumed that different free nerve endings possess different receptor molecules in their axon membrane and thus differ in their sensitivity to either noxious or non-noxious stimuli.

Nerve fibers are classified according to their fiber thickness (FT), their coating/myelination (Myel.) and the associated nerve conduction velocity (NCV) (see Tab. 2.1). In the classification according to Erlanger and Gasser, the nerve fibers are divided into afferent, vegetative, and efferent fibers (Aα, Aβ, Aγ, Aδ, B, C), according to Loyd and Hunt only into afferent fibers (I, II, III, IV). According to Erlanger and Gasser, the nociceptors represent the Aδ and C fibers and according to Loyd and Hunt the class III and IV fibers. The heterogeneity of nerve fiber structures is of functional relevance and the basis for understanding neurobiological mechanisms.

Tab. 2.1 Nerve fiber classification according to Erlanger & Gasser and Loyd & Hunt, own creation

Erlanger and Gasser	Loyd and Hunt	a = afferent e = efferent	FT (μm)	Myel.	NCV (m/s)
Aα	I	a = Proprioception from muscle spindles (Ia) and tendon spindles/Golgi organ (Ib)	15	Yes Yes	70–120
		e = alpha motor neurons			
Aβ	II	a = Touch and pressure sense of the skin	8	Yes	30–70
Aγ	–	a = Muscle spindles	5	Yes	
Aδ	III	a = nociceptive	5	Yes	12–30
B	–	e = sympathetic preganglionic visceral motor neurons	3	Light	2–12
C	IV	a = nociceptive	1	No	0,5–2
	–	e = sympathetic postganglionic visceral motor neurons			

Depending on the literature, one can find different information about the NCV of the respective nerve fibers. In summary, Aδ fibers are thicker and myelinated compared to C fibers and therefore faster. They are mainly sensitive to noxious thermal (Aδ-I) and mechanical (Aδ-II) stimuli and are responsible for the first, sharp, and short pain. The quality of pain is often described as *stabbing* or *sharp* and can be localized more precisely, as the receptive fields of the Aδ fibers are small. C fibers are thinner, unmyelinated, and thus slower. They respond to noxious mechanical, thermal, and chemical stimuli (such as after inflammation) and are known for the second, late, and long-lasting pain (Fig. 2.1). The quality of pain is often described as *dull, diffuse* or *burning* and cannot be clearly localized like signals from Aδ fibers, as their receptive fields are larger.

C fibers are stimulated secondary to Aδ fibers and if the noxious stimulus persists, the C fibers quickly adapt to the stimulus after its activation and lose their reactivity (Frias & Merighi, 2016; Tracey, 2017; Sneddon, 2018; Bista & Imlach, 2019).

Nociceptors can be divided according to their **location:**

- superficial somatic: the highest density of nociceptors is in the skin.
- deep somatic: muscle, tendon, ligament, bone, joint. There are no nociceptors in cartilage.
- Visceral: internal organs. Visceral nociceptors do not respond to cut or burn injuries like somatic nociceptors. Instead, they are activated in response to pathological changes. Pain-inducing stimuli in the viscera include inflammation, tension and stretching of hollow organs such as the gastrointestinal tract, urinary tract and gallbladder, strong contractions of the muscle layers surrounding such hollow organs, chemical irritants or ischemia in organs, such as the heart.

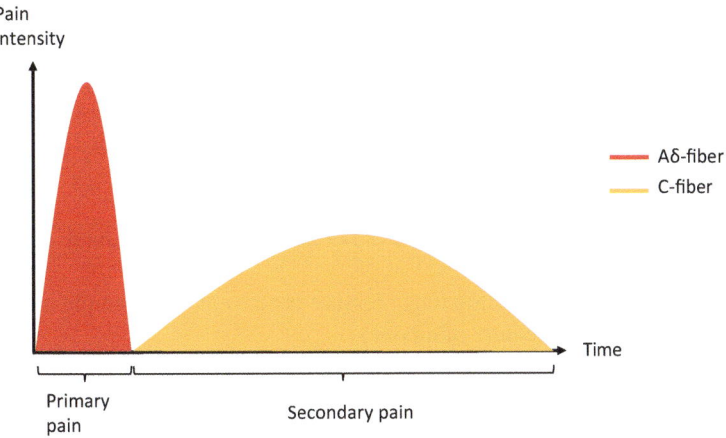

Fig. 2.1 Fiber type-dependent pain response, own production

In addition, each nociceptor, like every other somatosensory neuron, has a specific nociceptive or **receptive field.** Each somatosensory neuron responds specifically to stimuli of a certain modality that occur in a very specific region of the body. For example, a mechano-sensory axon that responds to tactile stimulation of the left index fingertip does not respond to tactile stimulation of the ulnar edge of the hand. The stimulated area that elicits a response is referred to as the receptive field of the neuron. This receptive field can also be anatomically defined as the area of the sensory organ (such as skin, muscles, or joints) that is directly or indirectly innervated by the neuron. Thus, a somatosensory neuron conveys information about the location and modality of the stimulus. The size of a neuron's receptive field is closely related to the innervated or represented body area. The receptive fields of neurons that innervate or represent the fingertips, lips, and tongue are the smallest, while neurons that innervate or represent shoulders, back, and legs have larger receptive fields. Smaller receptive fields are required for more precise localization of the stimulus contact. Fine motor activities, such as playing the piano or speaking, also require small proprioceptive receptive fields.

The **nozineuronal processes** can be divided from the peripheral noxious stimulus to the entry of signals in the cortex into **4 phases:**

1. Transduction (reception of noxious mechanical, thermal, or chemical stimuli and conversion into an electrical signal)
2. Transmission (transport of this signal to the brain)
3. Modulation (influence of this signal)
4. Perception (interaction of different brain structures with subsequent pain perception)

2.1 Transduction

The free nerve endings of Aδ and C fibers possess different receptor modalities, meaning different stimuli trigger different **nociceptive fibers**. Not every nociceptor responds to every noxious stimulus. Nociceptors can be divided into 3 groups according to their **receptor modality:**

1. Monomodal: can be activated by noxious mechanical, thermal or chemical stimuli
   a) mechanical (by strong noxious pressure or tension, for example after rupture of a ligament or fracture of a bone)
   b) thermal (by strong noxious heat or cold)
   c) chemical (by pH change due to acid exposure, for example after heart attacks or peripheral sensitization due to local inflammatory markers, such as bradykinin or histamine)
2. polymodal: can be activated by different noxious mechanical, thermal or chemical stimuli. The vast majority of Aδ and C fibers are polymodal
3. silent: a small proportion of Aδ fibers and a third of C fibers are silent nociceptors. This group of nociceptors has a very high activation threshold and is only excited by extremely high or prolonged stimulus intensities or as a result of peripheral sensitization. They are primarily not activated by noxious thermal or mechanical stimuli, but secondarily after inflammatory processes, which, for example, lead to redness around the irritated skin area after mosquito bites. The irritation results in a reduction of the activation threshold of silent nociceptors, making them also mechano- or thermosensitive. The activation of silent nociceptors contributes to the amplification of nociceptive signals towards the spinal cord, intensifying nociception and supporting the acute process of primary hyperalgesia.

All modalities can be found in both types of nociceptive fibers (Aδ and C). It should be critically noted that most study results suggesting a polymodality of nociceptors are electrophysiological studies. Calcium ion studies rather suggest that most nociceptors only have one modality, such as Aδ-I fibers, which can be activated by heat (thermal), but not by noxious pressure (mechanical). The impression of polymodality from electrophysiological studies could result from the fact that electrophysiological examinations are invasive and cause trauma and thus small inflammatory processes when the needle is inserted, which sensitizes other nociceptors, such as silent nociceptors or monomodal nociceptive neurons. Noxious stimuli can cause monomodal or silent nociceptors to become active and polymodal (Woller et al., 2017; St John Smith, 2018). Whether the nociceptors are mono- or polymodal, however, has no clinical-practical relevance.

Stimuli of different modalities (thermal, mechanical, chemical) lead to the activation of different receptors and the opening of their specific ion channels, which then cause a depolarization by the influx of cations such as calcium (Ca+) into the cell and contribute to the generation of an action potential. The depolarization is propagated by the opening of voltage-gated sodium channels, which generate new action potentials and transport them to the CNS (Tracey, 2017). The responsible ion channels of the mechanical receptors are not clearly described in the literature, but those of the thermal receptors are. One of the transduction mechanisms takes place significantly through the TRP ion channels (transient receptor potential channels) (Mickle et al., 2015). The free nerve endings possess TRPs, which are activated by specific stimuli. The activation of these TRPs occurs via the release of factors from damaged cells, which dock onto TRPs and open them. TRPs transduce particularly noxious thermal stimuli, and a few of them also noxious mechanical and chemical stimuli. TRPV1, for example, is a cation channel that is opened by protons and capsaicin at heat above 43 °C. The opening of the TRP channels leads to the influx of cations and depolarization of the nociceptor, hence they are also called the *transducers* of nociception. TRP channels are classified into different types depending on their temperature threshold (Fig. 2.2) and are found in both Aδ fibers and C fibers.

Nociceptors respond when a stimulus leads to tissue damage or can lead to it, e.g., through strong mechanical pressure or extreme heat. The tissue damage leads to the release of a variety of substances from damaged cells as well as new substances that are synthesized at the site of damage. Some of these substances activate the TRP channels, which in turn trigger action potentials and initiate primary afferents. These substances include, among others (Kendroud et al., 2022):

1. **Arachidonic acid** is an essential fatty acid that is released during tissue damage. After release, arachidonic acid is converted by enzymes such as cyclooxygenase (COX) into prostaglandins and cytokines. The prostaglandins, a group of lipid-like compounds, mediate their effect through a complex signal transduction cascade that includes the activation of G-proteins and the downstream activation of protein kinase-A. The prostaglandins act on various cell types, including nociceptors, and can increase their sensitivity. One mechanism by which prostaglandins do this is by blocking the potassium efflux that is normally released by the nociceptors after damage. This leads to an additional

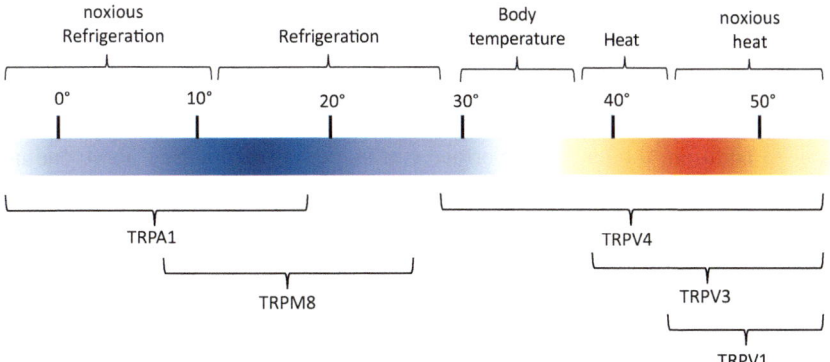

Fig. 2.2 Temperature-specific TRP types, own production

depolarization of the nociceptors and makes them more sensitive to noxious stimuli. A well-known example of a drug that targets this mechanism is aspirin. Aspirin inhibits the activity of the COX enzymes and thus prevents the conversion of arachidonic acid into prostaglandins. This reduces the inflammatory response and the sensitivity of the nociceptors, leading to pain relief.
2. It is suspected that damaged tissue releases **globulins and protein kinases.** Experiments have shown that subcutaneous injections of globulin can cause severe pain. This suggests that these substances could play a role in the onset of pain.
3. Tissue damage leads to the activation of mast cells, which release a variety of pro-inflammatory mediators, including **histamine.** Histamine is an important messenger that plays a key role in the inflammatory response and is also involved in the onset of pain. For example, subcutaneous injections of histamine can trigger severe pain by activating the nociceptors and thus sending danger signals to the central nervous system. The release of histamine is an important part of the inflammatory response and helps to activate the immune defense and protect the injured tissue.
4. Other classic pro-inflammatory markers such as **substance P and CGRP** (Calcitonin Gene-related Peptide) are released upon injury, thereby exciting nociceptors. Both peptides cause vasodilation, leading to the spread of edema around the original site of damage.
5. **NGF** (nerve growth factor) is also released during tissue damage. NGF then binds to TrkA (Tyrosine kinase-A) receptors on the surface of nociceptors, leading to their activation. A gene mutation that causes a lack of formation of TrkA receptors can result in NGF being unable to activate nociceptors. As a result, the person with this mutation may not perceive pain or perceive it very weakly. This illustrates the important role of NGF and TrkA receptors in the onset of pain.
6. Most tissue damage results in an increase in extracellular potassium cation (**K+**) levels. In the induction of acute noxious stimuli, there is a significant correlation between the local K+ concentration and the intensity of the pain.

These substances activate nociceptive channels. The activated channels close again when the harmful stimulus subsides. In addition, an excessive influx of calcium and sodium cations can stop the local inflammatory and nociceptive processes. Calcium overload in nociceptive neurons describes a situation where they take up too much calcium. This leads to the consumption of the originally present neuropeptides and the inhibition of the transport of new neuropeptides along the axon. In addition, the calcium overload causes the cutaneous free nerve endings to temporarily retract and withdraw. During this process, the TRPV cation channel enters a longer refractory period. During this time, the intracellular calcium gradient, i.e., the imbalance of calcium ions inside and outside the cell, is restored (Anand & Bley, 2011). This mechanism could be understood as one of the first modulations of the nociceptive afferents.

It is important to emphasize again at this point that the transduction of an external stimulus into a nociceptive signal is not the same as the onset of pain. The peripheral endings of the primary afferent are specialized in recognizing certain stimuli. However, the fibers are not specialized in the creation or production of specific perceptions. Nociceptors are specialized in recognizing harmful/noxious substances or stimuli and directing this danger signal into the central nervous system. This typically causes pain, but this is not always the case. In the heat of battle, the injury can go completely unnoticed despite nociceptor activation and thus the danger signal. Some soldiers of World War II had not noticed or only very faintly perceived gunshot wounds that were later identified (Beecher, 1946). On the other hand, the phenomenon of the *Thermo-Grill-Illusion* is known, where warm and cold rods (usually 40 and 20 °C) are arranged alternately like on a grill. These temperatures are not noxious and are below the activation threshold of the nociceptors, yet touching the grill triggers burning pain, even though no nociceptors were stimulated. This is suspected to be due to increased activation of special brain regions (thalamus, anterior insula, supramarginal gyrus), which are responsible for encoding emotions and new/unexpected stimuli (Lindstedt et al., 2011). These two examples illustrate that nociceptor activation is neither sufficient nor necessary for the onset of pain. Pain fibers do not exist.

2.2 Transmission

The image of Descartes, showing a man with his foot near a fire, is famous worldwide (Fig. 2.3). Upon closer inspection, 6 letters (a-f) can be seen, which he used to explain pain transmission and onset: "The fire (A) stirs up the cells of the foot (B). In this way, they open by pulling on the thread (c) over the entrance (e) the pore (d), where the thread ends; Just as one rings a bell by pulling on the end of a string that hangs at the other end." It continues: "When the entrance (e) of the pore (d) is opened, the souls flow in. These come from the cave F partly into the muscles, which serve to withdraw the foot from the fire, and partly into the muscles,

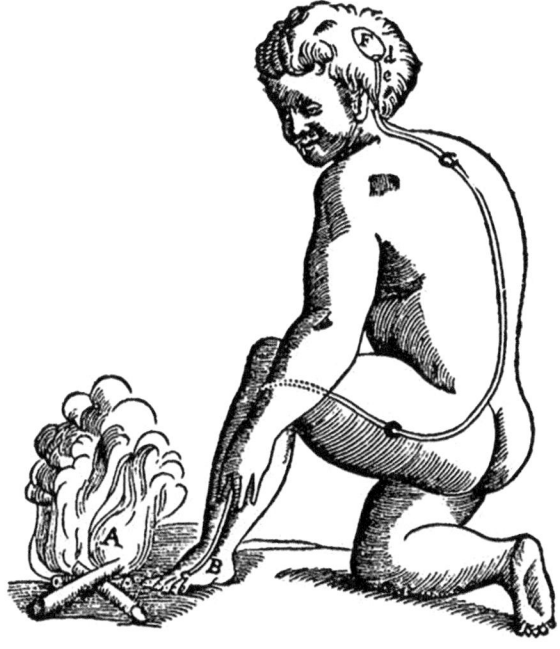

Fig. 2.3 Descartes pain pathway. (from the book "Traite de l'homme" 1664, public domain). https://upload.wikimedia.org/wikipedia/commons/8/8a/Descartes-reflex.JPG

which serve to turn the eyes and the head towards the fire (pain causer) and to look at it, and partly into the muscles, which serve to move the hands forward and to turn the whole body for its defense." (Descartes, 1664). Descartes describes nothing other than a motor protective reflex. Let's now use some more recent findings: the *thread* postulated by Descartes from the foot to the *bell* in the head, also understood as a conduction pathway, actually consists of three pathways (Fig. 2.4). The primary neuron connects peripheral tissue such as muscles, bones or organs nociceptively with the spinal cord. It transports action potentials, which arise after the detection of noxious stimuli and their transduction, from the damaged or damage-threatened tissue to the spinal cord. The secondary neuron transports the signals from the spinal cord towards the thalamus, where the signals are switched to the tertiary neuron before they reach the somatosensory cortex.

The pathways of the spinal cord run in the white matter and connect the spinal cord with the brain (connecting apparatus) on the one hand, and various spinal cord segments with each other (own apparatus) on the other hand. The connecting apparatus bundles the peripheral fiber types into different pathways at different locations in the spinal cord. They can be functionally divided into descending efferent (motor) and ascending afferent (sensory) pathways (Fig. 2.5).

The left-right division is only for better illustration. All red and blue pathways also exist on the contralateral side. (S = fibers from the sacral cord, L = lumbar cord, Th = thoracic cord, C = cervical pathway).

Fig. 2.4 Nociceptive transmission. primary neuron (yellow), secondary neuron (orange) and tertiary neuron (red)

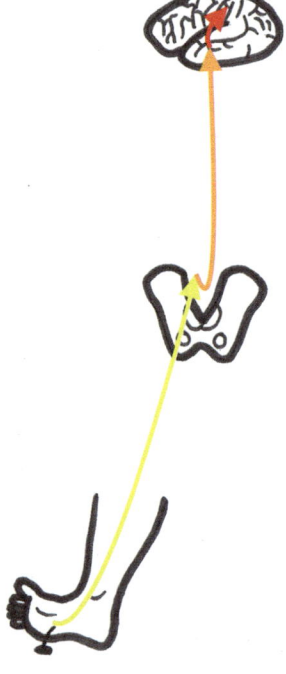

2.2 Transmission

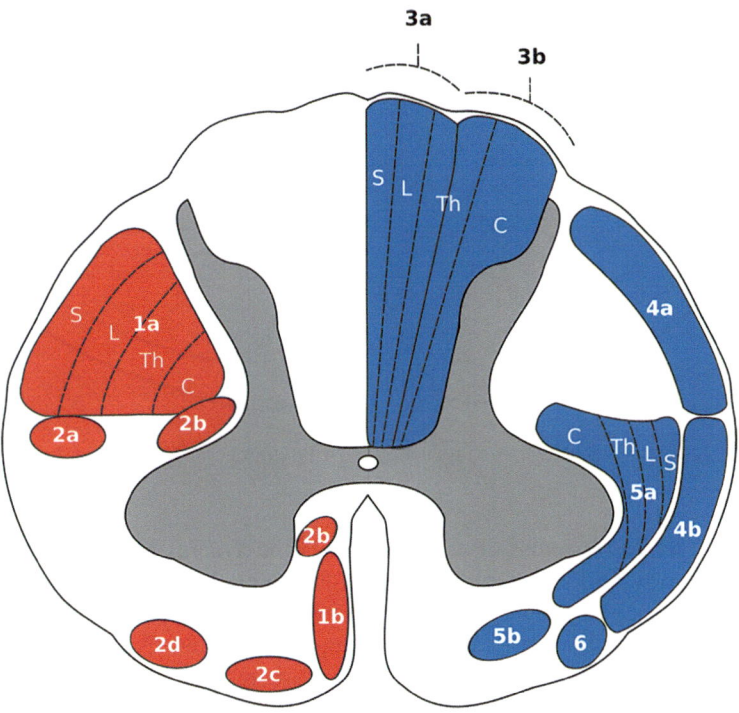

Fig. 2.5 Pathways of the spinal cord (by Polarlys, 05.06.2006, unchanged)

Efferent pathways (in red):	
1. Pyramidal tract 1a. Tractus corticospinalis lateralis 1b. Tractus corticospinalis anterior	Aα-fibers, (fine-)motor
2. Extrapyramidal tract 2a. Tractus rubrospinalis 2b. Tractus reticulospinalis 2c. Tractus vestibulospinalis 2d. Tractus olivospinalis	Aα-fibers, (gross-)motor
Afferent pathways (in blue):	
3. Posterior column pathway 3a. Fasciculus gracilis 3b. Fasciculus cuneatus	Aα-fibers, proprioceptive Aβ-fibers, mechano-sensory
4. Cerebellar lateral column pathway 4a. Tractus spinocerebellaris posterior 4b. Tractus spinocerebellaris anterior	Aγ-fibers, proprioceptive
5. Anterolateral column pathway 5b. Tractus spinothalamicus lateralis 5a. Tractus spinothalamicus anterior	Aβ-fibers, mechano-sensory Aδ-fibers, nociceptive C-fibers, nociceptive

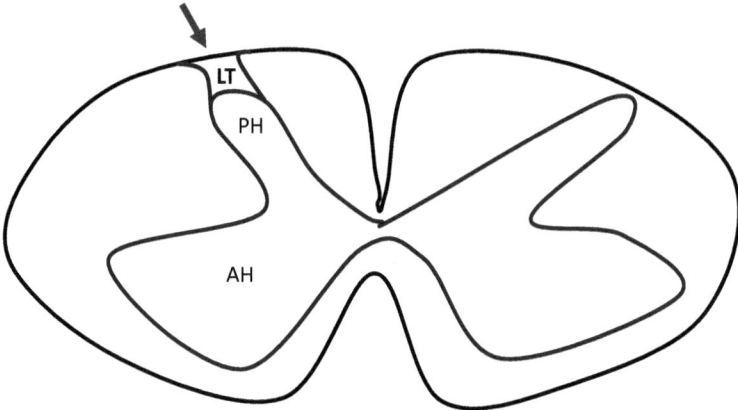

Fig. 2.6 Lissauer's tract (LT), own production. PH = posterior horn, AH = anterior horn

The nociceptive transmission takes place via the Tractus spinothalamicus lateralis (pathway 5b.). Prior to this, the action potentials of the primary neurons, whose frequency is proportional to the intensity of the noxious stimulus, are transmitted along the axons of the nociceptive Aδ- and C-fibers via the spinal nerve through the dorsal root ganglion, where they have their cell body, to the axon endings in the posterior horn of the spinal cord. Afferent fibers of the primary nociceptive neuron end via the posterolateral tract (also: Lissauer's tract, LT) in the posterior horn of the spinal cord (Fig. 2.6). The ends of these primary neurons cause a release of excitatory/amplifying amino acids (such as glutamate), neuropeptides (such as substance P and CGRP) and neurotrophins (such as NGF and BDNF).

Depending on the fiber type, the primary neurons end in different laminae, also called Rexed zones (Fig. 2.7). The posterior horn consists of laminae I–VI, where afferent fibers of the primary neuron are switched. The lateral and anterior horn consists of laminae VII–X and has efferent motor fibers.

Excursus
Posterior horn:
  The posterior horn contains 4 different types of neurons.

1. Terminations of afferent primary neurons from the periphery (the cell bodies are located in the spinal ganglion)
2. Interneurons
3. Dendrites of afferent secondary neurons, which direct signals to the brain via various tracts outside the posterior horn
4. Descending pathways from various parts of the brain, especially the brainstem (modulatory effect on nociceptive interconnection)

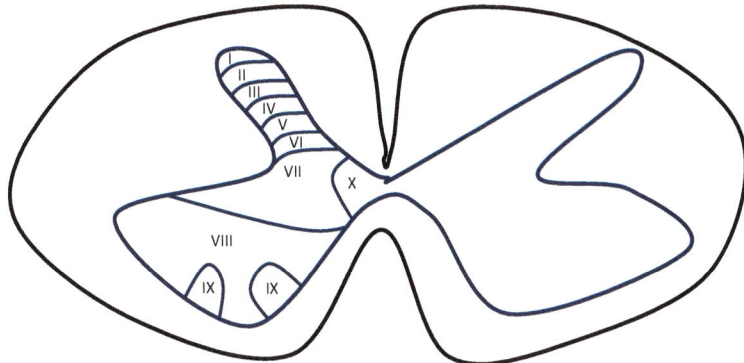

Fig. 2.7 Laminae of the spinal cord, own production

The nociceptive Aδ and C fibers primarily end in the superficial laminae I and II, the substantia gelatinosa. The mechanosensory Aβ fibers transport touch information to the deeper layers III–VI, some nociceptive fibers also end in lamina V. From the laminae, the nociceptive signals from Aδ and C fibers are switched to the secondary neuron (posterior horn neuron), of which there are two types: Either to a nociception-specific neuron (from laminae I–II) or a WDR (wide dynamic range) neuron (from laminae III–V), which modality-unspecifically receive and transmit various somatosensory stimuli (from Aβ, Aδ and C fibers). As the name suggests, WDR neurons are capable of transmitting signals of a wide range—nociceptive and subnociceptive. In both secondary posterior horn neurons (nociception-specific and WDR), the excitatory neurotransmitter glutamate is released from the primary neuron, which is recognized by glutamatergic receptors on the dendrites of the secondary neuron. After its excitation, the secondary neuron crosses diagonally towards the contralateral anterior horn and ascends via the lateral spinothalamic tract towards the brain. Not to be confused: The anterior spinothalamic tract transports touch and pressure sensation, whereas the lateral spinothalamic tract transports nociceptive afferents from Aδ and C fibers. As the name suggests, this tract connects the spinal cord and the thalamus, where most fibers of the secondary neuron end, specifically in the ventroposterolateral (VPL) and ventroposteroinferior (VPI) nucleus of the thalamus.

It should be noted that nociceptive signals from the body periphery take this standard path to the thalamus, while nociceptive signals from the head area take an alternative path. While the spinal nerve represents the primary neuron for the nociceptive afferents from the body periphery (limbs and trunk), nociceptive afferents from the head area are transported to the CNS via the N. trigeminus. This primary neuron for the cranial nerves is not switched to a secondary neuron via the spinal cord. It enters via the trigeminal ganglion, the medulla and pons in the spinal trigeminal nucleus (Nucleus spinalis nervi trigemini, Ncl. spin. N. trig.), crosses there contralaterally to the Tractus trigeminothalamicus, which joins the lateral spinothalamic tract. From there, fibers of this secondary neuron also lead to the thalamus. Signals from Aδ fibers go to the ventroposteromedial (VPM) area, while signals from C fibers end in the CM-PF (Centrum medianum and Ncl. parafascicularis thalami) complex in the intralaminar nuclei (IL-N). Thus, nociceptive afferents from the head area bypass the spinal cord and pass through brainstem structures to the thalamus (Fig. 2.8).

From the thalamus, tertiary neurons extend to the somatosensory cortex, which is located in the postcentral gyrus in the parietal lobe of the brain. These tertiary neurons, which extend from the thalamus to the cortex, can be divided into two types and thus into two differentiated pathways. One pathway is responsible for the precise transmission of information about the location and intensity of the stimulus, while the other pathway integrates the nociceptive stimuli into emotional and affective responses.

The first pathway, which provides information about the location and intensity of the stimulus, leaves the thalamus and continues to its final destination in the somatosensory cortex. Here, the sensory information is processed and allows the stimulus to be localized and its intensity to be recognized. Here, the pain receives its sensory-discriminative component. The somatosensory cortex can be divided into two areas. On the one hand, into the primary somatosensory cortex S. 1 (Brodmann areas 1, 2, and 3), where nociceptive afferents converge simultaneously with other non-nociceptive mechano-sensory afferents, and on the other hand, into a smaller area adjacent to the dorsal, the secondary somatosensory cortex S. 2 (Brodmann areas 40 and 43), which lies behind the postcentral gyrus on the parietal lobe and contributes to the interpretation of incoming sensory information.

The second pathway leaves the brainstem via the medial and ventro-medial thalamus and ends in other brain regions than the somatosensory cortex, such as the limbic system. In these brain regions, the nociceptive stimuli are linked with emotional components, which influences our response to pain and, among other things, allows pain to be perceived as unpleasant or threatening and to be avoided. Here, the pain receives its affective-cognitive component (Frias & Merighi, 2016; Woller et al., 2017). These neuroanatomical insights provide initial explanations for emotional aspects of pain and the inter-individual different perception of sensory information.

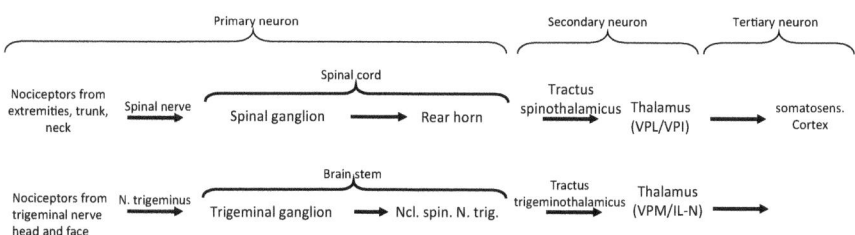

Fig. 2.8 Transmission path of nociceptive signals, own production

2.3 Modulation

> **Excursus**
> For a long time, it was assumed that the different cortical projections could be explained by the different pathways originating from the thalamus. However, this variation is not only due to the different course of tertiary neurons, but also to the different course of nociceptive afferents of the secondary neurons, which do not only ascend via the lateral spinothalamic tract. The neospinothalamic pathway is not the only pathway that transports nociceptive afferents to the brain according to the latest findings (Sengul & Watson, 2015; Kendroud et al., 2022). There are two more pathways.
>
> 1. Neospinothalamical Pathway ascends from Lamina I in a diagonal contralateral direction to the thalamus (VPL/VPI). From there, the signals are projected ipsilaterally onto the primary somatosensory cortex (S1) via the tertiary neuron. This tract quickly supplies the brain with the basic data of the noxious stimulus, i.e., the sensory-discriminative component (localization, intensity, quality).
> 2. Paleospinothalamic Pathway is evolutionarily older than the spinothalamic tract and is located ventrally in the spinal cord and ascends from Laminae II and IV–VIII from anterior, bilaterally and uncrossed via secondary WDR neurons to brainstem structures, such as the CM-PF complex and the PAG (Periaqueductal Gray). From there, the signals are projected bilaterally onto the secondary somatosensory cortex (S2) and limbic structures via the tertiary neuron. Fibers of this pathway mediate visceral, emotional, and autonomic reactions to pain. The paleospinothalamic pathway also activates brainstem nuclei, which are the starting point for descending inhibition (see Sect. 2.3, Modulation).
> 3. Archispinothalamic Pathway is phylogenetically the oldest ascending nociceptive pathway and starts from Lamina II, connects Laminae IV–VII and ascends from there (central in the spinal cord) also to brainstem structures, such as the CM-PF complex, the PAG, and the IL-N. From there, the signals are projected onto the secondary somatosensory cortex (S2) and limbic structures bilaterally via the tertiary neuron, similar to the paleospinothalamic pathway. Fibers of this pathway also mediate visceral, emotional, and autonomic pain reactions.

2.3 Modulation

The noxious stimulus that generates nociceptive signals is modulated by different mechanisms on its way to the brain. The modulation of nociceptive transmission in the nervous system can occur in the form of facilitation (enhancement) as well as inhibition (suppression) (Staud, 2013). Neurons thus either act:

1. enhancing (facilitating, also called excitatory) or
2. inhibiting (inhibitory)

Facilitation
Various neurotransmitters play a central role in nociceptive transmission. The most significant include peptides, purines, and excitatory amino acids (EAAs). In particular, glutamate, the most prominent EAA, triggers the first excitatory response at the postsynaptic secondary neuron. Glutamate binds to glutamate receptors, such as AMPA receptors and NMDA receptors, leading to the depolarization of the postsynaptic membrane. This depolarization causes the postsynaptic neuron to be activated and to relay nociceptive signals. Following the initial glutamatergic excitation, peptides such as substance P are released. These peptides bind to neurokinin-1 (NK-1) receptors on the postsynaptic neuron and cause a prolonged depolarization. This extended depolarization contributes to sustained nociceptive transmission. Substance P is particularly known for its role in enhancing nociceptive signals in both the spinal cord and the brain. The combination of glutamate and peptides, such as substance P, leads to the maintenance and enhancement of nociceptive signal transmission, contributing to the intensification of pain perception. The body wants to ensure that the nociceptive signals reach the brain, so nociception is a self-exciting phenomenon.

Inhibition
In addition to facilitation, inhibition also plays a crucial role in the modulation of nociceptive signals. Inhibitory neurotransmitters, such as gamma-aminobutyric acid (GABA) and glycine, cause a reduction in nociceptive transmission. These neurotransmitters bind to their respective receptors on the postsynaptic neuron and cause a hyperpolarization of the membrane, which prevents the activation of the neuron and thus inhibits the transmission of nociceptive signals. The balance between excitatory and inhibitory signals is crucial for pain perception. In chronic pain conditions, this balance can be disturbed, leading to an overactivation of nociceptive pathways and thus to an enhanced pain perception.

Examples of Modulation
The phenomenon of **peripheral sensitization,** which triggers primary hyperalgesia induced by trauma, is a facilitating modulation. Peripheral sensitization causes a reduction in the activation threshold of nociceptors and an increase in the frequency of action potentials towards the spinal cord. The inflammation-induced peripheral sensitization is physiological. Nociceptors and primary afferents have the ability to release neuropeptides (substance P or CGRP) from their endings in the spinal cord. These neuropeptides are transported from the cell body to the periphery and released there upon stimulation. They cause a so-called neurogenic inflammation. It is nociceptively self-exciting, enhancing, and thus contributes to acute regeneration through the compulsion to rest or conserve.

2.3 Modulation

In addition to these local and peripheral reactions that influence nociceptive signals, central mechanisms play a role in pain modulation. Mainly **interneurons** of the substantia gelatinosa of the dorsal horn of the spinal cord and **descending pathways** play a crucial role in the modulation of nociceptive signals by either facilitating or inhibiting them (Mitsi & Zachariou, 2016).

At the spinal cord level, excitatory and inhibitory neurotransmitters are involved in the connection from the primary to the secondary neuron:

1. Excitatory transmitters of nociceptors: Glutamate, substance P and CGRP (activation of AMPA and NMDA receptors in the postsynaptic membrane)
2. Inhibitory transmitters of interneurons: GABA, glycine, and endogenous opioids/endorphins (activation of opioid receptors at the pre- and postsynaptic membrane). These transmitters are released from the interneurons onto the secondary neuron.

Interneurons can be divided into two groups.

1. Facilitatory/excitatory interneurons: glutamatergic amplification
2. Inhibitory interneurons: GABA and glycinergic inhibition

It is suspected that interneurons not only act between primary nociceptive (Aδ fibers) and secondary nociceptive neurons (tractus spinothalamicus), but also between primary nociceptive and primary sensory neurons (Aβ fibers). Thus, sensory stimuli, such as rubbing the painful area, can activate inhibitory interneurons via Aβ fibers and weaken or block the nociceptive signals of the Aδ fibers. Interneurons form the largest population of all neurons in the dorsal horn of the spinal cord and under physiological conditions establish a finely tuned balance between facilitation and inhibition (Todd, 2010). However, this balance can be disturbed in chronic pain, leading to increased pain perception. In particular, various subtypes of glutamatergic interneurons play a crucial role in acute, inflammatory, and neuropathic pain conditions by influencing the intensity, frequency, and duration (Wang et al., 2013). A well-documented phenomenon is the reduced GABAergic and glycinergic inhibition, which contributes to the development of neuropathic hyperalgesia (Moore et al., 2002; Lu et al., 2013). This inhibition is normally crucial to control the activity of the nociceptors and prevent excessive nociceptive influx.

The inhibition of nociceptive signals (endogenous pain inhibition) is achieved by the release of endogenous **opioids.** Exogenous opioids are well known:

Opioids are drugs that are very effective for short-term pain relief and act through the CNS, while non-opioid analgesics mainly exert their effect peripherally. Opioids are derived from the poppy plant. These include opium, morphine, codeine or heroin; these opioids bind to various types of opioid receptors located throughout the brain, with receptor density particularly high in areas such as the midbrain and spinal cord. The brain also produces its own (endogenous) opioids, including endorphins or enkephalins, which bind to the same receptors in the brain and have an analgesic effect, like the exogenous opioids. When opioids (exogenous or endogenous) bind to their receptors, they modulate the incoming nociceptive signals and provide temporary pain relief by inhibiting these signals. It is known that opioids have effects on mood and can induce euphoric feelings. Unfortunately, they also have several side effects, especially drug dependence and abuse.

The release of endogenous opioids is achieved through the activity of **descending pathways.**

Opioid receptors are found at various locations at the level of the spinal cord and in cortical structures, such as the PAG, the raphe nuclei (nuclei raphes) and the habenula (in the brainstem), the nucleus caudatus (in the cerebrum), the nucleus septalis (in the limbic system), the hypothalamus and the hippocampus. At the level of the spinal cord, these receptors are located at the presynaptic ends of the nociceptive neurons in laminae IV to VII. Beta-endorphins, enkephalins, and dynorphins serve as ligands (substances that bind to receptors and trigger reactions) that activate these receptors and cause hyperpolarization of the cells through the activation of potassium channels and the blocking of calcium influx. The subsequent inhibition of substance P leads to a blocked or reduced nociceptive transmission. The descending modulation consists of a circuit that includes, among other things, brainstem structures, their descending pathways, interneurons, and opioid receptors. Especially the PAG and the structures associated with it are responsible for the modulation of the body's response to stress, especially pain, via opioid receptors. It suppresses information transmitted via C-fibers (not via Aδ fibers) by inhibiting local GABAergic interneurons (Kendroud et al., 2022).

Brainstem structures can influence nociceptive signals at the spinal cord level via descending pathways (top-down). Important involved brainstem structures are structures close to the rostral ventromedial medulla (RVM), the raphe nuclei, and the PAG. The neurons in the PAG have axons that descend to the raphe nuclei. These raphe nuclei are located in the medulla oblongata and contain serotonin. The neurons of the raphe nucleus send their axons to the spinal cord, where they release serotonin to the secondary neuron (in addition to opioids, another way to modulate nociceptive signals). These brainstem structures can thus either inhibit or facilitate nociceptive signals in the dorsal horn during the afferent interconnection from the primary to the secondary neuron via descending pathways (Ossipov et al., 2010). Modulating cells of these brainstem structures are divided into three categories. Into on-, off- or neutral cells, depending on how they influence nociception (Marinelli et al., 2002).

1. On-cells enhance nociceptive action potentials and are thus facilitating/amplifying. These cells are also called pro-nociceptive. For example, they show increased activity during central sensitization processes.
2. Off-cells reduce nociceptive action potentials and are thus inhibitory/suppressive. These cells are also called anti-nociceptive. For example, they are activated by morphine.

2.3 Modulation

3. Neutral cells: have no influence on nociceptive afference.

These cells project via descending pathways either through amplifying or inhibitory processes to the dorsal horn, where signals from the primary neuron are switched to the secondary neuron. The secondary neuron thus has synaptic connections both to the primary neuron, which transmits nociceptive signals from the periphery, and to the descending neuron of the PAG and the raphe nuclei. These neuronal connections are mediated via the interneurons in the dorsal horn. The released serotonin inhibits the activity of the secondary neuron and thus prevents the nociceptive signal from ascending to the brain or weakens its signals.

However, it is not yet conclusively clarified in which exact situations the PAG neurons prevent nociceptive signals from ascending to the brain. In certain stress situations, pain relief can occur, which is referred to as stress-induced analgesia (SIA). SIA provides insights into the psychological and physiological mechanisms that activate the body's own pain control and opiate systems. An example of this are athletes who injure themselves in competitions, do not feel pain during the acute stress situation, but the pain sets in after the end of the stress situation. In addition, animal experiments have shown that electric shocks can cause SIA. It is assumed that endogenous opiates are released under stress, which inhibit nociception by activating the descending pain control system in the brainstem (Kurrikoff et al., 2008; Liao & Lin, 2021). The underlying descending pain inhibition by painful stimuli is called DNIC (diffuse noxious inhibitory control by painful stimuli). Already in antiquity, there were practices based on this principle. Here, new pain stimuli were set with hot metal at body sites distant from the pain area to alleviate pain in another area. A new, stronger pain stimulus alleviated the pain of the old pain area. Now the question would have to be answered whether the old pain is perceived less strongly despite the same nociceptive influx, or whether the nociceptive influx is reduced and therefore less pain is perceived. In fact, the latter is the case: with a new noxious stimulus with strong nociceptive influx, the previous weaker nociceptive influx is actively attenuated (Fig. 2.9). Researchers conducted experiments in which they induced a noxious painful stimulus in rats and observed the electrical neurophysiological activity in a nociceptive neuron of the spinal cord. They found that they could inhibit this nociceptive reaction by setting noxious painful stimuli at other sites. Non-nociceptive mechano-sensory stimuli were ineffective in this regard and the degree of inhibition was proportional to the intensity and duration of the noxious painful stimulus. The SIA and suppression of the old less intense nociceptive influx represents a stronger contrast, which makes it easier for the brain to interpret the information of the new more intense (acutely more important) nociceptive influx (Le Bars et al., 1979; Sirucek et al., 2023). When conducting an intense and painful therapy in clinical practice with a subsequent reduction in pain in a patient, in addition to possible biomechanical changes, neurophysiological overlay and modulation effects of the SIA should also be considered for its explanation.

SIA and DNIC should not be confused with the mechanosensory overlay effect via Aβ fibers, for example when touching or rubbing oneself in pain. The pain relief through mechano-sensory stimuli takes place directly at the level of the dorsal horn via inhibitory interneurons. In the case of pain relief through noxious stimuli, brainstem structures in the midbrain are involved, which in turn inhibit nociceptive signals at the level of the dorsal horn via the release of opioids.

Descending pathways, which originate from the Raphe nuclei and the PAG, are not the only modulation pathways. The PAG not only sends descending pathways to the dorsal horn, but also ascending pathways to the thalamus, which in addition to spinal modulation can presumably also modulate supraspinally. In addition, the descending pathways are not only inhibitory (Heinricher et al., 2009; Staud, 2013). The fact that descending pathways can both facilitate and inhibit, but are better known for their inhibitory effect, is due to the fact that descending facilitation is not as well researched as descending inhibition. Facilitating phenomena shape sensitization processes that can lead to chronic pain conditions. These are discussed in more detail in Chap. 3.

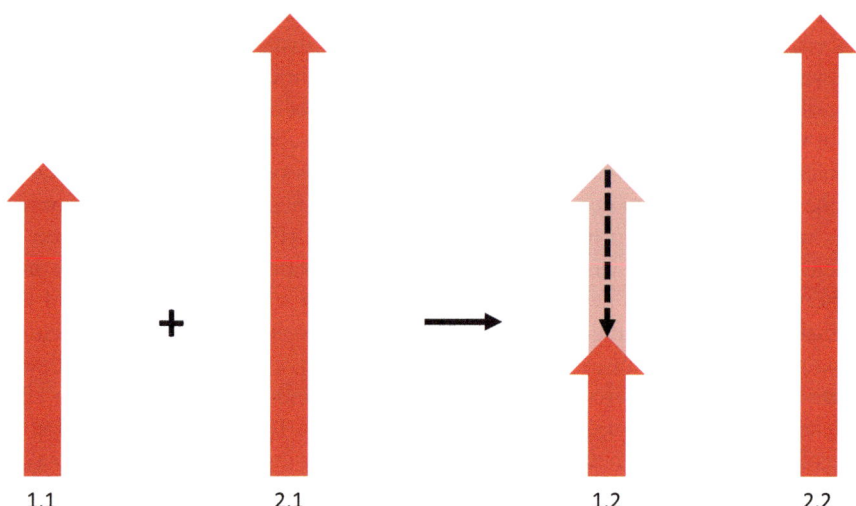

Fig. 2.9 Nociceptive inhibition, own production
1.1 = Nociceptive influx through a noxious stimulus,
2.1 = New stronger nociceptive influx through a larger noxious stimulus in another area,
1.2 = Attenuation of the weaker nociceptive influx,
2.2 = Constant, but in relation stronger, nociceptive influx of the second stimulus.

2.4 Perception

The entry of nociceptive information via the tertiary neuron, even after its modulation by dorsal horn or brainstem structures, is not the final step in the genesis of pain. At the cortical level, the incoming stimulus is never evaluated purely in sensory terms. The second type of tertiary neuron has already been introduced, which does not carry nociceptive information directly to the somatosensory cortex, but to the limbic system. This is followed by an interaction of different brain structures and the summary of all available information, which results in the perception of the noxious stimulus with an individual signature. Pain is a perception that contains different dimensions. Melzack and Casey were the first to distinguish dimensions and assigned three dimensions to pain (Melzack & Casey, 1968):

1. The **sensory-discriminative** dimension identifies the location, characteristics (including mechanical sharp, flat, thermal, chemical) and intensity of the noxious stimulus. With sufficient intensity, it leads to acute avoidance (withdrawal reflex) to prevent or limit tissue damage. The sensory-discriminative dimension not only includes the identification of the location of the noxious stimulus, but also the precise characterization of its properties. These properties can encompass various modalities, such as mechanical, thermal or chemical stimuli, and manifest in whether the stimulus is perceived as sharp, flat, piercing or burning. In addition, the intensity of the painful stimulus plays a crucial role in this dimension. With sufficient intensity, the noxious stimulus often leads to an immediate withdrawal reflex aimed at preventing or limiting tissue damage. This withdrawal reflex is an evolutionary response of the organism aimed at protecting the body from potential dangers. The sensory-discriminative dimension contributes to the organism's ability to respond quickly and effectively to noxious stimuli by precisely locating them, recognizing their properties, and assessing their intensity to initiate protective mechanisms.
2. The **affective-motivational** dimension refers to emotional aspects of pain. This includes both the emotions triggered by the painful stimulus and the emotional state of the person, which influences the interpretation of the stimulus. Noxious stimuli and pain often trigger a variety of unpleasant emotions, such as fear, anger, or frustration. These emotions can intensify the experience of pain and increase subjective suffering. At the same time, a person's emotional state before or during the experience of pain can influence the way the noxious stimulus is perceived and interpreted. A person who is in a state of anxiety or depression, for example, may perceive the pain as more intense or react more negatively to it than a person who is in a more positive emotional state. This reciprocal relationship between nociceptive sensation and emotions reflects the complex nature of the pain experience. The affective-motivational dimension of pain therefore encompasses emotional reactions and the motivation to cope with the painful state beyond the sensory experience.

3. The **cognitive-evaluative** dimension of the pain experience concerns the significance attributed to a painful stimulus and the consequences derived from it. Here, awareness of potential dangers plays a crucial role, as does the learning of behaviors that serve to avoid these dangers in the long term and thus ensure survival. By evaluating the noxious stimulus and assessing its potential consequences, the brain can develop adequate responses to protect itself. This evaluation also includes remembering past experiences and learning behaviors that help cope with future noxious/potentially pain-causing situations. The behaviors developed in response to painful stimuli often stem from the negative emotions associated with pain. These emotions thus serve as a drive for cognitive evaluation, which is why the cognitive and affective dimensions are closely intertwined and cannot be clearly separated from each other.

The IASP postulates 5 dimensions of pain (Merskey & Bogduk, 1986). In addition to the sensory-discriminative, affective-motivational, and cognitive-evaluative components, a motor and a vegetative component were also described.

4. The **motor** dimension of pain experience refers to the body's motor responses to a noxious stimulus. This includes, on the one hand, automatic and involuntary protective reflexes that occur in response to pain (such as withdrawing the hand) to avoid the noxious stimulus source, and on the other hand, pain-related changes in posture and movement aimed at relieving the painful area or avoiding pain. Melzack had combined the motor dimension of pain experience with the sensory-discriminative dimension. However, the IASP considers the motor dimension as a separate aspect of pain experience.
5. The **vegetative** dimension of pain experience, which Melzack does not explicitly name, refers to the body's autonomic or vegetative responses to a noxious or painful stimulus. These responses are part of the autonomic nervous system and include a variety of physiological changes aimed at preparing the body for the threat of pain or dealing with it. Typical vegetative responses to pain include, for example, an increase in blood pressure, an acceleration of heart rate, an increase in respiratory rate, which is due to the increased activity of the sympathetic nervous system, also known as the *fight-or-flight*-response.

In summary, pain perception has 5 different dimensions. Starting with the noxious stimulus, the brain receives sensory information, which is of an **informative** nature. This is followed by **reactive** dimensions, which include the motor protective response, response of the autonomic nervous system, and change in emotional state. The last dimension is **interpretive,** in which stimuli and responses are interpreted and influence future behavior patterns. In Fig. 2.10 the 5 dimensions are represented as a linear sequence, but a more likely scenario is an interaction between reactive and interpretive aspects (Fig. 2.11), as reactions, especially emotions, also rely on cognitive interpretation.

Fig. 2.10 Pain dimensions 1, own illustration

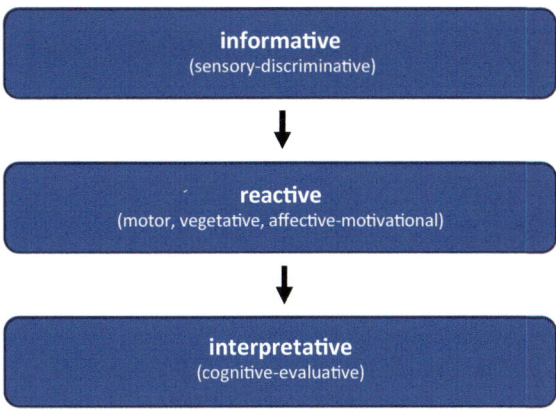

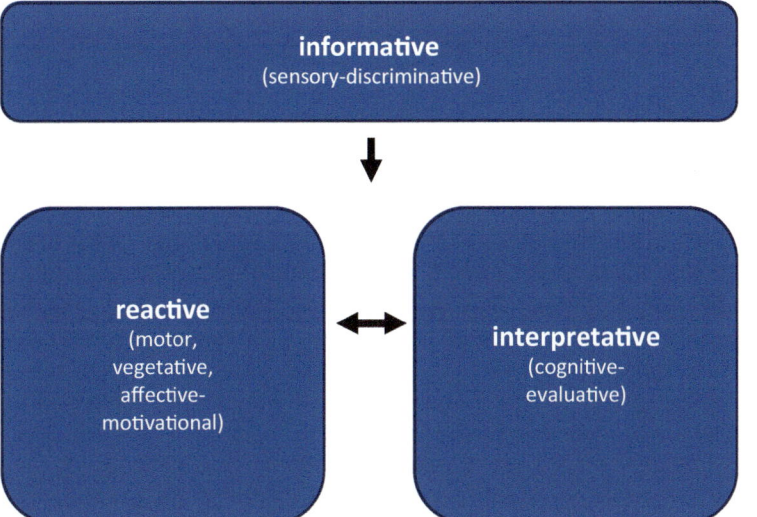

Fig. 2.11 Pain dimensions 2, own illustration

2.5 Forms of Pain

Pain can be divided into 3 different forms depending on their origin or driver.

1. Nociceptive: Pain that arises from actual or threatened damage to somatic and visceral (non-neuronal) tissue and is due to the activation of nociceptors.
2. Neuropathic: Pain caused by an injury or disease of the somatosensory nervous system (neuronal tissue).

3. Nociplastic: Pain that arises from altered nociception, without clear evidence of actual or threatened tissue damage causing the activation of peripheral nociceptors, or without clear evidence of an injury or disease of the somatosensory system or neural tissue causing the pain. Although nociplastic pain can have nociceptive or neuropathic drivers/components, these are not solely responsible for the pain.

Nociceptive pain originates from (potential) damage to peripheral tissue. Somatic nociceptive pains are superficial or deep, originating in the skin, muscles, or bones. Visceral pains originate in the abdominal cavity or in certain organs. Visceral pains often manifest as referred pain, whose location does not correspond with the pain-causing tissue/organ. An example of this is left-sided shoulder and upper arm pain during a heart attack. This phenomenon can be explained by the fact that nociceptive visceral afferents (C-fibers) converge at the spinal cord level in the posterior horn with mechanosensory afferents of the skin (Aβ-fibers), leading to co-activation and the brain including this skin area, which neurally attaches to the visceral fibers, in the pain interpretation, because the endings of the nociceptors from the organs in the spinal cord end at the same neurons that receive the input from the skin (Jin et al., 2023).

Neuropathic pain is also understood as a type of nociceptive pain, but it does not originate from somatic or visceral tissue, but from the somatosensory nervous system, the neural tissue. The dysfunction or damage can either be in the peripheral nervous system (peripheral neuropathic pain), as in diabetic neuropathy or postherpetic neuralgia, or in the central nervous system (central neuropathic pain), as in CNS damage following spinal cord injuries, strokes, or multiple sclerosis (Treede et al., 2008). These damages generate ectopic signals: increased and spontaneous impulses or discharges of nociceptive afferents, which occur without external peripheral stimulation. This is a typical characteristic of nerve injuries. These ectopic signals can lead to tingling or pain in the innervated area (positive symptoms), while damages (advanced stage) can cause sensory or even motor deficits in the innervated area (negative symptoms). In clinical testing, for example, pinpricks or temperature sensation in the pain area are tested. If the sensation on the affected side is significantly reduced compared to the unaffected side, one can assume damage to the spinothalamic tract and thus central neuropathic pain. Neuropathic pain, unlike nociceptive pain, has stronger central/spinal components, such as synaptic plasticity, which triggers enhanced neuronal reactions in the form of temporal and spatial summation. One of the causes for this is the loss of inhibitory modulation ability, which would normally apply in nociceptive pain. Other components are the enlargement and expansion of the receptive fields of primary neurons (nociceptors) and secondary neurons (spinothalamic tract), as well as an increased excitability of ascending nociceptive neurons. These neuroplastic changes occur along the nociceptive pathways in the spinal cord and in various brain regions (Cohen & Mao, 2014). Nerve damage and resulting neuropathic pain have a worse prognosis compared to muscle or bone damage and resulting nociceptive pain and are more prone to chronicity (Ciaramitaro et al., 2010).

Nociplastic pain is a new term for chronic pain. Terms like acute or chronic pain refer to the duration of the pain. The terms nociceptive or nociplastic refer to the cause/drivers/mechanisms of the pain. Nociplastic pain can be considered a form of primary chronic pain, which according to the IASP is defined as a pain that 1.) "lasts or recurs for more than 3 months", 2.) "is associated with significant emotional distress" and 3.) has symptoms that "cannot be better explained by another diagnosis" (Nicholas et al., 2019). While chronic secondary pain is defined as a symptom/consequence of another disease, such as cancer, in chronic primary pain the pain itself can be considered a disease. Some of the conditions in this classification include Chronic widespread pain (CWP) such as fibromyalgia, irritable bowel syndrome or chronic nonspecific back pain. These conditions often go hand in hand with central sensitization and can be associated with psychological stress, fear avoidance behavior and pain catastrophizing. Patients can benefit from appropriate cognitive and behavioral strategies (Nicholas et al., 2019).

It is important to mention: Nociceptive pain describes a correlation or a relationship between pain perception and the health status of the peripheral tissue. However, the nociceptive/nocineuronal system is also involved in every other non-nociceptive form of pain. In nociplastic pain, however, nociception does not occur due to peripheral tissue damage, activation of the primary neuron, or peripheral inflammation, but due to changes and independent impulse generation of the CNS. Thus, nociception does not always occur due to a peripheral noxious stimulus, but nociceptive pain does.

In some literature, **inflammatory pain** is considered a distinct form of pain (Prescott & Ratté, 2017). However, inflammatory processes play a role in almost every nociceptive transduction, transmission, and modulation. It is known that a nociceptive signal can be directly rerouted via a spinal reflex loop, leading to a rapid, reflex-like motor response (such as ducking away or pulling away) before it reaches the areas of the brain responsible for linking these signals with other information and triggering a pain perception. In addition to spinal afferent transmission to the CNS, however, nociceptive neurons also independently respond to harmful stimuli by secreting chemical reactions from their peripheral nerve endings. These reactions mediate local effects on neighboring neuronal and non-neuronal cells through the release of vesicles containing pro-inflammatory mediators (Woller et al., 2017), such as substance P, neurokinin-A, and CGRP. These pro-inflammatory cytokines activate surrounding immune cells, smooth muscle cells, epithelial cells, and the endothelium, leading to a further release of pro-inflammatory cytokines such as IL-1β, IL-6, IL-8, TNF-α, and extracellular ATP. These mediators activate additional (also silent) nociceptors that extend beyond the original stimulus induction site (also called the primary nociceptive field). This peripheral sensitization leads to a secondary nociceptive field through the amplification of nociceptive afferents and is part of the modulatory system. The spread of inflammation triggered by a nociceptor over an area larger than that of the originally involved nociceptor is referred to as *neuroinflammation*. This complex phenomenon is of particular interest as it exhibits a self-amplifying dynamic. The spread of nociceptive neurons to surrounding cells, which in turn can sensitize nearby nociceptive neurons, contributes to this amplification. The released pro-inflammatory molecules play a key role by not only activating local inflammatory cells but also achieving the direct activation of other nociceptive nerve endings. Almost all nociceptive nerve endings have receptors for the pro-inflammatory markers they release themselves. Thus, the molecules released by a directly stimulated nociceptive neuron can bind to a local adjacent, but originally completely unaffected by the noxious stimulus, nociceptive neuron and activate it. This mechanism of indirect activation further amplifies the response, as the pro-inflammatory molecules bind to the receptors on the nociceptive nerve endings and depolarize the cell. This depolarization triggers a cascade of reactions, including the activation of mitogen- and protein-activated kinases, which in turn phosphorylate other transducer proteins such as TRPV1. This activation further amplifies the depolarization, recruiting voltage-dependent sodium channels and ultimately depolarizing the nerve fiber. This complex sequence of events illustrates the ability of neuroinflammation to amplify itself (Miller et al., 2014; Frias & Merighi, 2016; Woller et al., 2017).

Inflammatory processes result from noxious stimuli that amplify nociceptive or neuropathic mechanisms and should therefore not be considered separately as a distinct form of pain.

This chapter began with the question *Why is there pain?*. Nociceptive pain has a clear function and is adequate. Nociception teaches us to avoid danger and motivates us through pain and functional restriction to regenerate, to become resilient again. Awareness and reaction to pain are fundamental aspects of survival behavior, which can significantly influence the well-being and survival chances of a living being. Pain perceptions serve as a vital alarm mechanism that alerts us, among other things, that an injury or potential damage to the body is present. This awareness of pain allows us to take timely measures to protect the injured area and prevent further damage. People **with congenital insensitivity to pain** (congenital insensitivity to pain with anhidrosis, CIPA) do not feel pain due to a gene defect. The CIPA syndrome can be based on two different gene defects. On the one hand, the NGF gene can be mutated. Normally, NGF binds to a specific TrkA receptor, leading to the formation of nociceptors during prenatal development. If this does not occur, no nociceptors are formed. Here, tissue-damaging stimuli cannot be perceived as such (Indo et al., 1996). On the other hand, the SCN9A gene can be mutated. This gene encodes the voltage-dependent sodium channel protein of the NaV1.7 channel in the parafall. This channel is probably less involved in the transduction of noxious stimuli at nociceptive endings than in the transmission of action potentials (Cox et al., 2006). Thus, due to these two gene mutations, noxious stimuli can either not be recognized or not transmitted. Congenital insensitivity to pain is an extremely rare syndrome. People with CIPA syndrome are unable to perceive pain, no matter how strong it is. Affected individuals have a significantly shorter life expectancy because they do not feel that their body could be injured and cannot learn to avoid harmful stimuli. Due to the insensitivity to pain, serious burns or other injuries often occur. The disease becomes apparent in the first year of life and is associated with a lower life expectancy (Nagasako et al.,

2003). These molecular biological findings show that in addition to cognitive factors, which are currently strongly focused on in science, specific groups of peripheral nerve fibers are also important for the onset of pain.

The physiology and neurobiology of pain are complex fields in which the terms *noxious* and *nociceptive* are frequently used. The question arises as to the exact relationship between pain and nociception and the role of noxious stimuli. Is pain nociception? Or the result of noxious stimuli? Is there pain without nociception? It is often assumed that pain can be perceived even without nociception. The hypothesis that pain can occur without nociception requires a more precise formulation: Nociception can be triggered both by peripheral tissue damage and by sensitized neurons of the nociceptive system. The latter react without direct peripheral noxious stimuli. Although the classic nociceptor (primary neuron) is not activated by a noxious stimulus in this case, the nociceptive system shows nozineuronal activities. Therefore, the nociceptive system is always involved in pain experiences, while noxious stimuli do not necessarily have to be present. Pain can persist even if there is no longer any acute tissue damage or the affected tissue has already regenerated. This underscores the complexity of pain perception beyond mere nociception based on noxious stimuli. Another important aspect is the context-dependent perception and interpretation of nociceptive signals. Identical nociceptive stimuli can lead to varying pain perceptions in different situations. A comparison between a martial artist in training and a person who experiences an attack on the street illustrates this connection. The context significantly influences how nociceptive signals are processed and perceived as pain. These findings explain why individuals voluntarily expose themselves to activities associated with an increased likelihood of nociceptive stimulation, such as martial arts.

References

Anand, P., & Bley, K. (2011). Topical capsaicin for pain management: Therapeutic potential and mechanisms of action of the new high-concentration capsaicin 8% patch. *British Journal of Anaesthesia, 107*(4), 490–502. https://doi.org/10.1093/bja/aer260.

Beecher, H. K. (1946). Pain in men wounded in battle. *Annals of Surgery, 123*(1), 96–105.

Boring, E. G. (1942). Sensation and perception in the history of experimental. *Psychology.* D. Appleton-Century. https://ia801507.us.archive.org/12/items/in.ernet.dli.2015.52372/2015.52372.Sensation-And-Perception-In-The-History-Of-Experimental-Psychology_text.pdf. Accessed 23. Dec. 2023.

Bista, P., & Imlach, W. L. (2019). Pathological mechanisms and therapeutic targets for trigeminal neuropathic pain. *Medicines (Basel, Switzerland), 6*(3), 91. https://doi.org/10.3390/medicines6030091.

Ciaramitaro, P., Mondelli, M., Logullo, F., Grimaldi, S., Battiston, B., Sard, A., Scarinzi, C., Migliaretti, G., Faccani, G., Cocito, D., & Italian Network for Traumatic Neuropathies. (2010). Traumatic peripheral nerve injuries: epidemiological findings, neuropathic pain and quality of life in 158 patients. *Journal of the peripheral nervous system: JPNS, 15*(2), 120–127. https://doi.org/10.1111/j.1529-8027.2010.00260.x.

Cohen, S. P., & Mao, J. (2014). Neuropathic pain: Mechanisms and their clinical implications. *BMJ (Clinical research ed.), 348*, f7656. https://doi.org/10.1136/bmj.f7656.

Cox, J. J., Reimann, F., Nicholas, A. K., Thornton, G., Roberts, E., Springell, K., Karbani, G., Jafri, H., Mannan, J., Raashid, Y., Al-Gazali, L., Hamamy, H., Valente, E. M., Gorman, S., Williams, R., McHale, D. P., Wood, J. N., Gribble, F. M., & Woods, C. G. (2006). An SCN9A channelopathy causes congenital inability to experience pain. *Nature, 444*(7121), 894–898. https://doi.org/10.1038/nature05413.

Descartes, R. (1664) Treatise on Man. *angepasst von Clerselier C., übersetzt von Sloan P. R.* https://www.coretexts.org/wp-content/uploads/2010/08/DescartesTreatiseMnfin.pdf. Accessed 10. Feb. 2023.

Frias, B., & Merighi, A. (2016). Capsaicin, nociception and pain. *Molecules (Basel, Switzerland), 21*(6), 797. https://doi.org/10.3390/molecules21060797.

Goldberg, J. S. (2008). Revisiting the cartesian model of pain. *Medical Hypotheses, 70*(5), 1029–1033. https://doi.org/10.1016/j.mehy.2007.08.014.

Heinricher, M. M., Tavares, I., Leith, J. L., & Lumb, B. M. (2009). Descending control of nociception: Specificity, recruitment and plasticity. *Brain Research Reviews, 60*(1), 214–225. https://doi.org/10.1016/j.brainresrev.2008.12.009.

Indo, Y., Tsuruta, M., Hayashida, Y., Karim, M. A., Ohta, K., Kawano, T., Mitsubuchi, H., Tonoki, H., Awaya, Y., & Matsuda, I. (1996). Mutations in the TRKA/NGF receptor gene in patients with congenital insensitivity to pain with anhidrosis. *Nature Genetics, 13*(4), 485–488. https://doi.org/10.1038/ng0896-485.

Jin, Q., Chang, Y., Lu, C., Chen, L., & Wang, Y. (2023). Referred pain: Characteristics, possible mechanisms, and clinical management. *Frontiers in Neurology, 14*, 1104817. https://doi.org/10.3389/fneur.2023.1104817.

Kendroud S., Fitzgerald L. A., Murray IV, & Hanna A. (2022). Physiology, nociceptive pathways. In: *StatPearls [Internet]. Treasure Island (FL): StatPearls Publishing.* https://www.ncbi.nlm.nih.gov/books/NBK470255/.

Kurrikoff, K., Inno, J., Matsui, T., & Vasar, E. (2008). Stress-induced analgesia in mice: Evidence for interaction between endocannabinoids and cholecystokinin. *The European Journal of Neuroscience, 27*(8), 2147–2155. https://doi.org/10.1111/j.1460-9568.2008.06160.x.

Le Bars, D., Dickenson, A. H., & Besson, J. M. (1979). Diffuse noxious inhibitory controls (DNIC). II. Lack of effect on non-convergent neurones, supraspinal involvement and theoretical implications. *Pain, 6*(3), 305–327. https://doi.org/10.1016/0304-3959(79)90050-2.

Liao, H. Y., & Lin, Y. W. (2021). Electroacupuncture reduces cold stress-induced pain through microglial inactivation and transient receptor potential V1 in mice. *Chinese Medicine, 16*(1), 43. https://doi.org/10.1186/s13020-021-00451-0.

Lindstedt, F., Lonsdorf, T. B., Schalling, M., Kosek, E., & Ingvar, M. (2011). Perception of thermal pain and the thermal grill illusion is associated with polymorphisms in the serotonin transporter gene. *PLoS ONE, 6*(3), e17752. https://doi.org/10.1371/journal.pone.0017752.

Lu, Y., Dong, H., Gao, Y., Gong, Y., Ren, Y., Gu, N., Zhou, S., Xia, N., Sun, Y. Y., Ji, R. R., & Xiong, L. (2013). A feed-forward spinal cord glycinergic neural circuit gates mechanical allodynia. *The Journal of Clinical Investigation, 123*(9), 4050–4062. https://doi.org/10.1172/JCI70026.

Marinelli, S., Vaughan, C. W., Schnell, S. A., Wessendorf, M. W., & Christie, M. J. (2002). Rostral ventromedial medulla neurons that project to the spinal cord express multiple opioid receptor phenotypes. *The Journal of Neuroscience: The Official Journal of the Society for Neuroscience, 22*(24), 10847–10855. https://doi.org/10.1523/JNEUROSCI.22-24-10847.2002.

Melzack R., & Casey K. L. (1968). Sensory, motivational and central control determinants of chronic pain: A new conceptual model. *The Skin Senses.* In Kenshalo DR (Hrsg.). Thomas (S. 423–443). https://www.researchgate.net/profile/Kenneth-Casey/publication/285016812_Sensory_motivational_and_central_control_determinants_of_pain_Kenshalo_DR_editor_The_skin_senses_proceedings_Springfield_Illinois_Charles_C/links/566ed69e08aea0892c52ac76/Sensory-motivational-and-central-control-determinants-of-pain-Kenshalo-DR-editor-The-skin-senses-proceedings-Springfield-Illinois-Charles-C.pdf. Accessed 12. Aug. 2024.

References

Merskey, H., & Bogduk, N. (1986). Classification of chronic pain. Descriptions of chronic pain syndromes and definitions of pain terms. *International Association for the Study of Pain, Subcommittee on Taxonomy, 3,* S1–226.

Moore, K. A., Kohno, T., Karchewski, L. A., Scholz, J., Baba, H., & Woolf, C. J. (2002). Partial peripheral nerve injury promotes a selective loss of GABAergic inhibition in the superficial dorsal horn of the spinal cord. *The Journal of Neuroscience : The Official Journal of the Society for Neuroscience, 22*(15), 6724–6731. https://doi.org/10.1523/JNEUROSCI.22-15-06724.2002.

Mickle, A. D., Shepherd, A. J., & Mohapatra, D. P. (2015). Sensory TRP channels: The key transducers of nociception and pain. *Progress in Molecular Biology and Translational Science, 131,* 73–118. https://doi.org/10.1016/bs.pmbts.2015.01.002.

Miller, R. E., Miller, R. J., & Malfait, A. M. (2014). Osteoarthritis joint pain: The cytokine connection. *Cytokine, 70*(2), 185–193. https://doi.org/10.1016/j.cyto.2014.06.019.

Mitsi, V., & Zachariou, V. (2016). Modulation of pain, nociception, and analgesia by the brain reward center. *Neuroscience, 338,* 81–92. https://doi.org/10.1016/j.neuroscience.2016.05.017.

Nagasako, E. M., Oaklander, A. L., & Dworkin, R. H. (2003). Congenital insensitivity to pain: An update. *Pain, 101*(3), 213–219. https://doi.org/10.1016/S0304-3959(02)00482-7.

Nicholas, M., Vlaeyen, J. W. S., Rief, W., Barke, A., Aziz, Q., Benoliel, R., Cohen, M., Evers, S., Giamberardino, M. A., Goebel, A., Korwisi, B., Perrot, S., Svensson, P., Wang, S. J., Treede, R. D., & IASP Taskforce for the Classification of Chronic Pain. (2019). The IASP classification of chronic pain for ICD-11: chronic primary pain. *Pain, 160*(1), 28–37. https://doi.org/10.1097/j.pain.0000000000001390.

Ossipov, M. H., Dussor, G. O., & Porreca, F. (2010). Central modulation of pain. *The Journal of Clinical Investigation, 120*(11), 3779–3787. https://doi.org/10.1172/JCI43766.

Polarlys. (2006). Bahnen des Rückenmarks. GNU-Lizenz für freie Dokumentation. https://de.m.wikipedia.org/wiki/Datei:Medulla_spinalis_-_Querschnitt_-_Bahnen_-_German.svg.

Prescott, S.A., & Ratté, S. (2017). Conn's translational neuroscience. Somatosensation and pain. *Academic Press* (S. 517–539). https://https://doi.org/10.1016/B978-0-12-802381-5.00037-3.

Raja, S. N., Carr, D. B., Cohen, M., Finnerup, N. B., Flor, H., Gibson, S., Keefe, F. J., Mogil, J. S., Ringkamp, M., Sluka, K. A., Song, X. J., Stevens, B., Sullivan, M. D., Tutelman, P. R., Ushida, T., & Vader, K. (2020). The revised International Association for the Study of Pain definition of pain: Concepts, challenges, and compromises. *Pain, 161*(9), 1976–1982. https://doi.org/10.1097/j.pain.0000000000001939.

Sengul, G. & Watson, C. (2015). Ascending and descending pathways in the spinal cord. The Rat Nervous System (Fourth Edition). *Academic Press (S. 115–130).* https://doi.org/10.1016/B978-0-12-374245-2.00008-5.

Sirucek, L., Ganley, R. P., Zeilhofer, H. U., & Schweinhardt, P. (2023). Diffuse noxious inhibitory controls and conditioned pain modulation: A shared neurobiology within the descending pain inhibitory system? *Pain, 164*(3), 463–468. https://doi.org/10.1097/j.pain.0000000000002719.

Sneddon L. U. (2018). Comparative physiology of nociception and pain. *Physiology (Bethesda, Md.), 33*(1), 63–73. https://doi.org/10.1152/physiol.00022.2017.

Tracey W. D., Jr. (2017). Nociception. *Current Biology: CB, 27*(4), R129–R133. https://doi.org/10.1016/j.cub.2017.01.037.

St John Smith E. (2018). Advances in understanding nociception and neuropathic pain. *Journal of Neurology, 265*(2), 231–238. https://doi.org/10.1007/s00415-017-8641-6.

Staud, R. (2013). The important role of CNS facilitation and inhibition for chronic pain. *International Journal of Clinical Rheumatology, 8*(6), 639–646. https://doi.org/10.2217/ijr.13.57.

Todd, A. J. (2010). Neuronal circuitry for pain processing in the dorsal horn. *Nature Reviews. Neuroscience, 11*(12), 823–836. https://doi.org/10.1038/nrn2947.

Treede, R. D., Jensen, T. S., Campbell, J. N., Cruccu, G., Dostrovsky, J. O., Griffin, J. W., Hansson, P., Hughes, R., Nurmikko, T., & Serra, J. (2008). Neuropathic pain: Redefinition and a grading system for clinical and research purposes. *Neurology, 70*(18), 1630–1635. https://doi.org/10.1212/01.wnl.0000282763.29778.59.

Woller, S. A., Eddinger, K. A., Corr, M., & Yaksh, T. L. (2017). An overview of pathways encoding nociception. *Clinical and Experimental Rheumatology, 35 Suppl 107*(5), 40–46. https://www.ncbi.nlm.nih.gov/pmc/articles/PMC6636838/pdf/nihms-1021663.pdf.

The Neurobiology of Pain   3

Abstract

Pain is a complex experience that goes beyond mere nociception and represents a subjective perception. The perception of pain can be influenced by various factors with identical nociceptive input, including attention, emotions, and other cognitive processes. Imaging studies have identified a widespread network of brain areas involved in pain processing, including the limbic system and the prefrontal cortex. In chronic pain, neuroplastic changes play a significant role, which can lead to central sensitization. These include structural and functional adaptations of the nervous system. Central sensitization is characterized by an increased excitability of neurons in the spinal cord and brain, leading to heightened pain sensitivity. This process can be amplified by the interaction of bottom-up and top-down mechanisms and contribute to the chronification of pain.

Typically, it is assumed that physical pain is associated with damage in the body. However, many people suffer from pain where no correlating damage/pathology can be identified and thus few or no nociceptive drivers (as far as clinically assessable) are detected. In the past, these patients were dismissed as therapy-resistant or mentally ill (see Chap. 1). However, with the progress of neuroscience, additional pain mechanisms, such as nociplastic pain, coupled with specific cortical activity patterns, have been identified, which correlate with individual pain perception and chronic pain. The relevance of sensory and nociception receded in the interpretation of pain, and perception and its individual influencing factors came to the fore. How is perception created? What influences perception? And how can perception be made visible? Smart questions, to which there are already many answers today.

Sensory information is detected by the sensory organs and transmitted to the brain. There, this sensory information is first received (reception), processed in several dimensions, and embedded into a sensory impression or perception. Perception describes the subjective and individual result of information processing, which encompasses far more than just sensation. This, mostly unconscious, information processing is situational, influenced by context factors, and varies inter-individually. This applies not only to nociception but also to other senses. If two people perceive the same pod as differently spicy or the smell of an old piece of clothing as differently unpleasant, this cannot be explained solely by biological or organic explanatory approaches, such as the colloquially often mentioned *better developed* sensory organs or receptors. Rather, the dualism of sensation and perception plays a central role: While sensation is defined as the immediate, unprocessed sensory experience, perception refers to the interpretation and processing of this sensory information by the brain (Fig. 3.1). These

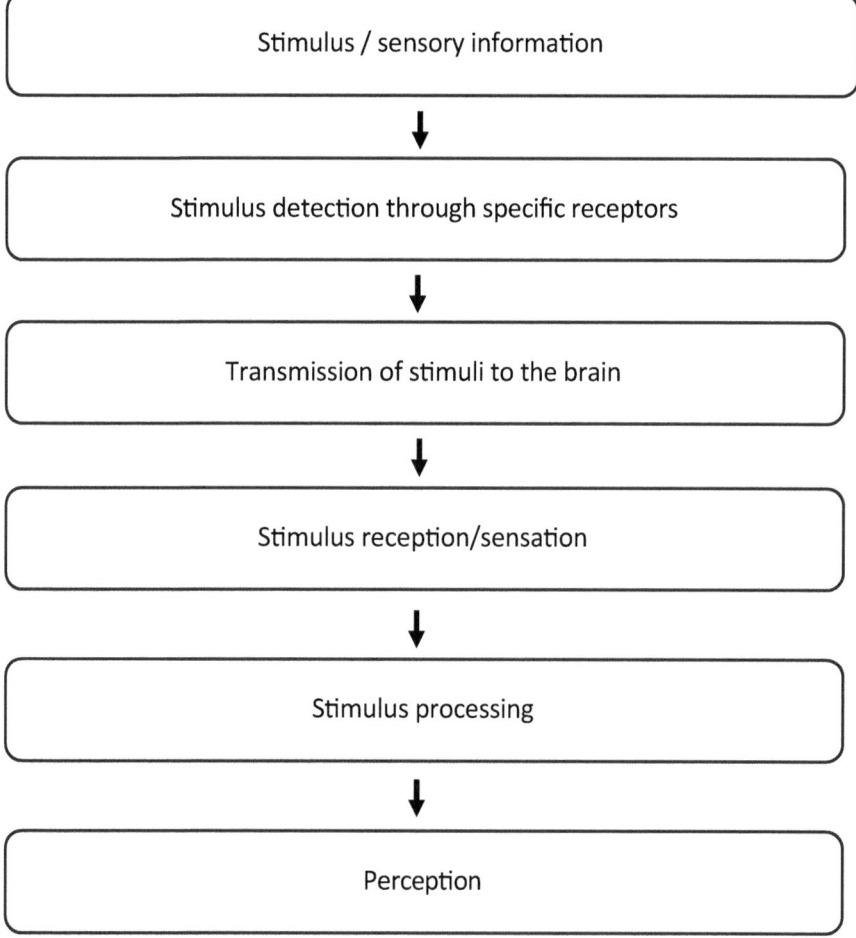

Fig. 3.1 Perception formation

perception processes are influenced by a multitude of individual factors, including psychological, cultural, social aspects, and other context factors, such as experiences and expectations. Thus, the perception of different people regarding the same information can differ from each other. Moreover, the perception of the same person to identical stimuli can vary depending on the situation and context. This discrepancy between sensation and perception illustrates the complexity of human sensory perception and emphasizes that the subjective experience is not solely determined by the sensory information content. However, it should be noted that sensation and perception are difficult to separate from each other and serve as abstract constructs for illustration. Sensation alone cannot be measured or expressed, as the individual contribution of central processing and thus perception cannot be isolated and separated.

The body is constantly exposed to different stimuli. The processing and perception of external environmental information is defined as exteroception and that of internal/bodily information as interoception.

Examples of exteroceptive perception:

- Daylight/Brightness
- Noise
- Weather, wind, and temperature

Examples of interoceptive perception:

- Vital functions such as heartbeat or breathing
- Joint position/Proprioception
- Muscle contraction/Movements

Nociception or pain is difficult to assign to either of these two forms of perception. Nociceptive signals can include both exteroceptive and interoceptive aspects (Ma, 2022). On the one hand, the detection of the noxious stimulus leads to the acquisition of information about the quality and intensity of the external stimulus acting on the body, which results in a motor withdrawal response to avoid this external source of danger (exteroceptive). On the other hand, both the injury of a body's own structure can impair physical functions and the perception of pain can disrupt trust in one's own physical integrity, which can lead to self-healing measures, such as touching the injured area, to rest and avoidance (interoceptive). Ultimately, persistent pain, in the absence or subsiding of the external stimulus, is an exclusively interoceptive perception, while acute nociceptive pain includes both exteroceptive and interoceptive aspects.

Pain is a complex experience that encompasses somatosensory, psychological, and affective factors and includes different aspects (Figs. 3.2 and 3.3). Nociception represents the somatosensory component, which is triggered by noxious stimuli and transmits danger signals to the brain. This process includes the phases of transduction, transmission, and modulation. In contrast, pain not only

Fig. 3.2 Aspects of pain perception (graphically)

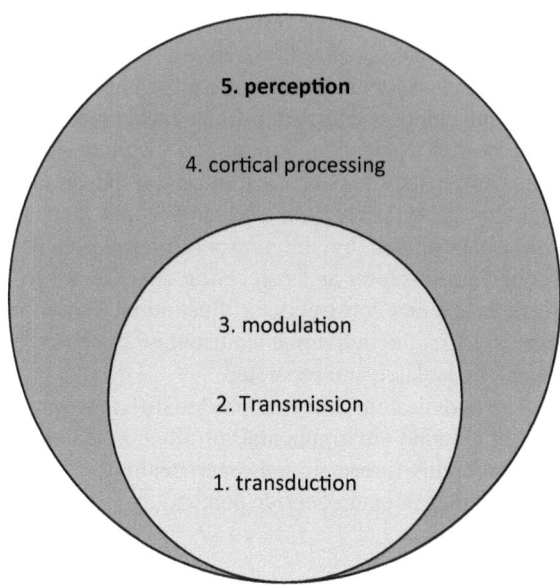

Fig. 3.3 Aspects of pain perception (anatomically). The arrows for point 3. (Modulation) represent the influences by the interneurons and descending pathways

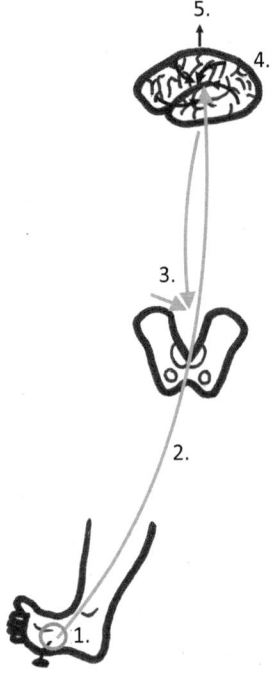

involves the processes of nociception (when present), but also cortical processing and perception.

In Fig. 3.2, the light circle includes points 1–3 and represents nociception. The large circle includes the light circle and the two additional points of processing and perception, which define the entire pain picture. Perception is not to be understood as an independent phase, but rather as the result of the preceding processes (1–4). In summary, nociception includes steps 1 to 3, while pain integrates points 1 to 5. Ultimately, it is perception that constitutes and defines pain. This model should not be misinterpreted and nociception seen as a prerequisite for every pain perception. Nociception or a noxious stimulus is not necessarily always a component of pain. People can perceive pain without a noxious/nociceptive input being present (Derbyshire et al., 2004; Raij et al., 2005).

Pain perception is a conscious perception, which is usually the product of subconscious/unconscious mechanisms. However, it can also be influenced by conscious attention and perception strategies (Merikle et al., 2001). The subjective severity of pain does not correlate with the extent of tissue damage, but with central processing processes. These central processing processes and perception factors exist not only in chronic pain, but also in acute/nociceptive pain. Each type of pain (whether nociceptive, neuropathic or nociplastic) involves inter-individually varying processing and perception processes. The 5 dimensions of pain according to the IASP (sensory-discriminative, affective-motivational, cognitive-evaluative, motor, vegetative) apply to every form of pain. Only the *signature* is different for each person, which is why pains vary so much, even though the cause and stimulus intensity appear the same. Before some examples are explained of how the brain can interpret and perceive identical stimuli differently (Sect. 3.2), an introduction to the functional pain-related neuroanatomy of the cortex follows. Earlier research focused mainly on afferent sensory inputs, spinal reorganization, and changes in descending modulation pathways. It was assumed that the brain plays a passive role in pain processing. The opposite has now been proven. New findings from brain imaging studies show an active role of the brain in pain processing.

3.1 Pain-Relevant Brain Areas

In contrast to other sensory perceptions such as vision, touch, and hearing, which are assigned to clearly defined brain regions, there is no isolated cortical area exclusively responsible for pain processing. Instead, imaging studies reveal a widespread network of various brain areas involved in pain processing, due to technological advancements and the use of functional magnetic resonance imaging (fMRI); also referred to as the *Pain Matrix*.

This network includes multiple cortical and subcortical structures that together enable the complex sensory, emotional, and cognitive dimensions of pain perception and processing. This finding underscores the multifactorial and comprehensive nature of pain processing in the brain. The most significant brain areas involved in pain processing include the thalamus and the somatosensory system

(S. 1 and S. 2), particularly the structures of the limbic system, such as the anterior cingulate cortex (ACC) and the amygdala, and the prefrontal cortex (PFC) (Apkarian et al., 2005; Peyron et al., 2000; Tracey & Mantyh, 2007). These activation patterns reflect the complex processing of nociceptive signals at various levels of the brain and illustrate the integration of sensory and emotional components.

Thalamus

The thalamus is a region of the diencephalon that, although often unmentioned in the interpretation and processing of sensory processes, already demonstrates at this level how different pain dimensions can be traced back to different areas. The thalamus is the last area during the transmission of nociceptive afferents to the brain where the signals are switched. The secondary neuron transports nociceptive afferents from the spinal cord to the thalamus, where they are switched to the tertiary neuron before reaching the somatosensory cortex. Depending on whether the signals are projected from the medial or lateral thalamus to the cortex, they differ in their functions and responses.

From the lateral thalamus, the signals are forwarded to the somatosensory cortex, which is responsible for the sensory-discriminative interpretation of the nociceptive signals (lateral pain system), and from the medial thalamus to limbic structures, which are responsible for emotion encoding (medial pain system). Fibers of this medial pathway mediate visceral, emotional, and autonomic pain responses. It should not be overlooked in these distinctions that limbic structures, although not directly, do receive information from the lateral thalamic nuclei via the somatosensory cortex (Price, 2002). This is described as neuronal convergence.

Brain lesion studies underline these functional differences from an anatomical and neurobiological perspective (Bushnell et al., 2013; Head & Holmes, 1911; Price, 2002). On the one hand, patients with lesions of the lateral thalamus can neither perceive the type, intensity, and location, nor the sensory quality (e.g., stabbing, sharp, burning) of noxious stimuli. However, these patients responded with excessive discomfort and emotional stress when inducing intense or long-lasting noxious stimuli. On the other hand, patients with lesions in the medial thalamic regions showed opposite reactions: They had neither strong discomfort nor emotional stress after intense noxious stimuli, but they could identify the type, quality, and location of the noxious stimulus. These observations suggest a functional subdivision of the lateral and medial thalamic systems in the emergence of various components and dimensions of pain perception.

The Limbic System

The limbic system is a complex and widely branched functional network of structures in the brain, responsible for emotions, behavior, motivation, long-term memory, and perceptual processes. The main pain-processing areas of the limbic system are:

Cingulate gyrus/ACC
The cingulate gyrus (cingulate cortex) is involved in the regulation of emotions and behavioral control. In pain processing, the anterior part of the cingulate gyrus, the anterior cingulate cortex (ACC), plays a crucial role and is probably the most frequently mentioned and studied brain region in pain research. Unlike in the somatosensory cortex, affective aspects of pain are processed here, not sensory-discriminative ones (Rainville et al., 1997). The ACC is of central importance for the processing of affective, emotional, and motivational aspects of external and internal stimuli, especially in the evaluation of the unpleasant properties of pain (Fuchs et al., 2014; Phelps et al., 2021; Xiao & Zhang, 2018).

Amygdala
The amygdala encodes emotions, especially exteroceptive fear (Adolphs et al., 2005; Broks et al., 1998). A patient with bilateral lesions of the amygdala lost the fear of exteroceptive influences, such as spiders or snakes, but still feared inhaling air with high carbon dioxide content (Feinstein et al., 2011). This illustrates the encoding of specific perception elements in specific brain areas. The amygdala shows increased activity in response to painful stimuli, especially in fear-induced pain perception (Neugebauer, 2015).

Hippocampus
The hippocampus is important for the formation, organization, and storage of memories. This area shows increased activity during fear-induced pain increase, possibly due to anticipatory behavior preparation. This area can be dampened in its activity by education and clarification before an intervention or stimulus induction, resulting in lower pain perception (Ploghaus et al., 2001). Particularly in chronic pain, neuroplastic changes are found here, which are caused by long-term potentiation and result in a change in architecture and reduction of memory function (Smallwood et al., 2013; Tajerian et al., 2018).

Entorhinal Cortex
The entorhinal cortex forms the interface between the neocortex and the hippocampus and is grouped with the hippocampus to form the hippocampus formation. This area is important for memory and the association of memory contents and the encoding of (fear-induced) expectations. The entorhinal cortex reacts differently to identical noxious stimuli, depending on whether the perceived pain intensity was amplified by fear (Ploghaus et al., 2001). This varying response suggests that emotional factors such as fear play a significant role in the modulation of pain perception. During this emotional pain modulation, the reactions of the entorhinal cortex could predict the activity of closely connected brain regions. These include areas responsible for encoding pain intensity, such as the insula.

Insula
The insula is one of the 5 major lobes of the cerebrum and can be divided into an anterior and posterior part, which have different connections to other brain areas. Due to its central location, it has an integrative function in various cortical processes. It is heavily involved in the conscious perception of bodily interoceptive states and mediates (especially via the anterior insula) emotional aspects of pain

(Craig, 2009; Livneh & Andermann, 2021). People with lesions of the insula can recognize and discriminate noxious stimuli, but do not perceive any threat or emotional stress (Berthier et al., 1988). In general, the insula shows increased activity during pain perception, which occurs very early in time (Bastuji et al., 2016). In chronic pain, this area shows tonically increased activity (Hsieh et al., 1995; Lu et al., 2016). The anterior insula also shows increased activity in other non-pain-related emotional states, such as anxiety or depression. In contrast, the activity of the posterior insula correlates with the intensity of peripheral stimulus induction, suggesting its function in intensity encoding (Labrakakis, 2023). Selective electrical stimulation of the insula alone, without peripheral stimulus induction, causes pain (Mazzola et al., 2009).

The PFC
The prefrontal cortex is located in the frontal lobe of the cerebral cortex. This area is involved in higher cognitive functions, such as problem-solving, decision-making, action planning, behavioral control, and emotional evaluation of pain. Imaging studies show increased activity of the PFC in both experimental and clinical pain conditions (Ong et al., 2019). Prefrontal brain activity during pain perception is associated with cognitive and attention-related processing of painful stimuli. The PFC may play an important role in coordinating pain modulation with goal-directed behavior, as electrical stimulation of the fiber connections from the PFC to the midbrain shows antinociceptive effects. The PFC is a heterogeneous brain area, in which various subareas play specific roles in different cognition, emotion, and memory functions (Apkarian et al., 2005). In this context, the dorsolateral PFC (DLPFC) is particularly relevant, which modulates the neuronal signals between the midbrain and thalamus as well as the midbrain and ACC (Lorenz et al., 2003). Another important area of the PFC in pain perception is the orbitofrontal cortex (OFC). The activity of the OFC correlates with the presence and intensity of chronic pain (Shirvalkar et al., 2023). In one study, fine electrodes were implanted under the skull, which recorded the activity in both the ACC and OFC over a period of three to six months. In addition, the intensity of pain was to be documented several times a day. The results showed that stronger intensities of chronic pain were associated with higher activity in the OFC. The ACC also showed activation, but to a lesser extent and more in acute pain. The combination of these measurements made it possible to determine the pain state of the subjects with over 80% sensitivity and specificity. Acute and chronic pain generate different activity patterns in the brain. Acute pain primarily activates the ACC, while chronic pain shows increased activity in the OFC. As already mentioned above, the ACC is a central region in the processing of acute pain stimuli.

The discovery of these specific activity patterns opens up the possibility of making chronic pain (partially) objectively measurable.

3.2 Acute Pain Interpretation

While it is known that many cortical processes shape chronic pain, less is debated about cortical processes in the interpretation of acute nociceptive stimuli.

Not only the noxious-sensory content determines the perception of the acute noxious stimulus, but also a number of emotional (mood, anxiety, anger) and cognitive (experiences, expectations, beliefs) factors.

Acute pain perception can be influenced by changes in **attention** in response to identical noxious stimuli (Villemure & Bushnell, 2002). Pain is perceived less intensely when individuals are distracted from the pain. This was achieved in a study by asking the test subjects to focus on another sensory stimulus, such as a visual, auditory, or tactile stimulus. These observations could also be demonstrated in a single-case study in which a subject was exposed to noxious laser stimuli under two conditions (Ohara et al., 2004). Once with an attention strategy, which consisted of counting the induced noxious stimuli, and once with a distraction strategy, by reading a newspaper article while receiving the noxious stimuli. The experimental chronology was as follows: 1.) Attention, 2.) Distraction, 3.) Distraction, 4.) Attention. The subject was asked to count during the induction of the stimuli in the first and fourth run and subsequently reproduce the correct number of laser stimuli (attention strategy) and in the second and third run read a newspaper article and subsequently answer questions about the content of the newspaper article correctly (distraction strategy). The average pain intensity for the laser stimulus was 5/10 with the attention strategy and only 1/10 during the distraction strategy. In addition, the pain was correctly counted during attention (38 times, but only perceived 2 or 3 times during distraction). This shows the influence of contextual and attention-related aspects on pain perception. Intracranial electrodes showed significantly higher activity of the primary somatosensory cortex (S. 1) during the attention strategy. Studies in monkeys show that pain-related neuronal activity in the spinal cord and medial thalamus decreased when the animals were distracted by visual tasks during noxious stimuli (Villemure & Bushnell, 2002). In addition, the distraction-related reduced pain perception correlates with reduced activities of the insula, the anterior and middle cingulate cortex (ACC, MCC) and the hippocampus (Bantick et al., 2002). These observations can explain the lower pain perception through distraction.

The **frequency** of pain assessment also seems to be related to the perception of pain intensity: In a study by Levine et al. (1982), patients were asked to document their pain more frequently or less frequently after surgery. Those who documented their pain more frequently reported stronger pain. This suggests that focusing on the pain can intensify pain perception.

These examples illustrate that manipulating attention can have a significant impact on pain perception. It seems as if evolution does not punish humans who divert focus from pain with even more pain.

In addition to attention and focus, **emotions** play a major role in pain perception. Pain can not only trigger unpleasant emotions, but can also be influenced by emotions and mood (Tracey & Mantyh, 2007). How easily mood and pain perception can be influenced is shown in studies where different images are shown just before the identical noxious stimulus induction, which are supposed to serve as positive or negative emotion triggers. Images with negatively associated emotions (mutilated bodies, attack scenes) reduced pain tolerance and increased pain perception, whereas images with positive emotion triggers (babies, extreme sports scenes or erotica) increased pain tolerance and reduced pain perception (Roy et al., 2011). Negative emotions generally intensify pain perception. These include fear, depression, and anger (Peters, 2015).

It has been shown numerous times that **fear** can significantly intensify the intensity of perceived pain (George et al., 2006; Horn et al., 2014). The anticipation of pain is a natural and protective human reaction that teaches people from an early age to avoid potentially harmful situations, such as touching hot surfaces or flames. However, for people who suffer from chronic pain, for example, this anticipation can become a burden and cause significant problems. Affected individuals often avoid movements or activities that could trigger pain, which can lead to social isolation and a restricted lifestyle. This constant fear and avoidance not only intensify pain perception, but also lead to a vicious cycle of increasing fear and pain intensity. The connection between fear and chronic pain will be discussed in more detail in the next subchapter (Sect. 3.3).

Also, **anger** can negatively influence and intensify pain perception (Bruehl et al., 2002; van Middendorp et al., 2010). In the study by van Middendorp and colleagues (2010), participants were asked to recall an event that made them angry or sad. They described the event in detail until they strongly felt the emotion. Then they thought quietly about their feelings for 2 minutes, after which an electrical stimulation on the forearm was supposed to cause pain. Anger and sadness lowered the pain tolerance threshold and increased the pain intensity ratings. The activation of pain-related brain areas by emotions and their influence on pain perception underscores the connection between emotional status and pain. While negative emotions have a negative impact on pain perception and intensify it, **positive emotions** can have a reverse effect on pain perception. This is less researched, but the data from research agree that positive emotions can have an analgesic effect (Finan & Garland, 2015). For example, joy or laughter can make both subjects perceive noxious stimuli less intensely and also alleviate existing pain in patients (Berk et al., 1989; Dunbar et al., 2012; Stuber et al., 2009; Zweyer et al., 2004). One of the suspected mechanisms is the release of endorphins and endogenous opioids, which activate descending pain inhibition, in addition to the deactivation of affect-related pain-enhancing brain areas. Positive emotions can also indirectly lower pain perception by reducing fear (a risk factor for stronger pain perception and chronicity) (Geschwind et al., 2015; Meulders et al., 2014; Sturgeon & Zautra, 2013; Vandael et al., 2022).

In this context, **optimism,** i.e., a positive attitude towards an action, can increase pain tolerance (Boselie & Peters, 2023). Higher optimism scores, which were collected using a general personality trait questionnaire, correlated with lower pain reports in cold application tests (Hanssen et al., 2014). Moreover, experimentally induced optimism, independent of personality, can increase pain tolerance. In a study with 96 young healthy students, two groups were formed (Hanssen et al., 2013). One group received a short optimism training before the stimulus induction, which consisted of 1.) thinking about their future *best possible self* for 1 minute, 2.) writing continuously about it for 15 minutes, and 3.) visualizing what they wrote as vividly as possible for 5 minutes. The control group performed a similar exercise, but focused on a typical daily routine, without reference to their best possible self. This method of experimentally inducing optimism is based on previous studies and aimed to promote positive future visions and thereby induce a more optimistic state in the participants. Unlike the previous study that measured optimism as a personality trait, this study actively tried to create an optimistic state. Here too, lower pain reports and higher pain tolerance were shown in the optimism group.

Both optimism and pessimism can be attributed more to the cognitive aspects than the emotional aspects of pain processing, as they represent a specific form of **expectation.** If a person expects a negative outcome, such as an intensification of pain, various studies have shown that this increases the activity of different brain areas, including ACC, PFC, insula, and hippocampus (Bott et al., 2023; Keltner et al., 2006; Lorenz et al., 2005). The level of expected pain intensity correlates both with the actual perceived pain intensity and with the activity level of these brain regions (Keltner et al., 2006). Surprisingly, not only the affective brain areas such as the PFC, ACC, or insula, but also the primary somatosensory cortex, which actually only processes sensory-discriminative information, are pre-activated in the expectation phase, even before a stimulus is induced (Porro et al., 2002).

You get what you expect: Positive expectations, where study participants anticipated a reduction in pain, can modulate both subjective experience and brain activation. Koyama and colleagues showed in 2005, for example, that a higher expectation of pain was associated with increased activation in the thalamus, PFC, ACC, and insula, and lower expectations of pain were associated with reduced activation. A study by Sipilä and colleagues (2017) showed that the higher patients rated their postoperative pain before surgery, the more pain they actually had after surgery. Another interesting study examined the influence of color on perceived temperature. Identical stimuli ($-20°$ C) were induced by rods with differently glowing lights (blue or red, see Fig. 3.4) (Moseley & Arntz, 2007). Participants were told that the blue light meant *cold* and the red light meant *hot*, although the actual stimulus was always cold.

Stimuli of the same temperature were rated 3.5 points warmer with red color than those with blue color. However, not only the visual processing of color, but also the verbal suggestion made by the study leaders probably plays a role here.

Fig. 3.4 Cold application with different colors, own production

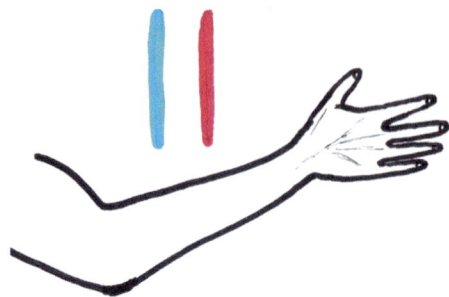

All these different modulations can influence pain perception both unconsciously through environmental and context factors and consciously through targeted strategies. Many of these modulations can occur through **placebo and nocebo effects.**

The placebo effect (from Latin: placere = to please) refers to the observable improvement of symptoms or conditions after the administration of an inert substance or treatment that has no specific (pharmacological or medical) effect on the target disease. This effect is based on the change in the patient's expectation that the treatment would be effective, which can lead to real physiological and psychological changes. It has been shown that placebo effects can be induced solely by verbal suggestions and can alleviate pain through both opioid and non-opioid mechanisms (Colloca & Benedetti, 2005). Key mechanisms of the placebo effect include the release of endogenous opioids, changes in the activity of certain brain areas, such as the ACC and PFC, as well as the activation of the brainstem and the descending pain-inhibiting pathways originating from the PAG (Zubieta et al., 2005; Zunhammer et al., 2021). In addition, the placebo effect can not only reduce pain perception, but also cause emotional modulation, such as the reduction of fear (Petrovic et al., 2005; Vase et al., 2005).

> **Excursion**
> The differentiation between a placebo and the placebo effect:
> It is a common misconception that placebos, i.e., certain substances themselves, have an effect. Rather, it is specific actions within a specific context that evoke placebo effects. This differentiation is of central importance, as the placebo effect is not attributable to the administered substance, but to a complex network of verbal, ritual, symbolic, and meaningful factors. These factors influence the neurobiological processes of the patient through subtle psychobiological mechanisms. The placebo effect is thus not the result of an inert substance, but the result of the entire treatment experience in its contextual framework (Benedetti et al., 2011). This insight underscores the importance of the doctor or therapist-patient relationship, the environment, and the patient's expectations for the healing process.

> Despite this important differentiation, the use of the term placebo to denote a medically and pharmacologically inert substance remains useful in professional discourse. It enables concise communication in clinical and research contexts, as long as awareness of the complexity of the placebo effect is maintained.

A classic example of the placebo effect is a study on postoperative pain, where the effect of Proglumid on pain was tested (Benedetti et al., 1995). It was found that Proglumid was more effective than the placebo, and the placebo was more effective than no treatment. These results initially seemed to suggest that Proglumid was an effective painkiller. However, it was also found that Proglumid had no effect when administered covertly, i.e., without the patients' knowledge. This suggests that Proglumid does not act directly on the nociceptive pathways, but on the expectation areas that encode the placebo effect. To investigate the pure pharmacological effect of a drug, administration can be done covertly. For example, a study showed that a covert administration of 6-8 mg of morphine after surgery was as effective as an open administration of saline solution. This underscores the importance of expectation in the effectiveness of treatments (Levine et al., 1981).

Whether placebo analgesia is caused by the inhibition of nociceptive afferents or by a reduced perception of these afferents is controversial. fMRI studies show that placebo analgesia is associated with decreased neural activity in pain-processing brain areas (Wager et al., 2004). Today, there is a large number of meaningful studies on the effectiveness of placebos and their effect on the activity of brain areas involved in pain processing. Some brain areas respond with negative interaction (activity reduction during analgesia), some with positive interaction (activity increase during analgesia) (Colloca & Benedetti, 2005; Price et al., 2007). Some studies contradict each other regarding positive or negative interaction of specific brain areas during placebo analgesia. However, the majority of studies show a decreased activity of specific brain areas ACC, Insula or Thalamus during placebo analgesia. Studies that show a positive interaction in these regions, i.e., increased activity, usually refer to the expectation phase or to their pain-inhibiting areas, whereas the negative interaction is observed during the stimulation phase, when the painful stimulus is applied. The expectation phase describes the period in which a person expects a certain effect due to verbal suggestions or conditioned stimuli, such as pain relief through a placebo. In this phase, the brain activates certain networks and biochemical mechanisms that respond to the expected effect, even before the placebo or the actual treatment is administered.

Negative Interaction:

- **Thalamus:** The thalamus is a central switching station where sensory and nociceptive signals are switched to the tertiary neuron and forwarded. During placebo analgesia, a decreased activity in the thalamus is observed. This suggests that fewer nociceptive signals are forwarded to higher brain regions.

- Both the primary and secondary somatosensory cortex (**S. 1, S. 2**) show, probably as a result of the reduced activation of the thalamus, a significant activity reduction, both through habituation and through placebo-induced analgesia. Fewer incoming nociceptive signals from the thalamus logically lead to a lower activation in these cortical areas.
- **Anterior Insula:** The anterior insula is involved in the processing of pain and the integration of sensory information. During placebo analgesia, the aINS shows a decreased activity. This could suggest that the processing of nociceptive signals is reduced by the expectation of pain relief.
- Middle and posterior insula: These areas also show a significant activity reduction during placebo analgesia. Their decreased activity could reflect the reduced processing and perception of pain during the placebo effect.
- **Dorsal ACC:** In the dorsal part of the ACC, affective components of pain are evaluated. Here, reductions in activity can be observed.
- **Caudal rostral ACC:** This area, like the dorsal ACC, shows decreased activity during placebo analgesia.

In summary, the activity reduction of these brain areas is associated with a reduced perception of pain. These neural correlates serve as a possible explanation for the analgesic effect of interventions triggering the placebo effect.

Positive Interaction:

- **Rostral anterior cingulate cortex (rACC):** The rACC likely mediates a descending pain control chain that includes the periaqueductal gray (PAG), the brainstem (pons), and the medulla. The activity of the rACC increases both during the administration of placebos and the administration of opioid agonists, indicating a common mechanism involvement.
- **Periaqueductal gray (PAG):** The PAG is a central pain control center in the midbrain that activates pain-modulating descending pathways. During placebo analgesia, increased activity in the PAG is observed, indicating the release of endogenous opioids.
- **Dorsolateral prefrontal cortex (DLPFC):** This region is involved in maintaining and updating internal representations of expectations. During placebo analgesia, the DLPFC shows increased activity. Stronger PFC activation during the expectation phase correlated with greater placebo-induced pain relief and reduction of neural activity within the stimulation phase. The activity of the DLPFC, like the rACC, correlates with that of the PAG. This shows that prefrontal mechanisms can also trigger the release of opioids in the brainstem during expectation to activate the descending pain-inhibiting system and subsequently modulate pain perception.
- **Rostral medial and anterior prefrontal cortex (rmAPFC and aAPFC):** The activity in these regions increases during the expectation phase, indicating their role in cognitive processing and expectation before placebo analgesia occurs.

- **Orbitofrontal cortex (OFC):** The OFC is part of the PFC and is involved in processing reward expectations and decisions. During placebo analgesia, increased activity is observed in the OFC.

The importance, almost a prerequisite, of prefrontal brain activities for a placebo effect becomes clear in Alzheimer's patients with degenerations of the prefrontal brain structures, in whom placebo effects cannot or can only be observed reduced (Benedetti et al., 2006; Thompson et al., 2003).

Beware of Placebo Misuse
Even though the placebo effect says something positive, namely the improvement of symptoms through positive change of expectation despite supposedly unspecific therapies, there is a risk of instrumentalizing this effect. Placebo research shows the susceptibility of the human mind to manipulation, especially through verbal suggestions. This seemingly easy influenceability of the human organism (psychologically and physiologically) could be exploited to legitimize any actions that alleviate complaints as effective therapies. There is a risk that sham therapies in a suitable psychosocial context positively influence the biochemistry of the brain, albeit only temporarily, and these interventions are propagated as effective. Both in science and in practice, efficiency should be sought to achieve the highest possible and as long-term changes as possible with the least possible effort. Otherwise, medicine and therapy sciences run the risk of spreading deceptions and errors about the supposedly specific healing mechanisms of placebos due to the placebo effect—which remains a good modulation instrument and should also be considered and used—especially since the explanation of supposed mechanisms or causes of pain in practice often borders on nocebos. Negative verbal suggestions can evoke nocebo effects that can intensify pain perception.

The nocebo effect (from Latin: nocere = harm), as the counterpart to the placebo effect, refers to the worsening of symptoms or the occurrence of negative effects after the administration of an inert substance or treatment that has no specific (pharmacological or medical) effect. This effect is based on negative expectations or fears of the patient towards the treatment, which can lead to real physiological and psychological changes. The mechanisms of the nocebo effect include the activation of stress and fear centers in the brain, such as the hippocampus and the amygdala, as well as the release of stress hormones like cortisol. The nocebo effect can also be amplified by previous negative experiences or by negative information about the treatment. Subjects reported pain (allodynia) with non-noxious tactile stimuli and strong pain (hyperalgesia) with noxious low-intensity stimuli when negative verbal suggestions (such as "This will hurt.") were previously expressed by third parties (Colloca et al., 2008).

All examples explained in this chapter underline the diverse modulation possibilities of pain and the variability of perception of identical noxious stimuli under different conditions. The nociception is thus evaluated and perceived differently depending on the context factor.

3.3 Chronic Pain Perception

Acute pain has a sudden onset, a short duration (maximum of several weeks) and is associated with a (presumably) clearly visible cause or trigger. The definition of chronic pain as suffering that extends beyond the actual or anticipated healing time (after injury) is often cited, but this criterion is difficult to apply to other conditions, such as chronic musculoskeletal or neuropathic pain. Thus, in recent years, the descriptive criterion of chronic pain lasting at least three months has become established (Treede et al., 2015; Wörz et al., 2022). However, this definition seems arbitrary and does not take into account the underlying mechanisms (Apkarian et al., 2009). The presence of chronic pain and its effects are of enormous significance. They not only impair the individual quality of life of those affected, but also burden the health system with significant socio-economic challenges required for the treatment of these persistent complaints (Bernfort et al., 2015; Hansen et al., 2015; Romanelli et al., 2017). Approximately 20% of Europeans suffer from chronic pain (Breivik et al., 2006; Reid et al., 2011). Data from the USA show a similar prevalence (Dahlhamer et al., 2018). Although mortality rates for heart attack and stroke are highest, chronic pain causes significant suffering and disability. Chronic pain and many associated diseases are not immediately life-threatening, but can plunge a large lifespan into suffering. The Global Burden of Disease Study assessed the *years lived with disability* (YLD) for many diseases and injuries in 188 countries, with chronic back pain being the leading cause of YLDs worldwide, followed by major depressive disorders (Rice et al., 2016). Other common causes of YLDs are: chronic neck pain, migraine, osteoarthritis, other musculoskeletal disorders, and headaches due to medication overuse. This sparked discussions about recognizing chronic pain as a disease in its own right.

The term chronic pain primarily says something about duration, not about the mechanism or cause. Due to these circumstances, the IASP developed a systematic classification for chronic pain syndromes, which distinguishes between primary and secondary pain syndromes, and uses the term *nociplastic pain*. If pain lasts longer than normal (if normal would be, for example, a few weeks, as after an ankle ligament sprain), a mechanism beyond the nociceptive, namely a nociplastic one, can be speculated. Here, the pain persists even though the original cause no longer exists; or even when a clear trigger has never existed. Nociplastic pain can be attributed to the reduction of nociceptive excitability (sensitization) and increased nociceptive excitation transmission (synaptic plasticity) and can be associated with psychosocial drivers. Nociplastic pain is considered a form of **primary chronic pain,** which according to the IASP is defined as a pain that 1.) lasts or recurs for more than 3 months, 2.) is associated with significant emotional distress, and 3.) has symptoms that cannot be better explained by another diagnosis (Nicholas et al., 2019). Primary chronic pain is considered a disease in its own right. Examples of some diseases in this classification include Chronic widespread pain (CWP) such as fibromyalgia, irritable bowel syndrome, migraine, or chronic

3.3 Chronic Pain Perception

nonspecific back pain. In contrast to primary chronic pain, **chronic secondary pain** is defined as a symptom or consequence of another disease (Treede et al., 2019). Examples of secondary chronic pain are cancer-related, postoperative, or neuropathic chronic pain. Here, the chronic pain has an (possibly) explainable pathology.

An overview of the **seven subcategories of chronic pain in ICD-11**

1. **Chronic primary pain (synonym: nociplastic pain):**

   - Definition: Pain in one or more anatomical regions that lasts or recurs for more than 3 months.
   - Associated with significant emotional distress or functional disability, not better explained by another chronic pain condition, characterized by nociplastic pain mechanisms.

Examples:

1.1 **CWP:** Chronic widespread pain is a diffuse musculoskeletal pain in at least 4 out of 5 body regions and must persist for at least 3 months and be associated with emotional distress and/or functional impairments (e.g., fibromyalgia). It is not based on any injury or damage.
1.2 **CRPS:** Complex regional pain syndrome often occurs after trauma, but is completely independent and has nothing to do with the healing of the originally damaged tissue. It shows autonomous and inflammatory changes in the affected region. In type 2, unlike type 1, a peripheral nerve is also injured.
1.3 **chronic primary headaches:** Headache or orofacial pain that occurs on at least 15 days per month for more than 3 months. Subtypes include chronic migraine, chronic tension headache, and trigeminal autonomic cephalalgias (e.g., cluster headaches).
1.4 **chronic primary visceral pain:** is localized in the head/neck, chest, abdomen, or pelvic region. They include chronic primary chest pain and irritable bowel syndrome. They are not based on any visceral pathologies.
1.5 **chronic primary musculoskeletal pain:** Pain lasting longer than 3 months in a specific region where neither an injury has occurred nor a specific pathology is found. An example is chronic nonspecific back pain.
2. Chronic secondary cancer-related pain:

   - Definition: Pain caused by the cancer itself or its treatment (surgery, chemotherapy, radiation therapy).
   - Note: Pain in long-term survivors of cancer often includes neuropathic and musculoskeletal pain.

3. Chronic secondary postoperative or posttraumatic pain:

   - Definition: Pain that persists longer than 3 months after surgery or trauma.
   - Examples: Pain after surgical procedures or after accidents.
   - Characteristic: Often of neuropathic nature.

4. Chronic secondary neuropathic pain:

   - Definition: Pain caused by a lesion or disease of the somatosensory nervous system.
   - Distinction: Chronic peripheral or chronic central neuropathic pain.
   - Detection: Requires a history of nervous system injuries and neuroanatomically plausible pain localization/distribution.

5. Chronic secondary headaches or orofacial pain:

   - Definition: Headaches or orofacial pain that occur for longer than 2 hours per day on at least 50% of the days for at least 3 months.
   - Including: Chronic secondary headaches and chronic orofacial pain, such as chronic toothache and temporomandibular disorders.
   - Demarcation: Chronic primary headaches are listed in the category of chronic primary pain.

6. Chronic secondary visceral pain:

   - Definition: Persistent or recurring pain originating from internal organs.
   - Causes: Mechanical factors (e.g., obstruction), vascular mechanisms (e.g., ischemia), or persistent inflammation.
   - Not included: Pain due to functional or unexplained mechanisms (these fall under chronic primary pain).

7. Chronic secondary musculoskeletal pain:

   - Definition: Persistent or recurring pain that results directly from a disease process of the bones, joints, muscles, or related soft tissues.
   - Causes: Inflammation, structural changes (e.g., in osteoarthritis), or secondary to diseases of the motor nervous system.
   - Delineation: Nociceptive pain, but not pain that is felt in musculoskeletal tissues but does not originate there (e.g., pain due to nerve compression).

Excursion

Diagnosis as a guide? Does the seemingly clear cause of secondary chronic pain syndromes hold potential for error? The treatment of secondary chronic pain might initially appear simpler, as its cause is supposedly known (e.g., cancer). In contrast, managing primary chronic pain is a greater challenge, as healthcare providers struggle to find cause-related treatment approaches and to provide patients with a plausible and tangible explanation for their pain. However, the supposed clarity of the cause in secondary chronic pain carries the risk of viewing the pain solely as a consequence of the disease and treating it purely symptomatically. Although pain and disease (like cancer) can occur simultaneously, the cancer as a pathology does not necessarily have to be the sole cause of the pain. Additional psychosocial,

3.3 Chronic Pain Perception

> cognitive, and emotional factors can significantly contribute to the onset, manifestation, and exacerbation of pain, which cannot be explained or need to be explained solely by the cancer. This could even be an obstacle to other treatment approaches in people with secondary chronic pain if the cause is defined per se and little could be done to alleviate the pain (the consequence) as long as the cancer (the cause) still exists.

Due to the numerous facets of a chronic pain syndrome and the associated difficulty in managing and treating it adequately as a therapist or doctor, several deficits arise in the care of chronic pain patients. These manifest firstly in an inadequate history and classification of clinical complaints (Piccoliori et al., 2013) and secondly (probably caused by the former) in an overuse and over-administration of painkillers and opioids, which are often fundamentally not indicated or their amount is not justified considering the side effects (Payne, 2000). Historically, chronic pain is classified as a syndrome (a group of symptoms resulting from a structural or functional disorder), but newer findings, mainly from brain imaging studies, suggest that chronic pain could be classified as a disease in its own right, as the symptoms are due to specific neuroplastic (functional and structural) and biochemical changes (Tracey & Bushnell, 2009). This perspective establishes chronic pain as a distinct pathology. It also questions the validity and usefulness of the term *nonspecific chronic back pain* and encourages a critical review of its use in clinical practice and research. A more differentiated classification and terminology may be required to adequately capture and describe the complex nature of chronic pain conditions.

Risk Factors and Drivers of Chronic Pain
Chronic and nociplastic pains can have different drivers, which can be divided into 3 categories (Fitzcharles et al., 2021; Tiemann et al., 2015).

1. **Bottom-up:** afferent nociceptive signals, which are based on damage or inflammation. These drivers are more likely to be found in patients with chronic secondary pain. Patients with mainly bottom-up drivers have few cognitive, affective, or nociplastic mechanisms.
2. **Top-down:** emotional and cognitive drivers of pain processing and perception. Patients with mainly top-down drivers have a higher activation of the affective pain-enhancing brain areas and a lower activation of the descending inhibitory pathways. Top-down drivers are more likely to be found in patients with primary chronic pain and include mood, emotions, beliefs, experiences, expectations.
3. **Central Sensitization:** Central sensitization describes changes in the CNS, such as the increased excitability of neurons in the spinal cord and brain (such as the insula, the PFC, and the ACC, which lead to increased pain sensitivity). An interaction between bottom-up and top-down processes can lead to an amplification and maintenance of pain and contribute to chronicity (see Sect. 3.5).

Possibly, both bottom-up and top-down drivers ultimately result in central sensitization during the chronification of pain, which is why central sensitization is worth discussing as a separate point. It is more likely the result of the interaction of bottom-up and top-down processes and a mechanism of pain chronification. After bottom-up mechanisms have been explained in Chap. 2, the following will focus on top-down mechanisms. Subsequently, the changes in neural networks/neuroplasticity (Sect. 3.4) caused by these and the associated central sensitization (Sect. 3.5) will be elucidated.

Top-Down Processes

A clear assignment of chronic pain patients to one of these categories is de facto not possible. Both primary and secondary chronic pains can be maintained by both bottom-up and top-down drivers. It is assumed that both driver categories interact with each other, but the top-down processes are dominant in chronic pain. Chronic pain often goes hand in hand with aversive states and psychological symptoms, such as anxiety and depression, which can contribute to the manifestation or worsening of pain (Bushnell et al., 2013; Kawai et al., 2017; Kroenke et al., 2013). A comprehensive understanding of the role of various brain areas, both in the sensory and affective components of pain, is therefore crucial. This not only contributes to the understanding of pain genesis but also to the development of effective therapeutic approaches. By exploring the neural mechanisms associated with both the perception and emotional processing of pain, targeted interventions can be developed that address not only the pain perception itself but also the associated psychological symptoms. Similar to acute pain perception, **anxiety** also influences the chronic pain experience. The fear-avoidance model explains how anxiety can contribute to the chronification of pain (Vlaeyen & Linton, 2012).

1. Fear of pain leads to avoidance behavior.
2. Avoidance behavior leads to reduced mobility and increased inactivity.
3. Inactivity worsens both the physical and psychological state.
4. This worsened state increases the likelihood of more pain and disability.

Pain-related anxiety can be a predictor of persistent pain and long-term disability. This has been demonstrated, for example, in studies where preoperative anxiety correlated with the development of postoperative chronic pain (Kehlet et al., 2006; Peters et al., 2007; Theunissen et al., 2012) or anxiety was identified as a predictor for the development of, for example, back pain (Linton et al., 2000; Picavet et al., 2002). Anxiety seems to exacerbate the subjective experience of pain, trigger maladaptive behavior in chronic pain patients, and promote the development of chronic pain conditions. In connection with anxiety, those affected often have **catastrophic thoughts.** Catastrophizing is a negative emotional state in which a pessimistic narrative is used. Patients with catastrophic thoughts tend to overestimate pain, ruminate about it, and have a helpless attitude towards actual or expected pain (Sullivan et al., 2001). This leads to a stronger experience of pain, lower therapy success, and is a risk factor for the chronification of pain (France et al., 2004; Theunissen et al., 2012). Imaging studies indicate increased activity in affective-emotional pain-processing brain areas in patients with catastrophic thoughts (Galambos et al., 2019). It is suspected that similar mechanisms underlie this as in attention-related pain amplification.

Depression or depressive moods are often observed in chronic pain patients. Whether these depressions are the result of chronic pain or a possible cause or driver of chronification cannot be conclusively clarified. However, longitudinal studies show that people with depression develop back pain episodes more often and preoperative depression increases the risk of chronic postoperative pain (Hinrichs-Rocker et al., 2009; Jarvik et al., 2005). These indications suggest that depression may be a possible cause or driver of chronic pain and is also considered the strongest predictor for the development of chronic pain due to a prospective long-term study in which depression significantly increased the likelihood of pain chronification (Meyer et al., 2007; Reid et al., 2003). In addition, it has been shown that the activation of sensory-discriminative brain areas in depressive pain patients during noxious stimulus induction does not correlate with the extent of depression, but the activity of emotion-processing and affective brain areas, such as the insula or amygdala, does (Giesecke et al., 2005).

Other psychosocial aspects can be closely related to chronic pain and promote it, such as **working conditions** (Clays et al., 2007; Nicholas et al., 2011). A high perceived stress level at work, dissatisfaction with the job or colleagues, and perceived inadequate support at work increase the risk of chronic pain. These so-called blue and black flags may in turn result in poorer affective-cognitive states and yellow flags. In addition to affective-cognitive risk factors and drivers, some **lifestyle factors** also show a connection to pain chronification. Lack of sleep, obesity, and smoking seem to increase the risk of pain chronification (Apkarian et al., 2009; Tanguay-Sabourin et al., 2023). All these factors are modifiable, which should give hope to both the patient and the therapist. Age, gender, and other non-modifiable socio-demographic characteristics, such as origin or parents' educational level, have long been considered risk factors for pain chronification. Despite some evidence supporting this (van Hecke et al., 2013), these seem to be only weak drivers for pain chronification (Tanguay-Sabourin et al., 2023).

"It is not only the pain that determines life, but also life that co-determines the intensity and the evaluation of the pain." (Müller-Busch, 2019)

Is pain in the brain?
In the previous subchapters 3.1 to 3.3, numerous cortical activity patterns were described that correlate with individual and chronic pain perception and influence it. This could give the impression that pain is exclusively a phenomenon of the brain. An article frequently used in German teaching titled *The pain is in the brain* summarizes various aspects of cortical activity in the onset and chronicity of pain (Pfeiffer & Luomajoki, 2015). Although the content of the article is sound, the title is potentially misleading. Undoubtedly, the processing of noxious stimuli and pain perception occur in the brain. However, the oversimplified statement *the pain is in the head* carries significant risks for misunderstandings:

1. Patient perspective: Affected individuals could interpret this as an insinuation that their pain is imagined, which can lead to frustration and a feeling of not being taken seriously.
2. Therapist perspective: There is a risk that therapists may dismiss pain as a purely psychological phenomenon. This could lead to an inappropriate trivialization of the symptom of pain.

It is important to emphasize that pain is a complex sensory and emotional experience. Regardless of whether a noxious stimulus is present or not, pain is the result of signals from the entire nervous system. Neuronal changes or autonomizations that lead to pain can occur at both spinal and supraspinal levels. Therefore, the statement that pain is exclusively in the head is not only factually inaccurate, but also carries a significant potential for misinterpretations. Neurobiological observations can help to better understand mechanisms of pain, but should never serve as an explanatory code for pain. Because pain arises from a person and a person should never be reduced to their nervous system. Not even with the apparently so neurobiologically shaped phenomenon of pain. A holistic understanding of pain should acknowledge the complexity of the phenomenon and consider both physical and psychological factors, without neglecting or overemphasizing any of these aspects.

Neuronal and biochemical correlates

The presence of psychosocial factors and their significance in chronic pain can not only be demonstrated in studies that collect these factors through assessments and questionnaires and show their connection either through retro- or prospective studies with the occurrence of chronic pain, but also through the activity analysis of specific brain regions in chronic pain patients that encode these affective states. These activity patterns associated with chronic pain are also called neuronal correlates. The medial prefrontal cortex (mPFC), known for its role in emotional processing and self-perception, shows increased activity and correlates with pain intensity. This persistent mPFC activity could reflect the emotional burden and suffering in chronic pain. With increasing pain, the activity of the insula (important for interoceptive body perception and intensity coding) and the ACC (involved in pain modulation and emotional-affective evaluation) is also increased. Other brain areas, such as the thalamus, somatosensory cortex, hippocampus, and amygdala, show increased activity in chronic pain (Apkarian et al., 2009; Baliki & Apkarian, 2015). These activation patterns resemble those in acute pain and suggest enhanced emotional and cognitive processing in chronic pain. Moreover, this increased activity is not only a stronger response to painful stimuli, but can also be detected at rest in the absence of noxious stimuli. The brain of chronic pain patients is in a constant state of hyperexcitability, even when no acute painful stimulus is present (Baliki et al., 2008; Saab, 2013). It is important to note that the activity patterns can vary depending on the type of chronic pain, duration, and individual factors. In addition, some studies also show changes in the functional connectivity between these regions, indicating a comprehensive reorganization of pain processing in the brain in chronic pain conditions.

3.3 Chronic Pain Perception

To dismiss psychosocial risk factors and drivers of chronic pain as a psychological phenomenon despite these findings would not sufficiently account for the complexity of the underlying neurobiology. These supposed meta-discoveries can be objectified and made measurable. They include both the cortical activity patterns already discussed, as well as metabolic and **chemical biomarkers.** For example, abnormal brain chemistry has been found in patients with chronic back pain (Grachev et al., 2000). These include an increased glucose concentration in the thalamus, which correlated with pain intensity and duration. The increased glucose concentration in the thalamus could be a result of increased activity and the associated higher energy demand. In addition, the higher glucose concentration may also be due to increased inflammation and sensitization processes. High glucose concentrations can lead to increased oxidative stress, which can contribute to cell damage and neuronal dysfunction in the long term. In patients with chronic pain, a decreased N-acetylaspartate (NAA) concentration, especially in the DLPFC, is observed, which also correlated with pain characteristics and anxiety states. NAA is one of the most common amino acids in the brain and an important biomarker that shows a decreased concentration in patients with chronic pain. This decrease often correlates with the duration and intensity of the pain and indicates neuronal stress or damage. The NAA changes are consistent with observations of **brain atrophy** in these patients (Apkarian et al., 2004; Kuchinad et al., 2007) and could serve as objective biomarkers for chronic pain. These brain-based biomarkers show a stronger correlation with clinical features, such as pain duration and intensity, than previous approaches. Similar to neurodegenerative diseases, such as Alzheimer's, metabolic changes could serve as early indicators as a possible prediction of the predisposition for chronic pain.

Millions of people worldwide suffer from chronic pain, which often persists even after the original trigger has healed. Chronic pain represents a complex phenomenon closely linked to **learning and memory processes.** Chronic pain can be understood as a persistent memory of pain or as the inability to erase this memory. This perspective is based on the evolutionarily advantageous property of pain to promote rapid and long-term learning. In chronic pain conditions, a continuous learning process occurs in which negative emotional associations are formed with certain actions or events (Apkarian et al., 2009). As the pain thus becomes more frequent, the opportunity to erase these associations is lacking. Pain can thus be learned and stored. This leads to the development of a **pain memory,** in which negative associations are continuously reinforced. The resulting vicious cycle of pain, negative associations, and the inability to erase intensifies the suffering and contributes to chronicity. These insights open up new approaches to the therapy of chronic pain by emphasizing the role of learning and memory processes in pain perception and processing. In the formation of this pain memory, persistent changes in cell metabolism, signal transmission, and nerve activity in the spinal cord and brain occur. These changes lead to the pain becoming autonomous. The fact that pain manifests, becomes autonomous, and chronifies is due to the adaptability of the CNS, which is called neuroplasticity.

3.4 Neuroplasticity

Neuroplasticity is a process that encompasses adaptive structural and functional changes in the nervous system. It is defined as the ability of the nervous system to change its activity in response to intrinsic or extrinsic stimuli by reshaping its structure and function. Although the mechanisms of persistent and chronic pain are not yet fully understood, it is now known that repeated nociceptive stimulation in healthy subjects can lead to plasticity of both peripheral and central neurons (Bingel et al., 2008; Teutsch et al., 2008). This is called long-term potentiation (LTP). Plasticity can also be observed in glial cells (Eroglu & Barres, 2010; Streit et al., 1988). In patients with chronic pain, plasticity is associated with changes in some brain structures, functions, and activities (Baliki et al., 2011; Davis, 2011; Seifert & Maihöfner, 2011). These changes are discussed as one of the causes of chronic pain (Scholz & Woolf, 2007; Zhuo et al., 2011).

Neuroplasticity can manifest itself not only in the **functional changes** of cortical activity patterns already described (Sect. 3.3), but also at a **structural level** (Kuner & Flor, 2016). These structural changes include **dendritic remodeling** and **axonal sprouting.** For example, following a peripheral nerve injury, there is regeneration and growth of new dendrites and axons. Specifically, in the dorsal horn of the spinal cord, there is a restructuring of neuronal connections. Axonal sprouting in this area can lead to increased synaptic activity (Davis & Price, 2023; Zheng et al., 2022). The newly formed axons and dendrites create new synapses. These changes are often associated with increased excitability of the affected neurons. Through axonal sprouting and the associated **synaptic plasticity,** nociceptive afferents are enhanced and maintained, and through the induced LTP, they can be a potential driver for the chronification of pain. Increased levels of pro-inflammatory cytokines such as TNF- α, IL-1-β, and IL-6 in the spinal cord and in pain-processing brain regions are underlying mechanisms of synaptic plasticity and alter the dendritic structure (Fang et al., 2023). These inflammatory processes contribute to the sensitization and remodeling of pain-processing networks. BDNF (brain derived neurotrophic factor) is a neurotrophin that promotes dendritic remodeling and synaptic growth. It is often released in areas of increased neuronal activity and plays a key role in pain chronification by promoting synaptic plasticity (Golia et al., 2019).

In addition, chronic pain patients consistently show a reduction in gray matter compared to healthy individuals (Apkarian et al., 2004, 2009). Particularly affected brain areas are the DLPFC, ACC, and the insula. This phenomenon was initially discovered in patients with chronic back pain and later confirmed in various other chronic pain conditions (Tracey & Bushnell, 2009). The decrease in gray matter seems to be related to the severity and duration of the pain:

- Patients with neuropathic symptoms, which are often perceived as particularly intense, show a greater decrease.
- The longer the pain symptoms persist, the more pronounced is the reduction in gray matter.

The deeper-lying **white matter,** which normally connects pain-processing regions with each other, also shows changes in density and integrity. This suggests a reduction and loss of physiological connectivity in pain processing.

The understanding of neuroplastic changes in pain patients received a significant boost through the phenomenon of phantom pain. Here, the patient perceives pain in a no longer existing/amputated body part. For a long time, it was assumed that these pains are due to the remnants of free nerve endings and nociceptors of the amputated body part. Recent findings have shown that the neuroplasticity of cortical structures plays a crucial role in the development of phantom pain (Makin et al., 2013). In particular, it is believed that cortical plasticity in the somatosensory cortex is responsible for the perception of phantom pain. After an amputation, adjacent somatosensory fields in the cortex blur together, as the brain rewires itself in the absence of sensory information, leading to a restructuring of the somatosensory cortex. In the primary somatosensory cortex (S. 1), there is a body map, a division of the brain surface according to body region, also called somatotopy. This map is diffusely altered in chronic and amputation pain (Birbaumer et al., 1997). It is also assumed that phantom pain occurs because a person gives a motor command to move a phantom limb, but receives no proprioceptive or visual feedback that the phantom limb has moved. Through repeated experiences, the brain learns that the phantom limb does not move, which can lead to a blurring of neuronal fields in the cortex and cause pain. This assumption is strengthened by the effectiveness of mirror therapy, which was developed by neuroscientist Ramachandran in 1996 (Ramachandran & Rogers-Ramachandran, 1996). In this therapy, the amputee uses a mirror to create a mirror image of the intact limb (e.g., the hand) opposite the amputated limb. By viewing the mirror image of the intact hand, the person receives visual feedback that the amputated hand is intact and can move. Viewing the movement of the phantom limb in the mirror provides strong input to the nervous system and helps alleviate and effectively unlearn the pain associated with the phantom limb. This leads to a reorganization of the cortical sensory fields.

Neuroplasticity as a result or cause of chronic pain?
So far, neuroplastic changes have been seen as drivers/results of the chronification of pain. However, they may also play a preventive role in the onset of pain. Can neuroplastic features be a risk factor for the onset of pain? In an interesting study, the relationships between brain structure and pain sensitivity in healthy adults were examined (Boissoneault et al., 2020). Current back pain, muscle diseases, and even regular back muscle training were exclusion criteria. The participants underwent a screening, which included the analysis of brain structures by MRI and the thermal and mechanical pain tolerance of the lumbar spine. Subsequently, all participants underwent standardized high-intensity back muscle training. Then, two days later, the participants were asked to assess their pain intensity using visual analogue scales (VAS 0–100 mm). Based on the pain scores, the participants were divided into a pain-resistant (VAS 0), moderately painful (VAS < 20 mm), and clinically relevant painful group (>20 mm). The main goal of the study was to

investigate individual differences in pain response to a standardized exercise and to link these with structural brain features and pain sensitivity. A remarkable result was that participants in the pain-resistant group had significantly higher pressure pain thresholds in the lumbar area than the other groups. This suggests a generally lower pain sensitivity. The analysis of brain structure revealed significant differences in the gray matter density (GMD) between the groups. Pain-resistant participants showed a higher GMD in several brain regions, including parts of the frontal, occipital, and temporal lobes. Interestingly, participants with medium pain intensity also showed medium GMD values, suggesting a gradual relationship between brain structure and pain sensitivity.

These results suggest that structural differences in the brain, particularly in the gray matter, could be associated with the individual's ability to resist or develop pain.

Seemingly pathological neuroplastic changes in chronic pain patients can, however, be reversed through targeted therapies (Flor et al., 2001; Seminowicz et al., 2011). The realization that the brain has a high adaptability in both directions can and should give hope.

3.5 Sensitization

In imaging diagnostics, especially in magnetic resonance imaging (MRI), incidental findings or physiological tissue adaptations can be mistakenly interpreted as pathological and associated with the present pain symptoms (Brinjikji et al., 2015). In many cases, no clear etiological assignment of the pain can be made. In the absence of detectable tissue damage, patients are often recommended a convalescence phase. In the case of persistent pain, for example one year after a Weber-C fracture, persistent pain symptoms may be present despite radiologically confirmed healing of bone and ligament structures. This can lead to diagnostic uncertainties. In such cases, physiotherapeutic tests offer additional explanatory approaches at the biomechanical level, focusing on deficits in mobility, stability, strength, or resilience. However, it remains unclear whether these factors are the cause of the pain or occur as a consequence of it. Alternatively, in the case of incomplete tissue healing, detectable in imaging procedures, a longer period of rest is recommended. This implies a correlation between persistent pain and incomplete tissue regeneration. In clinical practice, a causal relationship between tissue damage and pain is often postulated. Either the etiology of the pain is considered unclear when healing is complete, or delayed healing is used as an explanation for persistent pain. An often neglected aspect in this context is the potential persistence of pain perception despite completed tissue healing, possibly due to neuronal sensitization processes. This mechanism deserves increased attention in the differential diagnostic consideration of chronic pain conditions. The course of pain intensity after acute injuries, such as a muscle tear or ligament tear, is often predictable, as this pain is usually nociceptive. If pain lasts longer than usual, or is stronger than expected, this is referred to as sensitization, which was already

3.5 Sensitization

described in 1893 (Head, 1893). Head describes different phenomena of radiating pain and touch sensitivities, which he attributes, among other things, to the sensitization of central neurons. Abnormal or diffuse pain locations or pains, whose healing and subsiding differ inter-individually, must have other causes and drivers than just the peripheral excitation of nociceptors. Louis Gifford, a world-renowned physiotherapist, distinguished three different pain mechanisms in his *Mature Organism Model* in the 20th century (Gifford, 1998):

1. Input mechanism
   Input pain is characterized by a mechanical-nociceptive, inflammatory, or peripherally neurogenic cause, which often occurs in acute injuries. The pain here has a warning function after previous stimulation of nociceptors.
2. Processing mechanism
   Processing pain is less based on mechanical or nociceptive causes, but is rather influenced by affective and cognitive factors. The pain event is no longer only peripherally conditioned, but also centrally.
3. Output mechanism
   Output pain is a phenomenon characterized by cognitive, vegetative, neuroendocrine, and immunological mechanisms and is not based on any peripheral noxious stimulus, but rather on experiences, context, and central processes.

Thus, it became clear about 25 years ago that more than just tissue damage or nociception triggered by noxious stimuli are involved in some forms of pain. These distinctions offered explanations for why pain does not always subside in the same way and can—contrary to expectations—persist for different lengths of time. Chronic pain in particular has a high affective component (Yang & Chang, 2019). This includes, among other things, fear-avoidance behavior, catastrophizing thoughts, and depressive moods (Nicholas et al., 2011). Central sensitization is one of the discussed causes for chronicity. This can manifest itself in allodynia (pain with non-noxious stimuli) or hyperalgesia (hypersensitivity to noxious stimuli). Primary hyperalgesia is characterized by hypersensitivity at the site of injury itself, which is caused by the sensitization of peripheral nerve endings, whereas secondary hyperalgesia extends over a larger spectrum than just the site of injury itself, due to the sensitization of central neurons in the dorsal horn of the spinal cord (Hardy et al., 1950). Sensitization is the result of neuroplastic changes and has a maladaptive character in chronic pain.

Injury-induced sensitization processes are initially normal and physiological. On a peripheral level, a sensitization of neurons occurs first as a response to any acute onset of inflammation of damaged tissue, where as a result the activation thresholds of the nociceptors are lowered and thus can also be excited by non-noxious stimuli, such as gentle touch of the skin (Campbell & Meyer, 2006). This physiological mechanism of increased nociceptive influx to the CNS has a protective and accompanying rehabilitative function, allowing the tissue to recover during the inflammation phase. This hyperprotection initiated by the body is appropriate to force the injured area to rest, thus avoiding even greater damage and increasing the chance of healing. Therefore, even gentle touches or movements at the acutely injured site can cause severe pain, which would not normally be the case, such as after a sunburn, where touching the skin lightly can cause pain. This is a form of allodynia, as touching the skin normally does not lead to pain, but it does after a sunburn. With each acute injury, central neurons temporarily change their activity. The influence of acute injuries on central neurons has been demonstrated in studies where, in mice, pain sensitivity increased after acute peripheral burn injuries and the triggerability of flexor reflexes changed (Woolf, 1983). However, if this mechanism of increased response persists beyond the inflammation phase, it is no longer physiological, it is referred to as *maladaptive* (Gifford, 1998). In acute cases, it is normal for the patient to react with increased sensitivity to a slight stimulus, such as when the patient screams or pulls away their foot due to the diagnostic palpation of the injured ankle. If palpation or slight movements still trigger similar reactions months after the injury, such maladaptation may be underlying. This persistent peripheral and central maladaptation can be facilitated by insufficient tissue regeneration, but especially by affective and cognitive components, such as fear of movement or conspicuous psychosocial factors (Nicholas et al., 2011). Increased activity of peripheral sensitized nociceptors leads to an increased release of glutamate and neuropeptides in the secondary neuron in the posterior horn, ultimately causing increased activity of these pathways and becoming independent of the peripheral stimulus. The formation of new nociceptive nerve fibers can accompany this (Hirth et al., 2013). So if the pain persists after the acute healing phase has subsided, this may be due to the sensitization of peripheral and central neurons, after which stimulus and response are not adequately related to each other.

> **Example**
>
> **The angry boyfriend:** a metaphorical explanation for sensitization.
>
> Imagine the following situation: A man argues with his girlfriend and goes angrily and annoyed into another room and closes the door. He tries to distract himself and opens his laptop (Figs. 3.5, 3.6, and 3.7).
>
> Two minutes later, the girlfriend (benevolently) tries to seek conversation and knocks on the door and opens it.

Fig. 3.5 Man at his PC, own creation

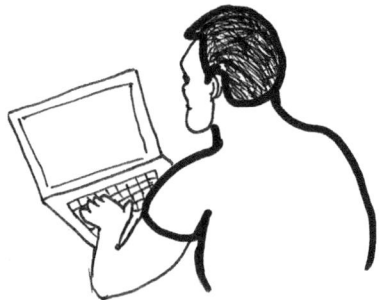

3.5 Sensitization

Fig. 3.6 Woman opening the door, own production

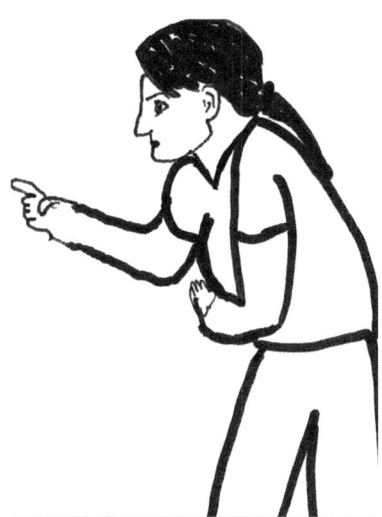

Fig. 3.7 Angry man, own production

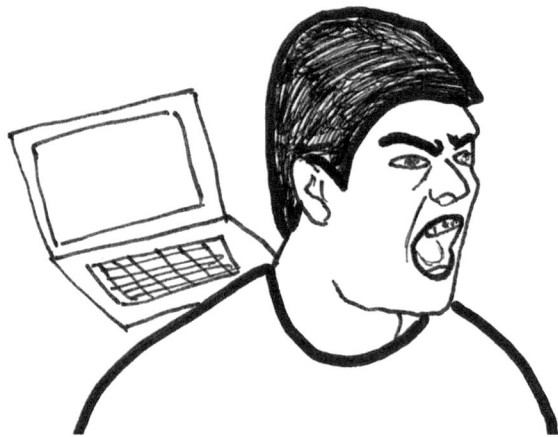

Normally this is not an action that would cause a great annoyance, if it had not occurred directly and shortly after an emotional dispute. The boyfriend reacts angrily and yells at her to leave him alone and close the door again.

What happened here? The reaction was undoubtedly not adequate to the input. The boyfriend was acutely sensitized and withdrew for recovery. Before the healing or subsiding of the inflammation stage was complete, there was a new input (acute attempt at conciliation), whereupon the output (screaming and anger) was inadequate and larger than it would normally be (allodynia, hyperalgesia). If the same stimulus (knocking and offering a conversation) still provokes the same reaction a few hours or days later (after the classic inflammation phase), this does not correspond to the expected healing process. Here, more factors would need to be examined and treated than just the trigger of the reaction. ◄

There are **two places** of sensitization: peripheral (also primary) sensitization refers to the primary neuron, central (secondary) sensitization to the secondary and tertiary neuron. In the acute phase, peripheral sensitization is the result of a neuroinflammatory response to a noxious stimulus. This has **two characteristics:**

1. Lowering the activation threshold of nociceptors
2. Activation of silent nociceptors

This increases the nociceptive influx; nociceptors can also be activated by non-noxious stimuli. This can result in hypersensitivity. This hypersensitivity can manifest itself in **two forms** in both peripheral and central sensitization (Fig. 3.8).

1. **Allodynia:** Pain response to non-noxious stimuli caused by inflammatory markers. Allodynia is present when a completely harmless stimulus (e.g., a light touch) causes pain. This is the basis for palpation tests or pressure tenderness from clinical practice. In allodynia, the nociceptors are so sensitized that they depolarize even with non-noxious stimuli (like normal pressure) (Tracey, 2017).
2. **Hyperalgesia:** Excessive pain response to a noxious stimulus. Hyperalgesia describes an excessive pain reaction to a noxious stimulus that goes far beyond the usual extent. Input and pain output are not adequate to each other due to the reduction of the stimulus threshold of the nociceptors. Primary hyperalgesia is due to increased input from the periphery, while secondary hyperalgesia involves changes in the CNS. In hyperalgesia, not only neurons of the medial (tactile) system but also of the lateral (nociceptive) system are activated more

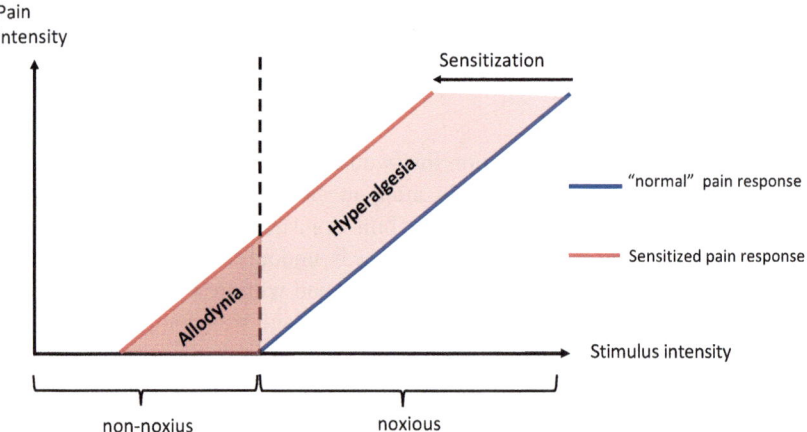

Fig. 3.8 Allodynia and hyperalgesia, own production

strongly. These changes lead to an increased perception of pain, which cannot be explained solely by the peripheral stimulus, but is also caused by central adjustments in the nervous system.

Normally, the sensitization states triggered by inflammation and tissue injuries (initially physiological) subside with the decline of inflammation and the progression of wound healing. If these states persist, they can be based on one hand on insufficient tissue healing and the maintenance of ongoing inflammations, but also on the other hand on the sensitization and autonomization of central neurons.

A central (or secondary) sensitization occurs when ascending nociceptive impulses are facilitated/amplified. Central sensitization is a complex process characterized by cumulative depolarization, known as wind-up. Wind-up is a measurable phenomenon that occurs in nociceptive C-fibers, but not in nociceptive A-fibers. This process occurs when C-fibers repeatedly fire in severe or untreated injuries, leading to an enhanced response of the dorsal horn neurons. In this case, a series of afferent signals, although low in intensity and moderately fast, but constant and repetitive, lead to ever-increasing depolarizations of the activated nerve fibers. These high-frequency signals increase the extent of depolarization, in which the nociceptor is permanently kept in a state of partial depolarization. The membrane potential is much closer to the depolarization threshold than usual, so it is easier to excite. Therefore, each subsequent stimulus leads to a stronger depolarization of the membrane than the previous one. With increasing depolarization, more local voltage-dependent sodium channels are recruited, leading to an increased intensity of the generated afferent action potential (Woller et al., 2017).

The wind-up phenomenon strongly depends on the release of glutamate, an important neurotransmitter that binds to NMDA (N-Methyl-D-Aspartate) receptors on the postsynaptic membrane and enhances neuronal activity. The complex cascade of central facilitation includes the following points:

1. Phosphorylation of the NMDA receptor and removal of the magnesium blockade
2. Activation of metabotropic glutamate and substance P receptors, which lead to an increase in intracellular calcium
3. Activation of voltage-gated calcium channels
4. Activation of various kinases to increase excitability
5. Activation of non-neuronal cells to release pro-excitatory molecules such as prostaglandins or interleukins
6. Afferent activation of the excitatory feedback on nociceptive neurons of the dorsal horn
7. Decreased activation of the inhibitory regulation of GABA and glycine; the secondary neuron is quasi disinhibited, leading to an increase in nociceptive afferents (Woller et al., 2017)

In mice, it was observed that the spinal ganglion expresses the activating transcription factor 3 more frequently in allodynia after healing of the peripheral wound healing (post-inflammatory phase), a marker associated with nerve injuries and neuropathic pain (Christianson et al., 2010). Together with the occurrence of GAP 43 (growth associated protein), a marker for axonal neurite formation and regeneration (Ghilardi et al., 2012), these observations suggest that there is a transition from an acute inflammation to a post-inflammatory neuropathic pain type, leading to central sensitization and a persistent pain state.

Another mechanism of central sensitization involves the induction of long-term changes in synaptic transmission, referred to as long-term potentiation (LTP). This LTP leads to an enhanced synaptic transmission between the involved neurons through the multiplication of action potentials, thus contributing to the amplification of nociceptive signals. In addition, there are changes in gene expression in the spinal cord, including an increased expression of genes such as c-fos. These changes contribute to the restructuring of neuronal networks and are part of the mechanism that leads to the development of a pain memory. Pain memory refers to the ability of the nervous system to store nociceptive signals and to amplify them over a longer period of time, even after the original noxious stimulus has subsided (Ji et al., 2003; Woolf & Slater, 2000).

Simply put, the nociceptive system becomes autonomous, without existing or persistent noxious stimulus, and sends danger information to the brain. If these changes persist permanently, this can lead to the development of chronic pain. The term pain memory was coined to describe this persistent state.

Chronic pain or non-specific low back pain (NSLBP), although not attributable to a specific peripheral tissue, the term *non-specific* seems increasingly inappropriate. Many specific activity and change patterns have been identified in the CNS, which correlate with individual pain perception variability and chronic pain. The specificity of a pain condition is not necessarily tied to a peripheral cause in muscle, ligament, or bone structures. Rather, the primary pathomechanism can be located in the nervous system, without this negating the specificity of a pain syndrome.

Adequate patient education about the mechanisms of peripheral and central sensitization can potentially help to reduce unfounded concerns about delayed tissue healing or persistent structural damage (Moseley, 2002). This could lead to improved pain management and increased physical activity. In this context, the therapeutic focus shifts from accelerating tissue healing, for example of a previously ruptured ligament, to desensitizing the nervous system. On the other hand, it is essential to avoid simplification in communication with patients that presents pain as a purely psychogenic phenomenon. Such simplification could lead to a loss of trust and thus a strain in the therapist-patient relationship.

3.6 The Bio-psycho-social Model as a Solution?

It is recommended that examinations and assessments, especially in patients with chronic pain, should not only focus on the physical structure, but should be bio-psycho-socially oriented in order to capture, understand and possibly explain dominant drivers and influencing factors to the patient (Wijma et al., 2016). Every therapist should be aware in patients with pain how much the phenomenon of pain is influenced by cultural-social norms beyond individual experience and this should be taken into account in therapy. However, the much-propagated BPSM may not be sufficient to fully capture the complex pain phenomenon, which is why the importance of a further understanding of chronic pain in the context of pain research should be emphasized. The currently prevailing BPSM, although widely used in pain therapy, is not sufficient to capture the full complexity and existential dimension of chronic pain (Kieselbach et al., 2023). Chronic pain goes far beyond physiological and psychological aspects and can fundamentally shake up the entire life, including life wishes and goals, and evoke existential despair and questions of meaning. This is illustrated by self-statements of those affected, which show how pain shakes the foundations of life. These include:

- Experiences of loss of control: A person reports feeling helpless and alienated from their own body due to the pain.
- Loss of life goals and wishes: An affected person expresses that chronic pain has destroyed his life plans and goals, and he no longer knows what he should live for.
- Existential despair: Another person describes how constant pain has plunged her into deep despair and she finds no joy or meaning in life anymore.
- Questions of meaning: An affected person wonders why he has to endure this pain and what the meaning of his suffering is.

Common therapy concepts, however, often do not sufficiently take into account these existential aspects. Even though the BPSM has emerged from the striving for wholeness, the dimensioning of chronic pain in particular still needs the existential character of pain. The IASP also recommends that pain management should be oriented towards the patient-reported severity of pain. The uniqueness of each individual's pain experience should be recognized and not schematized. The spiritual dimension can also be taken into account, as it is already established in palliative medicine (Hindmarch et al., 2022).

References

Adolphs, R., Gosselin, F., Buchanan, T. W., Tranel, D., Schyns, P., & Damasio, A. R. (2005). A mechanism for impaired fear recognition after amygdala damage. *Nature, 433*(7021), 68–72. https://doi.org/10.1038/nature03086.

Apkarian, A. V., Sosa, Y., Sonty, S., Levy, R. M., Harden, R. N., Parrish, T. B., & Gitelman, D. R. (2004). Chronic back pain is associated with decreased prefrontal and thalamic gray matter density. *The Journal of Neuroscience: The Official Journal of the Society for Neuroscience, 24*(46), 10410–10415. https://doi.org/10.1523/JNEUROSCI.2541-04.2004.

Apkarian, A. V., Bushnell, M. C., Treede, R. D., & Zubieta, J. K. (2005). Human brain mechanisms of pain perception and regulation in health and disease. *European journal of pain (London, England), 9*(4), 463–484. https://doi.org/10.1016/j.ejpain.2004.11.001.

Apkarian, A. V., Baliki, M. N., & Geha, P. Y. (2009). Towards a theory of chronic pain. *Progress in neurobiology, 87*(2), 81–97. https://doi.org/10.1016/j.pneurobio.2008.09.018.

Bantick, S. J., Wise, R. G., Ploghaus, A., Clare, S., Smith, S. M., & Tracey, I. (2002). Imaging how attention modulates pain in humans using functional MRI. *Brain: A Journal of Neurology, 125*(Pt 2), 310–319. https://doi.org/10.1093/brain/awf022.

Baliki, M. N., Geha, P. Y., Apkarian, A. V., & Chialvo, D. R. (2008). Beyond feeling: Chronic pain hurts the brain, disrupting the default-mode network dynamics. *The Journal of Neuroscience: The Official Journal of the Society for Neuroscience, 28*(6), 1398–1403. https://doi.org/10.1523/JNEUROSCI.4123-07.2008.

Baliki, M. N., Baria, A. T., & Apkarian, A. V. (2011). The cortical rhythms of chronic back pain. *The Journal of Neuroscience: The Official Journal of the Society for Neuroscience, 31*(39), 13981–13990. https://doi.org/10.1523/JNEUROSCI.1984-11.2011.

Baliki, M. N., & Apkarian, A. V. (2015). Nociception, pain, negative moods, and behavior selection. *Neuron, 87*(3), 474–491. https://doi.org/10.1016/j.neuron.2015.06.005.

Bastuji, H., Frot, M., Perchet, C., Magnin, M., & Garcia-Larrea, L. (2016). Pain networks from the inside: Spatiotemporal analysis of brain responses leading from nociception to conscious perception. *Human Brain Mapping, 37*(12), 4301–4315. https://doi.org/10.1002/hbm.23310.

Benedetti, F., Amanzio, M., & Maggi, G. (1995). Potentiation of placebo analgesia by proglumide. *Lancet (London, England), 346*(8984), 1231. https://doi.org/10.1016/s0140-6736(95)92938-x.

Benedetti, F., Carlino, E., & Pollo, A. (2011). How placebos change the patient's brain. *Neuropsychopharmacology: Official Publication of the American College of Neuropsychopharmacology, 36*(1), 339–354. https://doi.org/10.1038/npp.2010.81.

Berk, L. S., Tan, S. A., Fry, W. F., Napier, B. J., Lee, J. W., Hubbard, R. W., Lewis, J. E., & Eby, W. C. (1989). Neuroendocrine and stress hormone changes during mirthful laughter. *The American Journal of the Medical Sciences, 298*(6), 390–396. https://doi.org/10.1097/00000441-198912000-00006.

Benedetti, F., Arduino, C., Costa, S., Vighetti, S., Tarenzi, L., Rainero, I., & Asteggiano, G. (2006). Loss of expectation-related mechanisms in Alzheimer's disease makes analgesic therapies less effective. *Pain, 121*(1–2), 133–144. https://doi.org/10.1016/j.pain.2005.12.016.

Bernfort, L., Gerdle, B., Rahmqvist, M., Husberg, M., & Levin, L. Å. (2015). Severity of chronic pain in an elderly population in Sweden–impact on costs and quality of life. *Pain, 156*(3), 521–527. https://doi.org/10.1097/01.j.pain.0000460336.31600.01.

Berthier, M., Starkstein, S., & Leiguarda, R. (1988). Asymbolia for pain: A sensory-limbic disconnection syndrome. *Annals of Neurology, 24*(1), 41–49. https://doi.org/10.1002/ana.410240109.

Bingel, U., Herken, W., Teutsch, S., & May, A. (2008). Habituation to painful stimulation involves the antinociceptive system–a 1-year follow-up of 10 participants. *Pain, 140*(2), 393–394. https://doi.org/10.1016/j.pain.2008.09.030.

Birbaumer, N., Lutzenberger, W., Montoya, P., Larbig, W., Unertl, K., Töpfner, S., Grodd, W., Taub, E., & Flor, H. (1997). Effects of regional anesthesia on phantom limb pain are mirrored in changes in cortical reorganization. *The Journal of Neuroscience: The Official Journal of the Society for Neuroscience, 17*(14), 5503–5508. https://doi.org/10.1523/JNEUROSCI.17-14-05503.1997.

Boissoneault, J., Penza, C. W., George, S. Z., Robinson, M. E., & Bishop, M. D. (2020). Comparison of brain structure between pain-susceptible and asymptomatic individuals following experimental induction of low back pain. *The Spine Journal : Official Journal of the North American Spine Society, 20*(2), 292–299. https://doi.org/10.1016/j.spinee.2019.08.015.

Boselie, J. J. L. M., & Peters, M. L. (2023). Shifting the perspective: how positive thinking can help diminish the negative effects of pain. *Scandinavian journal of pain, 23*(3), 452–463. https://doi.org/10.1515/sjpain-2022-0129.

Bott, F. S., Nickel, M. M., Hohn, V. D., May, E. S., Gil Ávila, C., Tiemann, L., Gross, J., & Ploner, M. (2023). Local brain oscillations and interregional connectivity differentially serve sensory and expectation effects on pain. *Science Advances, 9*(16), 7572. https://doi.org/10.1126/sciadv.add7572.

Breivik, H., Collett, B., Ventafridda, V., Cohen, R., & Gallacher, D. (2006). Survey of chronic pain in Europe: Prevalence, impact on daily life, and treatment. *European Journal of Pain (London, England), 10*(4), 287–333. https://doi.org/10.1016/j.ejpain.2005.06.009.

Brinjikji, W., Luetmer, P. H., Comstock, B., Bresnahan, B. W., Chen, L. E., Deyo, R. A., Halabi, S., Turner, J. A., Avins, A. L., James, K., Wald, J. T., Kallmes, D. F., & Jarvik, J. G. (2015). Systematic literature review of imaging features of spinal degeneration in asymptomatic populations. *AJNR. American Journal of Neuroradiology, 36*(4), 811–816. https://doi.org/10.3174/ajnr.A4173.

Broks, P., Young, A. W., Maratos, E. J., Coffey, P. J., Calder, A. J., Isaac, C. L., Mayes, A. R., Hodges, J. R., Montaldi, D., Cezayirli, E., Roberts, N., & Hadley, D. (1998). Face processing impairments after encephalitis: Amygdala damage and recognition of fear. *Neuropsychologia, 36*(1), 59–70. https://doi.org/10.1016/s0028-3932(97)00105-x.

Bruehl, S., Burns, J. W., Chung, O. Y., Ward, P., & Johnson, B. (2002). Anger and pain sensitivity in chronic low back pain patients and pain-free controls: The role of endogenous opioids. *Pain, 99*(1–2), 223–233. https://doi.org/10.1016/s0304-3959(02)00104-5.

Bushnell, M. C., Ceko, M., & Low, L. A. (2013). Cognitive and emotional control of pain and its disruption in chronic pain. *Nature Reviews. Neuroscience, 14*(7), 502–511. https://doi.org/10.1038/nrn3516.

Campbell, J. N., & Meyer, R. A. (2006). Mechanisms of neuropathic pain. *Neuron, 52*(1), 77–92. https://doi.org/10.1016/j.neuron.2006.09.021.

Christianson, C. A., Corr, M., Firestein, G. S., Mobargha, A., Yaksh, T. L., & Svensson, C. I. (2010). Characterization of the acute and persistent pain state present in K/BxN serum transfer arthritis. *Pain, 151*(2), 394–403. https://doi.org/10.1016/j.pain.2010.07.030.

Clays, E., De Bacquer, D., Leynen, F., Kornitzer, M., Kittel, F., & De Backer, G. (2007). The impact of psychosocial factors on low back pain: Longitudinal results from the Belstress study. *Spine, 32*(2), 262–268. https://doi.org/10.1097/01.brs.0000251884.94821.c0.

Colloca, L., & Benedetti, F. (2005). Placebos and painkillers: Is mind as real as matter? *Nature reviews. Neuroscience, 6*(7), 545–552. https://doi.org/10.1038/nrn1705.

Colloca, L., Sigaudo, M., & Benedetti, F. (2008). The role of learning in nocebo and placebo effects. *Pain, 136*(1–2), 211–218. https://doi.org/10.1016/j.pain.2008.02.006.

Craig, A. D. (2009). How do you feel-now? The anterior insula and human awareness. *Nature Reviews. Neuroscience, 10*(1), 59–70. https://doi.org/10.1038/nrn2555.

Dahlhamer, J., Lucas, J., Zelaya, C., Nahin, R., Mackey, S., DeBar, L., Kerns, R., Von Korff, M., Porter, L., & Helmick, C. (2018). Prevalence of chronic pain and high-impact chronic pain among adults—United States, 2016. *MMWR. Morbidity and Mortality Weekly Report, 67*(36), 1001–1006. https://doi.org/10.15585/mmwr.mm6736a2.

Davis, K. D. (2011). Neuroimaging of pain: What does it tell us? *Current Opinion in Supportive and Palliative Care, 5*(2), 116–121. https://doi.org/10.1097/SPC.0b013e3283458f96.

Davis, O. C., & Price, T. J. (2023). Tiam1 creates a painful link between dendritic spine remodeling and NMDA receptors. *Neuron, 111*(13), 1993–1995. https://doi.org/10.1016/j.neuron.2023.06.001.

Derbyshire, S. W., Whalley, M. G., Stenger, V. A., & Oakley, D. A. (2004). Cerebral activation during hypnotically induced and imagined pain. *NeuroImage, 23*(1), 392–401. https://doi.org/10.1016/j.neuroimage.2004.04.03.

Dunbar, R. I., Baron, R., Frangou, A., Pearce, E., van Leeuwen, E. J., Stow, J., Partridge, G., MacDonald, I., Barra, V., & van Vugt, M. (2012). Social laughter is correlated with an elevated pain threshold. *Proceedings. Biological Sciences, 279*(1731), 1161–1167. https://doi.org/10.1098/rspb.2011.1373.

Eroglu, C., & Barres, B. A. (2010). Regulation of synaptic connectivity by glia. *Nature, 468*(7321), 223–231. https://doi.org/10.1038/nature09612.

Fang, X. X., Zhai, M. N., Zhu, M., He, C., Wang, H., Wang, J., & Zhang, Z. J. (2023). Inflammation in pathogenesis of chronic pain: Foe and friend. *Molecular Pain, 19,* 17448069231178176. https://doi.org/10.1177/17448069231178176.

Feinstein, J. S., Adolphs, R., Damasio, A., & Tranel, D. (2011). The human amygdala and the induction and experience of fear. *Current Biology, 21*(1), 34–38. https://doi.org/10.1016/j.cub.2010.11.042.

Finan, P. H., & Garland, E. L. (2015). The role of positive affect in pain and its treatment. *The Clinical Journal of Pain, 31*(2), 177–187. https://doi.org/10.1097/AJP.0000000000000092.

Fitzcharles, M. A., Cohen, S. P., Clauw, D. J., Littlejohn, G., Usui, C., & Häuser, W. (2021). Nociplastic pain: Towards an understanding of prevalent pain conditions. *Lancet (London, England), 397*(10289), 2098–2110. https://doi.org/10.1016/S0140-6736(21)00392-5.

Flor, H., Denke, C., Schaefer, M., & Grüsser, S. (2001). Effect of sensory discrimination training on cortical reorganisation and phantom limb pain. *Lancet (London, England), 357*(9270), 1763–1764. https://doi.org/10.1016/S0140-6736(00)04890-X.

France, C. R., Keefe, F. J., Emery, C. F., Affleck, G., France, J. L., Waters, S., Caldwell, D. S., Stainbrook, D., Hackshaw, K. V., & Edwards, C. (2004). Laboratory pain perception and clinical pain in post-menopausal women and age-matched men with osteoarthritis: Relationship to pain coping and hormonal status. *Pain, 112*(3), 274–281. https://doi.org/10.1016/j.pain.2004.09.007.

Fuchs, P. N., Peng, Y. B., Boyette-Davis, J. A., & Uhelski, M. L. (2014). The anterior cingulate cortex and pain processing. *Frontiers in Integrative Neuroscience, 8,* 35. https://doi.org/10.3389/fnint.2014.00035.

Galambos, A., Szabó, E., Nagy, Z., Édes, A. E., Kocsel, N., Juhász, G., & Kökönyei, G. (2019). A systematic review of structural and functional MRI studies on pain catastrophizing. *Journal of Pain Research, 12,* 1155–1178. https://doi.org/10.2147/JPR.S192246.

George, S. Z., Dannecker, E. A., & Robinson, M. E. (2006). Fear of pain, not pain catastrophizing, predicts acute pain intensity, but neither factor predicts tolerance or blood pressure reactivity: An experimental investigation in pain-free individuals. *European Journal of Pain (London, England), 10*(5), 457–465. https://doi.org/10.1016/j.ejpain.2005.06.007.

Geschwind, N., Meulders, M., Peters, M. L., Vlaeyen, J. W., & Meulders, A. (2015). Can experimentally induced positive affect attenuate generalization of fear of movement-related pain? *The Journal of Pain, 16*(3), 258–269. https://doi.org/10.1016/j.jpain.2014.12.003.

Ghilardi, J. R., Freeman, K. T., Jimenez-Andrade, J. M., Coughlin, K. A., Kaczmarska, M. J., Castaneda-Corral, G., Bloom, A. P., Kuskowski, M. A., & Mantyh, P. W. (2012). Neuroplasticity of sensory and sympathetic nerve fibers in a mouse model of a painful arthritic joint. *Arthritis and Rheumatism, 64*(7), 2223–2232. https://doi.org/10.1002/art.34385.

Giesecke, T., Gracely, R. H., Williams, D. A., Geisser, M. E., Petzke, F. W., & Clauw, D. J. (2005). The relationship between depression, clinical pain, and experimental pain in a chronic pain cohort. *Arthritis and Rheumatism, 52*(5), 1577–1584. https://doi.org/10.1002/art.21008.

Gifford, L. (1998). Pain, the tissues and the nervous system: A conceptual model. *Physiotherapy, 84*(1), 27–36. https://doi.org/10.1016/S0031-9406(05)65900-7.

Golia, M. T., Poggini, S., Alboni, S., Garofalo, S., Ciano Albanese, N., Viglione, A., Ajmone-Cat, M. A., St-Pierre, A., Brunello, N., Limatola, C., Branchi, I., & Maggi, L. (2019). Interplay between inflammation and neural plasticity: Both immune activation and suppression impair LTP and BDNF expression. *Brain, Behavior, and Immunity, 81,* 484–494. https://doi.org/10.1016/j.bbi.2019.07.003.

Grachev, I. D., Fredrickson, B. E., & Apkarian, V. A. (2000). Abnormal brain chemistry in chronic back pain: An in vivo proton magnetic resonance spectroscopy study. *Pain, 89*(1), 7–18. https://doi.org/10.1016/S0304-3959(00)00340-7.

Hansen, A. B., Skurtveit, S., Borchgrevink, P. C., Dale, O., Romundstad, P. R., Mahic, M., & Fredheim, O. M. (2015). Consumption of and satisfaction with health care among opioid users with chronic non-malignant pain. *Acta Anaesthesiologica Scandinavica, 59*(10), 1355–1366. https://doi.org/10.1111/aas.12568.

Hanssen, M. M., Peters, M. L., Vlaeyen, J. W. S., Meevissen, Y. M. C., & Vancleef, L. M. G. (2013). Optimism lowers pain: Evidence of the causal status and underlying mechanisms. *Pain, 154*(1), 53–58. https://doi.org/10.1016/j.pain.2012.08.006.

Hanssen, M. M., Vancleef, L. M., Vlaeyen, J. W., & Peters, M. L. (2014). More optimism, less pain! The influence of generalized and pain-specific expectations on experienced cold-pressor pain. *Journal of Behavioral Medicine, 37*(1), 47–58. https://doi.org/10.1007/s10865-012-9463-8.

Hardy, J. D., Wolff, H. G., & Goodell, H. (1950). Experimental evidence on the nature of cutaneous hyperalgesia. *The Journal of Clinical Investigation, 29*(1), 115–140. https://doi.org/10.1172/JCI102227.

Head, H. (1893). On disturbances of sensations with specific reference to the pain of visceral disease. *Brain, 16*, 1–132.

Head, H., & Holmes, G. (1911). Sensory disturbances from cerebral lesions. *Brain, 34*, 102–254. https://doi.org/10.1093/brain/34.2-3.102.

Hindmarch, T., Dalrymple, J., Smith, M., & Barclay, S. (2022). Spiritual interventions for cancer pain: a systematic review and narrative synthesis. *BMJ Supportive & Palliative Care, 12*(1), 1–9. https://doi.org/10.1136/bmjspcare-2021-003102.

Hinrichs-Rocker, A., Schulz, K., Järvinen, I., Lefering, R., Simanski, C., & Neugebauer, E. A. (2009). Psychosocial predictors and correlates for chronic post-surgical pain (CPSP)—a systematic review. *European Journal of Pain (London, England), 13*(7), 719–730. https://doi.org/10.1016/j.ejpain.2008.07.015.

Hirth, M., Rukwied, R., Gromann, A., Turnquist, B., Weinkauf, B., Francke, K., Albrecht, P., Rice, F., Hägglöf, B., Ringkamp, M., Engelhardt, M., Schultz, C., Schmelz, M., & Obreja, O. (2013). Nerve growth factor induces sensitization of nociceptors without evidence for increased intraepidermal nerve fiber density. *Pain, 154*(11), 2500–2511. https://doi.org/10.1016/j.pain.2013.07.036.

Horn, M. E., Alappattu, M. J., Gay, C. W., & Bishop, M. (2014). Fear of severe pain mediates sex differences in pain sensitivity responses to thermal stimuli. *Pain Research and Treatment, 2014*, 897953. https://doi.org/10.1155/2014/897953.

Hsieh, J. C., Belfrage, M., Stone-Elander, S., Hansson, P., & Ingvar, M. (1995). Central representation of chronic ongoing neuropathic pain studied by positron emission tomography. *Pain, 63*(2), 225–236. https://doi.org/10.1016/0304-3959(95)00048-W.

Jarvik, J. G., Hollingworth, W., Heagerty, P. J., Haynor, D. R., Boyko, E. J., & Deyo, R. A. (2005). Three-year incidence of low back pain in an initially asymptomatic cohort: Clinical and imaging risk factors. *Spine, 30*(13), 1541–1549. https://doi.org/10.1097/01.brs.0000167536.60002.87.

Ji, R. R., Kohno, T., Moore, K. A., & Woolf, C. J. (2003). Central sensitization and LTP: Do pain and memory share similar mechanisms? *Trends in Neurosciences, 26*(12), 696–705. https://doi.org/10.1016/j.tins.2003.09.017.

Kawai, K., Kawai, A. T., Wollan, P., & Yawn, B. P. (2017). Adverse impacts of chronic pain on health-related quality of life, work productivity, depression and anxiety in a community-based study. *Family Practice, 34*(6), 656–661. https://doi.org/10.1093/fampra/cmx034.

Kehlet, H., Jensen, T. S., & Woolf, C. J. (2006). Persistent postsurgical pain: Risk factors and prevention. *Lancet (London, England), 367*(9522), 1618–1625. https://doi.org/10.1016/S0140-6736(06)68700-X.

Keltner, J. R., Furst, A., Fan, C., Redfern, R., Inglis, B., & Fields, H. L. (2006). Isolating the modulatory effect of expectation on pain transmission: A functional magnetic resonance imaging study. *The Journal of Neuroscience: The Official Journal of the Society for Neuroscience, 26*(16), 4437–4443. https://doi.org/10.1523/JNEUROSCI.4463-05.2006.

Kieselbach, K., Koesling, D., Wabel, T., Frede, U., & Bozzaro, C. (2023). Chronischer Schmerz als existenzielle Herausforderung. *Schmerz, 37,* 116–122. https://doi.org/10.1007/s00482-022-00632-2.

Koyama, T., McHaffie, J. G., Laurienti, P. J., & Coghill, R. C. (2005). The subjective experience of pain: Where expectations become reality. *Proceedings of the National Academy of Sciences of the United States of America, 102*(36), 12950–12955. https://doi.org/10.1073/pnas.0408576102.

Kuchinad, A., Schweinhardt, P., Seminowicz, D. A., Wood, P. B., Chizh, B. A., & Bushnell, M. C. (2007). Accelerated brain gray matter loss in fibromyalgia patients: Premature aging of the brain? *The Journal of neuroscience: The Official Journal of the Society for Neuroscience, 27*(15), 4004–4007. https://doi.org/10.1523/JNEUROSCI.0098-07.2007.

Kroenke, K., Outcalt, S., Krebs, E., Bair, M. J., Wu, J., Chumbler, N., & Yu, Z. (2013). Association between anxiety, health-related quality of life and functional impairment in primary care patients with chronic pain. *General Hospital Psychiatry, 35*(4), 359–365. https://doi.org/10.1016/j.genhosppsych.2013.03.020.

Kuner, R., & Flor, H. (2016). Structural plasticity and reorganisation in chronic pain. *Nature Reviews. Neuroscience, 18*(1), 20–30. https://doi.org/10.1038/nrn.2016.162.

Labrakakis, C. (2023). The Role of the Insular Cortex in Pain. *International Journal of Molecular Sciences, 24*(6), 5736. https://doi.org/10.3390/ijms24065736.

Levine, J. D., Gordon, N. C., Smith, R., & Fields, H. L. (1981). Analgesic responses to morphine and placebo in individuals with postoperative pain. *Pain, 10*(3), 379–389. https://doi.org/10.1016/0304-3959(81)90099-3.

Levine, J. D., Gordon, N. C., Smith, R., & Fields, H. L. (1982). Post-operative pain: Effect of extent of injury and attention. *Brain Research, 234*(2), 500–504. https://doi.org/10.1016/0006-8993(82)90894-0.

Linton, S. J., Buer, N., Vlaeyen, J., & Hellsing, A. L. (2000). Are fear-avoidance beliefs related to the inception of an episode of back pain? A prospective study. *Psychology & health, 14*(6), 1051–1059. https://doi.org/10.1080/08870440008407366.

Livneh, Y., & Andermann, M. L. (2021). Cellular activity in insular cortex across seconds to hours: Sensations and predictions of bodily states. *Neuron, 109*(22), 3576–3593. https://doi.org/10.1016/j.neuron.2021.08.036.

Lorenz, J., Minoshima, S., & Casey, K. L. (2003). Keeping pain out of mind: The role of the dorsolateral prefrontal cortex in pain modulation. *Brain: A Journal of Neurology, 126*(Pt 5), 1079–1091. https://doi.org/10.1093/brain/awg102.

Lorenz, J., Hauck, M., Paur, R. C., Nakamura, Y., Zimmermann, R., Bromm, B., & Engel, A. K. (2005). Cortical correlates of false expectations during pain intensity judgments–a possible manifestation of placebo/nocebo cognitions. *Brain, Behavior, and Immunity, 19*(4), 283–295. https://doi.org/10.1016/j.bbi.2005.03.010.

Lu, C., Yang, T., Zhao, H., Zhang, M., Meng, F., Fu, H., Xie, Y., & Xu, H. (2016). Insular Cortex is Critical for the Perception, Modulation, and Chronification of Pain. *Neuroscience bulletin, 32*(2), 191–201. https://doi.org/10.1007/s12264-016-0016-y.

Ma, Q. (2022). A functional subdivision within the somatosensory system and its implications for pain research. *Neuron, 110*(5), 749–769. https://doi.org/10.1016/j.neuron.2021.12.015.

Makin, T. R., Scholz, J., Filippini, N., Henderson Slater, D., Tracey, I., & Johansen-Berg, H. (2013). Phantom pain is associated with preserved structure and function in the former hand area. *Nature Communications, 4,* 1570. https://doi.org/10.1038/ncomms2571.

Mazzola, L., Isnard, J., Peyron, R., Guénot, M., & Mauguière, F. (2009). Somatotopic organization of pain responses to direct electrical stimulation of the human insular cortex. *Pain, 146*(1–2), 99–104. https://doi.org/10.1016/j.pain.2009.07.014.

Merikle, P. M., Smilek, D., & Eastwood, J. D. (2001). Perception without awareness: Perspectives from cognitive psychology. *Cognition, 79*(1–2), 115–134. https://doi.org/10.1016/s0010-0277(00)00126-8.

Meulders, A., Meulders, M., & Vlaeyen, J. W. (2014). Positive affect protects against deficient safety learning during extinction of fear of movement-related pain in healthy individuals scoring relatively high on trait anxiety. *The Journal of Pain, 15*(6), 632–644. https://doi.org/10.1016/j.jpain.2014.02.009.

Meyer, T., Cooper, J., & Raspe, H. (2007). Disabling low back pain and depressive symptoms in the community-dwelling elderly: A prospective study. *Spine, 32*(21), 2380–2386. https://doi.org/10.1097/BRS.0b013e3181557955.

Moseley L. (2002). Combined physiotherapy and education is efficacious for chronic low back pain. *The Australian Journal of Physiotherapy, 48*(4), 297–302. https://doi.org/10.1016/s0004-9514(14)60169-0.

Moseley, G. L., & Arntz, A. (2007). The context of a noxious stimulus affects the pain it evokes. *Pain, 133*(1–3), 64–71. https://doi.org/10.1016/j.pain.2007.03.002.

Müller-Busch, H.-C- (2019). Kulturgeschichte des Schmerzes. https://www.schmerzgesellschaft.de/patienteninformationen/entwicklung-der-schmerzmedizin/kulturgeschichte-des-schmerzes Zugigriffen: 12. 03.2024.

Neugebauer, V. (2015). Amygdala pain mechanisms. *Handbook of Experimental Pharmacology, 227,* 261–284. https://doi.org/10.1007/978-3-662-46450-2_13.

Nicholas, M., Vlaeyen, J. W. S., Rief, W., Barke, A., Aziz, Q., Benoliel, R., Cohen, M., Evers, S., Giamberardino, M. A., Goebel, A., Korwisi, B., Perrot, S., Svensson, P., Wang, S. J., Treede, R. D., Taskforce, I. A. S. P., & for the Classification of Chronic Pain,. (2019). The IASP classification of chronic pain for ICD-11: Chronic primary pain. *Pain, 160*(1), 28–37. https://doi.org/10.1097/j.pain.0000000000001390.

Ohara, S., Crone, N. E., Weiss, N., Vogel, H., Treede, R. D., & Lenz, F. A. (2004). Attention to pain is processed at multiple cortical sites in man. *Experimental Brain Research, 156*(4), 513–517. https://doi.org/10.1007/s00221-004-1885-2.

Ong, W. Y., Stohler, C. S., & Herr, D. R. (2019). Role of the prefrontal cortex in pain processing. *Molecular Neurobiology, 56*(2), 1137–1166. https://doi.org/10.1007/s12035-018-1130-9.

Payne, R. (2000). Limitations of NSAIDs for pain management: Toxicity or lack of efficacy? *The Journal of Pain, 1*(3 Suppl), 14–18. https://doi.org/10.1054/jpai.2000.16611.

Peters, M. L., Sommer, M., de Rijke, J. M., Kessels, F., Heineman, E., Patijn, J., Marcus, M. A., Vlaeyen, J. W., & van Kleef, M. (2007). Somatic and psychologic predictors of long-term unfavorable outcome after surgical intervention. *Annals of Surgery, 245*(3), 487–494. https://doi.org/10.1097/01.sla.0000245495.79781.65.

Peters, M. L. (2015). Emotional and cognitive influences on pain experience. *Modern Trends in Pharmacopsychiatry, 30,* 138–152. https://doi.org/10.1159/000435938.

Petrovic, P., Dietrich, T., Fransson, P., Andersson, J., Carlsson, K., & Ingvar, M. (2005). Placebo in emotional processing–induced expectations of anxiety relief activate a generalized modulatory network. *Neuron, 46*(6), 957–969. https://doi.org/10.1016/j.neuron.2005.05.023.

Peyron, R., Laurent, B., & García-Larrea, L. (2000). Functional imaging of brain responses to pain. A review and meta-analysis. *Neurophysiologie Clinique = Clinical Neurophysiology, 30*(5), 263–288. https://doi.org/10.1016/s0987-7053(00)00227-6.

Pfeiffer, F., & Luomajoki, H. (2015). The pain is in the brain : Die Rolle des Gehirns bei chronischen Rückenschmerzen. *pt Zeitschrift für Physiotherapeuten, 67*(10), 30–38. https://doi.org/10.21256/zhaw-4844.

Phelps, C. E., Navratilova, E., & Porreca, F. (2021). Cognition in the chronic pain experience: Preclinical insights. *Trends in Cognitive Sciences, 25*(5), 365–376. https://doi.org/10.1016/j.tics.2021.01.001.

Picavet, H. S., Vlaeyen, J. W., & Schouten, J. S. (2002). Pain catastrophizing and kinesiophobia: Predictors of chronic low back pain. *American Journal of Epidemiology, 156*(11), 1028–1034. https://doi.org/10.1093/aje/kwf136.

Piccoliori, G., Engl, A., Gatterer, D., Sessa, E., in der Schmitten, J., & Abholz, H. H. (2013). Management of low back pain in general practice—is it of acceptable quality: An observational study among 25 general practices in South Tyrol (Italy). *BMC Family Practice, 14,* 148. https://doi.org/10.1186/1471-2296-14-148.

Ploghaus, A., Narain, C., Beckmann, C. F., Clare, S., Bantick, S., Wise, R., Matthews, P. M., Rawlins, J. N., & Tracey, I. (2001). Exacerbation of pain by anxiety is associated with activity in a hippocampal network. *The Journal of Neuroscience: The Official Journal of the Society for Neuroscience, 21*(24), 9896–9903. https://doi.org/10.1523/JNEUROSCI.21-24-09896.2001.

Porro, C. A., Baraldi, P., Pagnoni, G., Serafini, M., Facchin, P., Maieron, M., & Nichelli, P. (2002). Does anticipation of pain affect cortical nociceptive systems? *The Journal of Neuroscience: The Official Journal of the Society for Neuroscience, 22*(8), 3206–3214. https://doi.org/10.1523/JNEUROSCI.22-08-03206.2002.

Price, D. D. (2002). Central neural mechanisms that interrelate sensory and affective dimensions of pain. *Molecular Interventions, 2*(6), 392–339. https://doi.org/10.1124/mi.2.6.392.

Price, D. D., Craggs, J., Verne, G. N., Perlstein, W. M., & Robinson, M. E. (2007). Placebo analgesia is accompanied by large reductions in pain-related brain activity in irritable bowel syndrome patients. *Pain, 127*(1–2), 63–72. https://doi.org/10.1016/j.pain.2006.08.001.

Raij, T. T., Numminen, J., Närvänen, S., Hiltunen, J., & Hari, R. (2005). Brain correlates of subjective reality of physically and psychologically induced pain. *Proceedings of the National Academy of Sciences of the United States of America, 102*(6), 2147–2151. https://doi.org/10.1073/pnas.0409542102.

Rainville, P., Duncan, G. H., Price, D. D., Carrier, B., & Bushnell, M. C. (1997). Pain affect encoded in human anterior cingulate but not somatosensory cortex. *Science, 277*(5328), 968–971. https://doi.org/10.1126/science.277.5328.968.

Ramachandran, V. S., & Rogers-Ramachandran, D. (1996). Synaesthesia in phantom limbs induced with mirrors. *Proceedings. Biological sciences, 263*(1369), 377–386. https://doi.org/10.1098/rspb.1996.0058.

Reid, M. C., Williams, C. S., & Gill, T. M. (2003). The relationship between psychological factors and disabling musculoskeletal pain in community-dwelling older persons. *Journal of the American Geriatrics Society, 51*(8), 1092–1098. https://doi.org/10.1046/j.1532-5415.2003.51357.x.

Reid, K. J., Harker, J., Bala, M. M., Truyers, C., Kellen, E., Bekkering, G. E., & Kleijnen, J. (2011). Epidemiology of chronic non-cancer pain in Europe: Narrative review of prevalence, pain treatments and pain impact. *Current Medical Research and Opinion, 27*(2), 449–462. https://doi.org/10.1185/03007995.2010.545813.

Rice, A. S. C., Smith, B. H., & Blyth, F. M. (2016). Pain and the global burden of disease. *Pain, 157*(4), 791–796. https://doi.org/10.1097/j.pain.0000000000000454.

Romanelli, R. J., Shah, S. N., Ikeda, L., Lynch, B., Craig, T. L., Cappelleri, J. C., Jukes, T., & Ishisaka, D. (2017). Patient characteristics and healthcare utilization of a chronic pain population within an integrated healthcare system. *The American Journal of Managed Care, 23*(2), e50–e56.

Roy, M., Lebuis, A., Peretz, I., & Rainville, P. (2011). The modulation of pain by attention and emotion: A dissociation of perceptual and spinal nociceptive processes. *European Journal of Pain (London, England), 15*(6), 641.e1–10. https://doi.org/10.1016/j.ejpain.2010.11.013.

Saab, C. (2013). Visualizing the complex brain dynamics of chronic pain. *Journal of Neuroimmune Pharmacology: The Official Journal of the Society on NeuroImmune Pharmacology, 8*(3), 510–517. https://doi.org/10.1007/s11481-012-9378-8.

Scholz, J., & Woolf, C. J. (2007). The neuropathic pain triad: Neurons, immune cells and glia. *Nature Neuroscience, 10*(11), 1361–1368. https://doi.org/10.1038/nn1992.

Seifert, F., & Maihöfner, C. (2011). Functional and structural imaging of pain-induced neuroplasticity. *Current Opinion in Anaesthesiology, 24*(5), 515–523. https://doi.org/10.1097/ACO.0b013e32834a1079.

Seminowicz, D. A., Wideman, T. H., Naso, L., Hatami-Khoroushahi, Z., Fallatah, S., Ware, M. A., Jarzem, P., Bushnell, M. C., Shir, Y., Ouellet, J. A., & Stone, L. S. (2011). Effective treatment of chronic low back pain in humans reverses abnormal brain anatomy and function. *The Journal of Neuroscience: The Official Journal of the Society for Neuroscience, 31*(20), 7540–7550. https://doi.org/10.1523/JNEUROSCI.5280-10.2011.

Shirvalkar, P., Prosky, J., Chin, G., Ahmadipour, P., Sani, O. G., Desai, M., Schmitgen, A., Dawes, H., Shanechi, M. M., Starr, P. A., & Chang, E. F. (2023). First-in-human prediction of chronic pain state using intracranial neural biomarkers. *Nature Neuroscience, 26*(6), 1090–1099. https://doi.org/10.1038/s41593-023-01338-z.

Sipilä, R. M., Haasio, L., Meretoja, T. J., Ripatti, S., Estlander, A. M., & Kalso, E. A. (2017). Does expecting more pain make it more intense? Factors associated with the first week pain trajectories after breast cancer surgery. *Pain, 158*(5), 922–930. https://doi.org/10.1097/j.pain.0000000000000859.

Smallwood, R. F., Laird, A. R., Ramage, A. E., Parkinson, A. L., Lewis, J., Clauw, D. J., Williams, D. A., Schmidt-Wilcke, T., Farrell, M. J., Eickhoff, S. B., & Robin, D. A. (2013). Structural brain anomalies and chronic pain: A quantitative meta-analysis of gray matter volume. *The Journal of Pain, 14*(7), 663–675. https://doi.org/10.1016/j.jpain.2013.03.001.

Streit, W. J., Graeber, M. B., & Kreutzberg, G. W. (1988). Functional plasticity of microglia: A review. *Glia, 1*(5), 301–307. https://doi.org/10.1002/glia.440010502.

Stuber, M., Hilber, S. D., Mintzer, L. L., Castaneda, M., Glover, D., & Zeltzer, L. (2009). Laughter, humor and pain perception in children: A pilot study. *Evidence-Based Complementary and Alternative Medicine: ECAM, 6*(2), 271–276. https://doi.org/10.1093/ecam/nem097.

Sturgeon, J. A., & Zautra, A. J. (2013). Psychological resilience, pain catastrophizing, and positive emotions: Perspectives on comprehensive modeling of individual pain adaptation. *Current Pain and Headache Reports, 17*(3), 317. https://doi.org/10.1007/s11916-012-0317-4.

Sullivan, M. J., Thorn, B., Haythornthwaite, J. A., Keefe, F., Martin, M., Bradley, L. A., & Lefebvre, J. C. (2001). Theoretical perspectives on the relation between catastrophizing and pain. *The Clinical Journal of Pain, 17*(1), 52–64. https://doi.org/10.1097/00002508-200103000-00008.

Tajerian, M., Hung, V., Nguyen, H., Lee, G., Joubert, L. M., Malkovskiy, A. V., Zou, B., Xie, S., Huang, T. T., & Clark, J. D. (2018). The hippocampal extracellular matrix regulates pain and memory after injury. *Molecular Psychiatry, 23*(12), 2302–2313. https://doi.org/10.1038/s41380-018-0209-z.

Teutsch, S., Herken, W., Bingel, U., Schoell, E., & May, A. (2008). Changes in brain gray matter due to repetitive painful stimulation. *NeuroImage, 42*(2), 845–849. https://doi.org/10.1016/j.neuroimage.2008.05.044.

Theunissen, M., Peters, M. L., Bruce, J., Gramke, H. F., & Marcus, M. A. (2012). Preoperative anxiety and catastrophizing: A systematic review and meta-analysis of the association with chronic postsurgical pain. *The Clinical Journal of Pain, 28*(9), 819–841. https://doi.org/10.1097/AJP.0b013e31824549d6.

Tiemann, L., May, E. S., Postorino, M., Schulz, E., Nickel, M. M., Bingel, U., & Ploner, M. (2015). Differential neurophysiological correlates of bottom-up and top-down modulations of pain. *Pain, 156*(2), 289–296. https://doi.org/10.1097/01.j.pain.0000460309.94442.44.

Thompson, P. M., Hayashi, K. M., de Zubicaray, G., Janke, A. L., Rose, S. E., Semple, J., Herman, D., Hong, M. S., Dittmer, S. S., Doddrell, D. M., & Toga, A. W. (2003). Dynamics of gray matter loss in Alzheimer's disease. *The Journal of Neuroscience: The Official Journal of the Society for Neuroscience, 23*(3), 994–1005. https://doi.org/10.1523/JNEUROSCI.23-03-00994.2003.

Tracey, I., & Mantyh, P. W. (2007). The cerebral signature for pain perception and its modulation. *Neuron, 55*(3), 377–391. https://doi.org/10.1016/j.neuron.2007.07.012.

Tracey, I., & Bushnell, M. C. (2009). How neuroimaging studies have challenged us to rethink: Is chronic pain a disease? *The Journal of Pain, 10*(11), 1113–1120. https://doi.org/10.1016/j.jpain.2009.09.001.

Tracey, W. D. Jr. (2017). Nociception. *Current Biology, 27*(4), R129–R133. https://doi.org/10.1016/j.cub.2017.01.037.
Treede, R. D., Rief, W., Barke, A., Aziz, Q., Bennett, M. I., Benoliel, R., Cohen, M., Evers, S., Finnerup, N. B., First, M. B., Giamberardino, M. A., Kaasa, S., Kosek, E., Lavand'homme, P., Nicholas, M., Perrot, S., Scholz, J., Schug, S., Smith, B. H., ... Wang, S. J. (2015). A classification of chronic pain for ICD-11. *Pain, 156*(6), 1003–1007. https://doi.org/10.1097/j.pain.0000000000000160.
Treede, R. D., Rief, W., Barke, A., Aziz, Q., Bennett, M. I., Benoliel, R., Cohen, M., Evers, S., Finnerup, N. B., First, M. B., Giamberardino, M. A., Kaasa, S., Korwisi, B., Kosek, E., Lavand'homme, P., Nicholas, M., Perrot, S., Scholz, J., Schug, S., ... Wang, S. J. (2019). Chronic pain as a symptom or a disease: The IASP classification of chronic pain for the International Classification of Diseases (ICD-11). *Pain, 160*(1), 19–27. https://doi.org/10.1097/j.pain.0000000000001384.
van Hecke, O., Torrance, N., & Smith, B. H. (2013). Chronic pain epidemiology—where do lifestyle factors fit in? *British Journal of Pain, 7*(4), 209–217. https://doi.org/10.1177/2049463713493264.
van Middendorp, H., Lumley, M. A., Jacobs, J. W., Bijlsma, J. W., & Geenen, R. (2010). The effects of anger and sadness on clinical pain reports and experimentally-induced pain thresholds in women with and without fibromyalgia. *Arthritis Care & Research, 62*(10), 1370–1376. https://doi.org/10.1002/acr.20230.
Vandael, K., Meulders, M., Mühlen, K. Z., Peters, M., & Meulders, A. (2022). Increased positive affect is associated with less generalization of pain-related avoidance. *Behaviour Research and Therapy, 158,* 104199. https://doi.org/10.1016/j.brat.2022.104199.
Vase, L., Robinson, M. E., Verne, N. G., & Price, D. D. (2005). Increased placebo analgesia over time in irritable bowel syndrome (IBS) patients is associated with desire and expectation but not endogenous opioid mechanisms. *Pain, 115*(3), 338–347. https://doi.org/10.1016/j.pain.2005.03.014.
Villemure, C., & Bushnell, C. M. (2002). Cognitive modulation of pain: How do attention and emotion influence pain processing? *Pain, 95*(3), 195–199. https://doi.org/10.1016/S0304-3959(02)00007-6.
Vlaeyen, J. W. S., & Linton, S. J. (2012). Fear-avoidance model of chronic musculoskeletal pain: 12 years on. *Pain, 153*(6), 1144–1147. https://doi.org/10.1016/j.pain.2011.12.009.
Wager, T. D., Rilling, J. K., Smith, E. E., Sokolik, A., Casey, K. L., Davidson, R. J., Kosslyn, S. M., Rose, R. M., & Cohen, J. D. (2004). Placebo-induced changes in FMRI in the anticipation and experience of pain. *Science (New York, N.Y.), 303*(5661), 1162–1167. https://doi.org/10.1126/science.1093065.
Wijma, A. J., van Wilgen, C. P., Meeus, M., & Nijs, J. (2016). Clinical biopsychosocial physiotherapy assessment of patients with chronic pain: The first step in pain neuroscience education. *Physiotherapy Theory and Practice, 32*(5), 368–384. https://doi.org/10.1080/09593985.2016.1194651.
Woller, S. A., Eddinger, K. A., Corr, M., & Yaksh, T. L. (2017). An overview of pathways encoding nociception. *Clinical and Experimental Rheumatology, 35 Suppl 107*(5), 40–46. https://www.ncbi.nlm.nih.gov/pmc/articles/PMC6636838/pdf/nihms-1021663.pdf.
Woolf, C. J. (1983). Evidence for a central component of post-injury pain hypersensitivity. *Nature, 306*(5944), 686–688. https://doi.org/10.1038/306686a0.
Woolf, C. J., & Salter, M. W. (2000). Neuronal plasticity: Increasing the gain in pain. *Science (New York, N.Y.), 288*(5472), 1765–1769. https://doi.org/10.1126/science.288.5472.1765.
Wörz, R., Horlemann, J., & Müller-Schwefe, G. H. H. (2022). Schmerz in der Sprache Konzeptionen und Definitionen. *Schmerzmedizin, 38*(3), 48–51. https://doi.org/10.1007/s00940-022-3351-2.
Xiao, X., & Zhang, Y. Q. (2018). A new perspective on the anterior cingulate cortex and affective pain. *Neuroscience and Biobehavioral Reviews, 90,* 200–211. https://doi.org/10.1016/j.neubiorev.2018.03.022.

References

Yang, S., & Chang, M. C. (2019). Chronic pain: Structural and functional changes in brain structures and associated negative affective states. *International Journal of Molecular Sciences, 20*(13), 3130. https://doi.org/10.3390/ijms20133130.

Zheng, Q., Dong, X., Green, D. P., & Dong, X. (2022). Peripheral mechanisms of chronic pain. *Medical Review, 2*(3), 251–270. https://doi.org/10.1515/mr-2022-0013.

Zhuo, M., Wu, G., & Wu, L. J. (2011). Neuronal and microglial mechanisms of neuropathic pain. *Molecular Brain, 4,* 31. https://doi.org/10.1186/1756-6606-4-31.

Zubieta, J. K., Bueller, J. A., Jackson, L. R., Scott, D. J., Xu, Y., Koeppe, R. A., Nichols, T. E., & Stohler, C. S. (2005). Placebo effects mediated by endogenous opioid activity on mu-opioid receptors. *The Journal of Neuroscience: The Official Journal of the Society for Neuroscience, 25*(34), 7754–7762. https://doi.org/10.1523/JNEUROSCI.0439-05.2005.

Zunhammer, M., Spisák, T., Wager, T. D., Bingel, U., & Placebo Imaging Consortium (2021). Meta-analysis of neural systems underlying placebo analgesia from individual participant fMRI data. *Nature Communications, 12*(1), 1391. https://doi.org/10.1038/s41467-021-21179-3.

Zweyer, K., Velker, B., & Ruch, W. (2004). Do cheerfulness, exhilaration, and humor production moderate pain tolerance? A FACS study. *Humor: International Journal of Humor Research, 17*(1–2), 85–119. https://doi.org/10.1515/humr.2004.009.

The Postural-Structural-Biomechanical (PSB) Model

4

Abstract

Physiotherapists and doctors traditionally use the postural-structural-biomechanical (PSB) model and often see in functional deficits, such as reduced mobility or postural and movement asymmetries, the cause and root of their patients' pain. The impression of causality arises when two simultaneously existing parameters, such as pain and, for example, excessive lumbar lordosis, are identified through examination. Contrary to popular belief, however, these supposed deficits are neither the cause nor a risk factor for the onset of pain. They are often either a driver or the result of a painful condition or a variable expression of the normal, which occurs as frequently in asymptomatic people as in symptomatic patients. The pathologization of normal things could lead to false conclusions and reduced explanatory and therapeutic effectiveness.

The PSB model plays a central role in physiotherapy and manual medicine. It is based on the assumption that postural errors, structural deviations, and biomechanical dysfunctions are the primary causes of pain and functional disorders of the musculoskeletal system.

- Postural factors: The body's posture at rest and in motion is considered crucial for avoiding overloads and incorrect loads. Deviations from an optimal posture are seen as risk factors for pain and injuries and should be corrected.
- Structural factors: Anatomical anomalies, such as joint misalignments, bone or tendon degenerations, herniated discs, and other abnormalities detectable in MRI, are seen as causes of pain.
- Biomechanical factors: Here, the focus is on movement patterns and loads that act on the joints and soft tissues. Incorrect biomechanics is considered a cause of wear and tear, injuries, and pain.

This model emphasizes the importance of correct alignment and balance of the body to ensure optimal function and prevent or minimize pain. However, in recent years, the evidence base has changed, leading to increasing criticism and a paradigm shift. Dr. Eyal Lederman, a prominent physiotherapist and researcher, has significantly contributed to this discussion (Lederman, 2011). In recent years, an increasing number of studies and clinical observations have raised doubts about the exclusive validity of the PSB model. Critics of the postural-structural-biomechanical approach argue that biomechanical factors may play a role but are not the sole or primary causes of pain. Instead, it is suggested that a variety of biological, psychological, and social factors contribute to these complaints. The biopsychosocial model (BPSM) calls for a holistic view of the patient, taking into account not only physical structures but also psychological states, social circumstances, and individual life stories. And even if the biological part of the BPSM is the dominant driver, it should be critically questioned whether the presumed postural, structural, and biomechanical deficits actually play a relevant role in the development of pain.

This chapter summarizes myths and research findings on different PSB factors. The aim is to develop a deeper understanding of why a holistic approach, which takes into account the complexity of the human body and its complaints, is gaining increasing importance in modern physiotherapy. Perhaps many abnormalities postulated as functional deficits are not deficient at all. The term *functional deficit* has a negative connotation for which there is initially no evidence. It often cannot be proven that an abnormality, e.g., reduced mobility, is good or bad. Nevertheless, hypotheses often turn out to be evaluative after thorough investigations. The term *functional difference* or *functional variance* would be recommended. This implies a difference, but it does not have to be negative, bad, or unhealthy. The term *asymmetry* also implies, even though it does not contain a direct negative connotation, a deviation from the norm. Since the word *symmetry* is changed by the prefix *A-,* the linguistic usage alone implies that asymmetry is a deviation and symmetry is the rule. Further examples would be *normal/un-normal* or *typical/a-typical.*

New research findings suggest that many supposed functional deficits are not a risk factor for the development of pain and are quite normal (Lederman, 2011). Thus, many assumptions and myths can be scientifically refuted. With the numerous abnormalities or side differences evaluated as functional deficits, a change of perspective could raise the question of whether asymmetry might not actually be the norm, and symmetry the exception.

> **The Alleged Deficit**
>
> Person A owns a car, Person B does not. At first glance, B seems to have a deficit. Both earn 2500 EUR net per month, but A pays 600 EUR for car maintenance. So who has a deficit? Person B may not have a car, but they have more financial flexibility. Does owning more of something not also mean having to use, even waste, more resources to maintain this possession? Does this resource use not possibly equate to a deficit? This raises the question: Is more possession

actually advantageous if it requires continuous resource use? The answer lies in individual needs. If Person A needs the car for work or their quality of life, the costs for them are resource-using, perhaps even resource-consuming, but not resource-wasting. For Person B, who does not need a car, the lack of possession is also not a deficit. Two people have different possessions here, but no deficit. This principle can be applied to sports. Athletes of different disciplines develop specific characteristics according to their requirements. A handball player, for example, does not need symmetrical shoulder internal rotation. Just like a sports car does not need a large interior—its *deficit* is actually an advantage for its speed. This specialization is not limited to competitive sports. Every person has side differences, often due to asymmetric loads in everyday life, work or sports. Asymmetries are not only normal and unavoidable, but often necessary for specific performances. What superficially appears as a deficit can in reality be an adaptation to individual requirements and thus an advantage. ◄

The following provides a complete analysis of alleged pain-causing or alleged pain-related biomechanical deficits (?), asymmetries (?), abnormalities (?), functional variances (!).

4.1 Postural Deficitsglenohumeral Internal Rotation Deficit

The topic of alleged incorrect posture receives special attention in physiotherapy. Therapists often identify a noticeable body posture as a potential cause of back or neck complaints. For example, when examining a patient with neck pain, a pronounced anteroposition of the head is identified as a possible cause of pain.

The fact that certain postures can be associated with complaints in certain situations under certain circumstances is evident from the individual experience of every person who has felt more comfortable after changing their posture at the computer. All alleged deficits, including postural deficits, can have three different levels of effect when correlated with pain.

The correlate can either be the cause, a driver, or the result, which should be formulated accordingly.

1. Cause: "This posture leads to pain."
2. Driver: "This posture maintains/promotes the pain."
3. Result: "This posture arises from the pain."

How likely are these statements each? Are possibly two parameters (posture and pain) described together, which do not directly relate to each other mechanistically, but the examination and simultaneous determination of which creates the impression of a situational connection? The assumption that a single body posture, such as a pronounced anteroposition of the head, is the sole cause of pain, can be critically questioned by the following thought experiment:

If we consider a model that only includes six domains: musculoskeletal, neurophysiological, cognitive, motivational, social, and genetic factors. Within each of these domains, ten potential abnormalities could be defined. In the musculoskeletal area, for example, strength, mobility, flexibility, endurance, posture, axis, movement control, stability, load, and regeneration deficits could be mentioned. This hypothetical construct already opens up 60 possible sources of pain. If we now consider that each of these causes can occur in different degrees—for simplicity's sake three—the spectrum expands to 180 potential pain-triggering anomalies.

Under the simplifying assumption of an equal weighting of all factors, the following insight emerges: The probability that the anterior position of the head is the sole cause of pain is only 1/180, or less than one percent. This quantitative consideration exposes the statement "Your pain results from your head posture." as logically untenable, as it disregards the multifactorial nature of pain development. There is a risk that an excessive focus on individual factors, which may only contribute marginally, distorts and clouds the view of the overall picture. While the examination of individual components can help to complete the complex puzzle of pain piece by piece, it is crucial to step back after analyzing the individual parts and look at the overall picture. It is important to internalize that the examination of individual factors is valuable, but often of limited significance for the overall understanding. This thought experiment warns against monocausal explanatory approaches and underlines the necessity of a holistic approach in pain therapy.

What is good posture?
An upright and straight posture is often considered good posture (Korakakis et al., 2019). However, considering the anatomical features, this does not correspond to the natural curvature of the double S-shape of the spine. Humans naturally have a cervical and lumbar lordosis and thoracic kyphosis. A very upright posture without thoracic kyphosis or cervical/lumbar lordosis could therefore already be considered unnatural. So what is good posture? One that corresponds as closely as possible to the natural double S-shape? This varies anatomically and is differently pronounced in every person. The search for a norm for body posture brings various challenges. The question arises as to who or what the patients' posture is compared with and when a deviation is rated as too strong, too crooked, or too straight. Even if a norm existed and deviations from the norm could be identified, it remains unclear whether a deviation is actually to be rated negatively. The dichotomization of posture into good and bad can be problematic as it disregards possible context factors.

The ancient Greeks saw the upright posture as that of the intellectual. An upright posture stood for a person who is closer to paradise and thus can think better and further (Gregorić, 2005). The upright posture as a positive characteristic of a person was a symbol of strength, health, and respect over the centuries. Whether this can be used to infer painlessness is questionable. However, some voices were raised nearly 60 years ago, such as that of American public health professor John Keeve, who critically views the dichotomization of good and bad posture in an

4.1 Postural Deficitsglenohumeral Internal Rotation Deficit

article (Keeve, 1967). He concludes that the scientific data at the time provided no evidence for the supposedly healthier upright posture and advocates that less attention should be paid to correcting supposedly bad posture. Nevertheless, the idea of the ideal posture, from which a large industry has emerged, persists to this day and is deeply ingrained in the thinking of physiotherapists. In a study with over 500 physiotherapists, over 90% state that they consider the upright thoracic lordotic posture to be ideal (Korakakis et al., 2019). In another study, three quarters of the 279 prospective German physiotherapists state that an increased cervical lordosis is bad and leads to headaches (Bassimtabar & Alfuth, 2024). However, there is no scientific evidence for these assumptions. Quite the contrary. A large-scale study with over a thousand teenagers examined the cervical posture and two other parameters: pain and depressive mood. It was shown that an anterior position of the head (Fig. 4.1) did not correlate with more neck or headaches (Richards et al., 2016). If two factors correlate, causality is not proven. But if two factors do not even correlate, a causal relationship is ruled out. A factor that did correlate with postural abnormalities, however, was depressive moods. A possible indication that posture can be an expression of emotional status. Interesting secondary results were that participants who sat more upright were significantly taller, and participants who sat more hunched had a higher weight. Girls sat significantly more upright compared to boys. Posture here seems to be related to

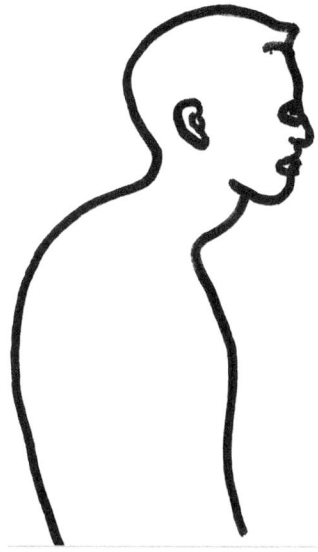

Fig. 4.1 Anterior position of the head, own illustration

emotional status as well as physical proportions and biological conditions, but not to pain.

In a meta-analysis, the results from 15 studies were examined, which investigated the relationship between a FHP (forward head posture) and pain (Mahmoud et al., 2019). It was shown that there is no connection between a FHP and pain. However, in older (>50 years) symptomatic participants, the intensity of neck pain seemed to correlate with the intensity of the FHP. Other studies, on the other hand, showed that there is no connection between posture and pain. When observing asymptomatic people, a FHP is just as prevalent as in symptomatic people (Ghamkhar & Kahlaee, 2019). The widespread belief that a FHP is an indication of a weakness or a strength deficit of the cervical flexors was also refuted in the study. Therefore, neither conclusions about the cause of pain nor about strength can be drawn from the posture. The data situation for lower back pain looks similar. If hyperlordosis were indeed a risk factor for lower back pain, this characteristic would have to occur more frequently in pain patients than in people without pain. If you compare people with and without pain and examine the occurrence of a *hyperlordosis* (Fig. 4.2), there is no difference between the two groups (Laird et al., 2016). In an attempt to find a possible causality between a postural abnormality (both sitting and standing) and lower back pain, a systematic review, which screened 41 systematic reviews (including 11 meta-analyses), concluded that the data situation diverges and there are both studies that show no connection between

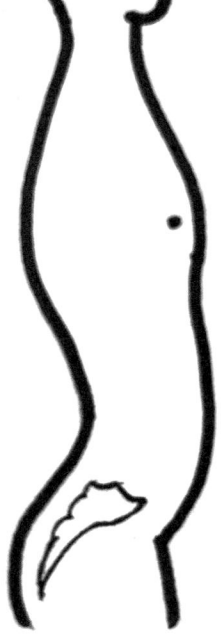

Fig. 4.2 Lumbar curvature, own production

back pain and posture, as well as studies that were able to show a connection (Swain et al., 2020). Causalities could not be derived.

In a meta-analysis, it was shown that the occurrence of an increased lordosis in back pain patients is not different from an asymptomatic group (Laird et al., 2014). A systematic review showed that out of 29 studies, 9 studies showed no connection and 10 studies showed a connection (Christensen & Hartvigsen, 2008). In another systematic review, in which 4 of the 8 analyzed studies were prospective, it was shown that there is no connection between supposedly poor posture and back pain, and the studies that found a connection could only show a weak and low correlation (Roffey et al., 2010). The tendency is that postural abnormalities and back pain have no direct connection with each other and certainly no causality. The idea of ergonomics or ideal posture fails at the latest when ergonomic interventions at the workplace, such as an ergonomic posture or an ergonomic adjustment of the screen/desk height, showed no significant influence on back pain (Driessen et al., 2010).

Now a study will be highlighted that found a supposed connection between posture and pain: This study examined the posture of 731 school children and asked them if they had had back pain recently (Sainz de Baranda et al., 2020). The main result of the study was that the lordosis was more pronounced in children who had had back pain in the previous week. In a comparison of genders, it was shown that a more pronounced lordosis occurs 2.5 times more frequently in girls. The authors' conclusion is that the measurement of the curvature can be used as a predictive value for the development of back pain and thus its detection in childhood is necessary. It should be noted that a retrospective study does not allow for prediction or forecasting models. At most, it allows the statement that the factor pain in the previous week correlates with the factor stronger lumbar curvature. It should be considered that the stronger lumbar curvature could be the result of the pain.

Posture varies greatly in the same person throughout the day, is hardly reproducible and thus very susceptible to misinterpretations in clinical examination (Dreischarf et al., 2016; Schmidt et al., 2018). Thus, posture, even when measured correctly and objectively, is not an indicator or risk factor for pain. A prospective study investigated whether the recording of PSB factors (posture, pelvic statics, mobility of the spine, etc.) and their abnormalities can predict future pain onset and its risk. This was not the case. No correlation could be found between PSB factors and pain episodes and intensities (Van Nieuwenhuyse et al., 2009). Now it should be added that a factor that does not seem to cause pain is rarely measured correctly in practice. Because posture analysis takes place in scientific studies with objective measurement methods (camera systems, markers, sensors). The reality is that posture analysis during daily work takes place as part of a visual inspection, which cannot be compared with an objective measurement, but rather with an estimate. Because the examiner orientates himself on anatomical landmarks, such as the sacrum and its inclination angle or the bone points SIAS and SIPS, whether they are at the same level or not. In an examination of asymptomatic people without pain, it was found that 80% have a so-called *anterior pelvic tilt,* i.e. lower SIAS than SIPS, with a significant difference between left and right (Herrington, 2011). Whether this is related to an ISG blockage is questionable, because an ISG is a wedged stable amphiarthrosis with very little displacement and almost non-existent range of motion (less than 1° at maximum hip flexion, measured with high-tech 3D technology) (Palsson et al., 2019). It is not possible to detect these marginal differences by inspection and palpation (McGrath, 2006; Goode et al., 2008; Holmgren and Waling, 2008). More likely are morphological asymmetries, i.e. differences in the constitution of the left and right pelvic bones, which lead to differences in anatomical landmarks in the left-right comparison. Studies also show that the position of these anatomical landmarks provides little information about the actual position of the lumbar vertebrae and they are individually variably proportioned in each individual, regardless of the actual expression of the lordosis, and this can also not be reliably recorded (Walker et al., 1987; Heino et al., 1990; Preece et al., 2008). This can lead to the fact that in the side comparison differently pronounced or naturally differently positioned bone protrusions imply an asymmetry in the transversal or sagittal plane, which however does not exist at all. Asymmetries in the frontal plane, i.e. different heights of the

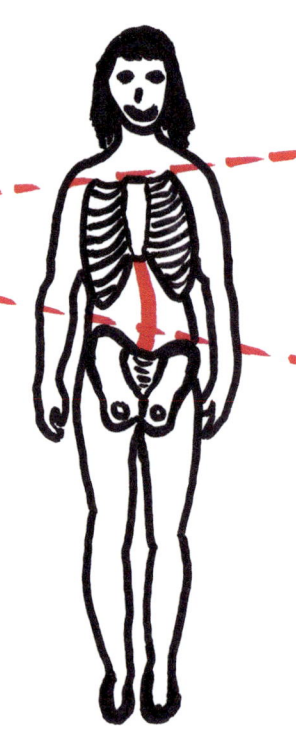

Fig. 4.3 Pelvic obliquity, own production

iliac crest, which are related to supposed leg length differences and result in pelvic obliquities (Fig. 4.3), are often used to explain pain, although these also occur just as frequently in asymptomatic people as in symptomatic ones (Grundy & Roberts, 1984; Pope et al., 1985; Nourbakhsh & Arab, 2002). 90% of all people have a leg length discrepancy (Knutson, 2005). Asymmetries are thus completely normal.

The prevention of the global back pain problem does not occur through the correction of postural factors or asymmetries. Pathologizing the normal creates a new, invented problem that is supposed to be related to back pain, but this is not the case and is only an additional burden for every back pain patient who is told this. Based on the data presented, there is no evidence of a causality between posture and pain. In correlations, the majority of the evidence speaks against a connection, as there seems to be no difference between symptomatic and asymptomatic people in terms of postural abnormalities. And if a correlation could be shown in studies, it is highly likely that the posture has changed due to the pain (protective posture), i.e. the postural abnormality is the result of the pain.

Despite all evidence against the thesis that posture is a cause or driver of pain, the topic of posture is not completely irrelevant. It cannot be ruled out that posture tips may be part of patient education. Sitting upright is not the savior, but it is also not bad, just as slouching is not bad. The blanket recommendation of sitting upright could potentially be counterproductive. The context is crucial. If the context is chronic nonspecific back pain, the data situation is clear. However, if the context is spinal stenosis, where patients usually perceive a worsening of symptoms in lordosis/extension and an improvement of symptoms in a rounded/flexed posture (Chung et al., 2000), the recommendation of sitting upright would not be in line with the patient's preferences and status and could therefore potentially be counterproductive. What could fall into the category of *blanket recommendations* are posture variation tips. Perhaps it is not a specific posture that is the problem, but the monotony behind each posture. Movement and dynamic posture variations can alleviate the risk of lower back pain (Booth et al., 2012; Foley et al., 2016; Gordon & Bloxham, 2016; Bontrup et al., 2019; Hanna et al., 2019). In summary, posture recommendations should focus on movement, position changes, and posture variation, and less energy should be wasted on finding the ideal posture and avoiding supposedly bad postures (Coenen et al., 2017).

Posture deficit? Posture abnormality? Posture diversity!

4.2 Movement Deficits

In addition to static postural factors, such as sitting and standing, dynamic-postural factors, i.e., during movement, also play a supposed role in pain prevention in practice. Sports scientists have also made it their task to determine the optimal movement. A topic that was created to investigate movement efficiency, for example in sprinting or lifting heavy weights (performance optimization), has now also found its way into medicine and physiotherapy (pain prevention). Rightly so? What does *optimal movement* actually mean? And what are supposed deficits? The following will present the relationships and levels of effect between dynamic-postural or kinematic factors and pain.

In kinematic tests, the following *movement deficits* are often observed: increased knee valgus in single-leg squats, increased foot valgus in jump landings, contralateral pelvic drop during running, scapular dyskinesis in shoulder movements, decreased mobility or a hunched back when lifting. These observations are often considered causes of pain in practice.

> **Excursus**
>
> A patient with unilateral knee pain comes for gait analysis. Examination result: The patient shows increased knee valgus on the painful side. Question: Does the patient have pain because the patient moves in this way? Or does the patient move the way they do because they have pain? It is clear: People who have pain or expect pain move differently (Kantak et al., 2022). This is normal. Possible underlying mechanisms are pain-related hyperactive muscles (Lund et al., 1991), pain-related inhibited or differently innervated/activated muscles (Hodges, 2011), pain-related task and environment-dependent movement change due to differences between the individual's resilience and the resilience required for the movement (Shumway-Cook & Woollacott, 2006) and/or a pain-related protective function to prevent painful movements. This can lead to movement control disorders, so-called *pain related movement dysfunctions* (PRMDs) (Kantak et al., 2022). PRMDs can be addressed and treated, but the PRMD or the movement abnormality here is not the cause of the complaints, but the consequence. These movement abnormalities are not irrelevant due to these findings, they simply have no preventive relevance. Movement analyses are not about cause research, but rather about finding solutions. Equating the solution (e.g., a corrective exercise or a movement modification) with the cause (pain due to a movement deficit) can negatively influence beliefs and promote kinesiophobia and avoidance behavior (Brox, 2018), which in turn is a risk factor for the chronicity of pain (Picavet et al., 2002). Patients are often told that bow legs are the cause of their knee pain and that, for example, exercises for the gluteus medius and the foot arch would correct the valgus. However, the assumption that changing the movement represents the solution can be deceptive, because the solution is not always synonymous with the cause. It has been shown that strength training of the gluteus medius and the leg axis can improve the symptoms of patellofemoral pain syndrome, which could lead to the assumption that bow legs were the problem. Interestingly, however, the valgus angle remains unchanged (Rabelo & Lucareli, 2018; Wilczyński et al., 2020). This suggests that the kinematic abnormality (here: bow leg) was not the actual cause and that the training relieves pain, but does not change the leg axis.

4.2 Movement Deficits

Is there an ideal leg axis? Knee valgus or varus, also known as X- and Bow-legs, are considered unphysiological and risk factors for meniscus and cartilage wear and osteoarthritis according to the load line theory of Johann von Mikulicz (Ruchholtz & Wirtz, 2013). Studies show that osteoarthritis patients with increased lateral cartilage loss also have increased knee valgus (Tanamas et al., 2009; Felson et al., 2013). Whether the knee valgus (Fig. 4.4) is the cause or the result of cartilage loss cannot be answered by this. It seems that in the management of osteoarthritis patients, the most important causes such as overweight, exercise, gender, genetics, and nutrition (Silverwood et al., 2015; Xu et al., 2022; Su et al., 2023) are overlooked and minor contributing factors, such as the leg axis, are given more attention. Moving away from osteoarthritis, a specific multifactorial pathology, whose deeper analysis is not the aim of this chapter, the

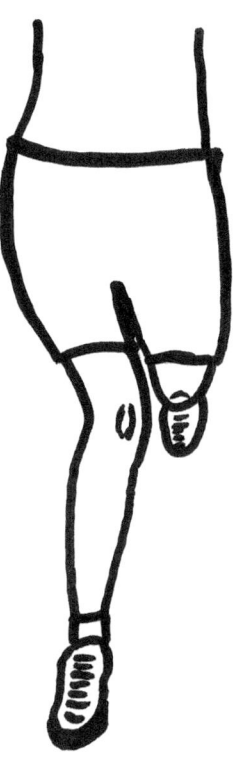

Fig. 4.4 Right knee valgus, own production

question arises whether deviations from the ideal leg axis increase the risk of knee pain. 85% of participants consisting of aspiring physiotherapists in Germany attribute a higher risk of developing pain to running technique with a knee valgus than when the leg axis is neutral (Bassimtabar & Alfuth, 2024). However, according to current evidence, no specific leg axis is a cause or a risk factor for the development of knee pain (Almeida et al., 2016; Wyndow et al., 2018). Knee valgus occurs in people without pain as often as in people with pain (Rees et al., 2019). And the pain intensities of knee patients do not correlate with the degree of knee valgus (Kudo et al., 2020). The clinical and preventive insignificance of the knee valgus applies not only to pain syndromes but also to cruciate ligament ruptures (Cronström et al., 2020; Nilstad et al., 2021), although it was long assumed that a strong valgus is a risk factor for cruciate ligament ruptures. That a single factor cannot predict the likelihood of pain or injury is clear. What about a multifactorial movement analysis? A prospective study conducted tests on 240 aspiring marine soldiers, consisting of 6 different movements, including deep squat, step-up, single-leg squat, and a jump test (Bunn et al., 2021). Depending on the quality of execution, the participants were classified into 4 different risk categories: high, moderate, medium, and low. Analysis criteria were classic biomechanical parameters and motor movement controls, such as the extent of hip adduction, trunk flexion, pelvic rotation or lateral flexion, Trendelenburg sign or heel lift. The participants were followed for one year. Pain and injuries were recorded, and it was analyzed whether the predictive categorization correlated with the pain and injuries that occurred. This was not the case. There was no significant correlation between the classification of injury risk based on biomechanical parameters and the actual occurrence of pain and injuries in the following 12 months.

Similarly, the scientific data on whether running technique and supposed deficits (such as increased hip adduction, knee and hip internal rotation, or foot eversion/flat foot) increase the risk of pain and injury are inconclusive. A review that examined 16 studies concluded that study results vary greatly, but there is no evidence that biomechanical deficits lead to more pain (Ceyssens et al., 2019). Another meta-analysis, consisting of 13 studies, which investigated the influence of foot axes on knee pain, came to similar results, that the studies make partly contradictory statements and there is no evidence for a connection between, for example, a foot valgus or flat foot and the risk of knee pain (Martinelli et al., 2022). And if a study highlights the influence of a single dimension, such as biomechanics, on pain, these results should still be treated with caution, because pain remains a symptom of multidimensional processes (biomechanics, cognition, psyche, sociality, and environment), which cannot be explained, influenced, or prevented by a single factor. And if a study identified a biomechanical deficit as a significant predictor, the result should always be analyzed more closely, as it may not have practical relevance, see the following example:

Even though there are some indications that there are correlations between biomechanical factors (such as flat and splay feet) and the risk of pain and injury, as shown in a meta-analysis of 29 studies, the correlations are weak. Moreover, these are subject to measurement errors due to their qualitative execution and visual assessment (Tong & Kong, 2013). The clinical relevance of these supposed deficits is therefore questionable. Another study, which was conducted prospectively, postulates a connection between abnormalities in biomechanical parameters during running and the injury probability of runners (Dillon et al., 2023). This includes, for example, a smaller distance between the ground and the navicular bone, so-called navicular drop (ND), clinically a flat foot (Fig. 4.5).

It turned out that the difference in ND between injured and non-injured participants is statistically significant but small (7.9 mm versus 9 mm), with the standard deviation being over 3 mm. The mean difference is 1.1 mm and is clearly smaller than the standard deviation, which makes the practical relevance of such measurements for preventive measures questionable.

In the examination of patients with shoulder pain, there are movement deficits that are specifically investigated. This includes the scapular kinematics during shoulder movements, such as during elevation or abduction. In an interesting study, 67 patients with and 68 patients without shoulder pain were examined regarding the posture and kinematics of the scapula (Plummer et al., 2017). The often postulated scapular dyskinesis (Fig. 4.6) or shoulder protraction, which is thought to cause pain, was as prevalent in the group of symptomatic participants as in the group of asymptomatic ones. No difference between the groups could be determined. Apparently, the movements of patients with shoulder pain are not different from those of asymptomatic people. Due to the lack of correlation, a connection between shoulder posture and kinematics and pain could be ruled out, and thus also causality.

In a prospective study, 140 elite soldiers were examined for their shoulder strength and scapular kinematics. These were observed over 12 months and pain and injuries were documented. No correlation could be found between strength deficits or kinematic abnormalities in the baseline examination and the complaints that occurred later. Biomechanical asymmetries were not predictors of future injuries (Johnson et al., 2019). Thus, scapular kinematic abnormalities are not a risk factor for pain. But could they be an important approach in the therapy of shoulder pain? An interesting study examined 25 participants with subacromial shoulder pain for pain, function and shoulder kinematics and the influence of kinematic training on these parameters. After 8 weeks, these parameters were examined

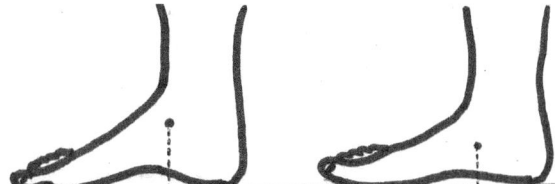

Fig. 4.5 Navicular Drop. Distance between the ground and the tuberosity of the navicular bone, own production

Fig. 4.6 Right scapular dyskinesis, own production

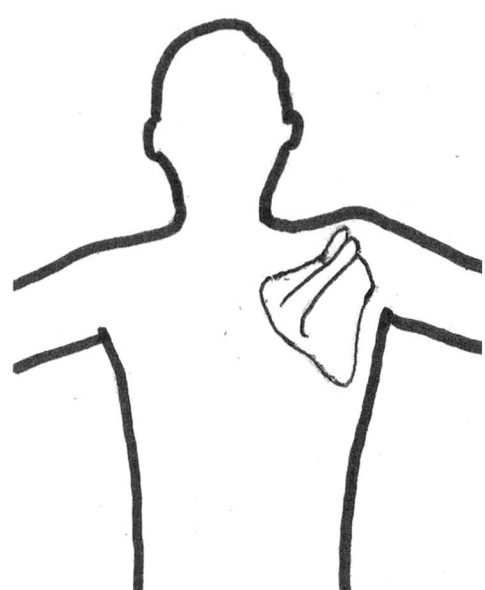

again. The pain could be alleviated, but there were no changes in scapular kinematics (Jafarian Tangrood et al., 2022). Thus, abnormalities in scapular kinematics do not seem to be a risk factor for pain and their actual correction does not seem to be an important therapeutic goal.

At the same time, there are studies that show a correlation between scapular kinematics and pain. Increased scapular dyskinesis was observed in patients with shoulder pain (Sanchez et al., 2016). Scapular kinematic abnormalities were examined at 6 different shoulder abduction angles (0°, 30°, 60°, 90°, 120°, 180°). A correlation of the abnormalities to pain and thus an accumulation in the pain group could be determined, but only at 2 of the 6 angles. The weight of this study is therefore rather low. In a meta-analysis, it was concluded from 7 studies that scapular dyskinesis did not show a significant correlation with shoulder complaints (Hogan et al., 2021). Scapular dyskinesis is therefore not a risk factor for pain, but a normal and frequently observed movement variability (Salamh et al., 2023). Possibly, a unilateral scapular dyskinesis, or better formulated a scapular kinematic difference in side comparison, is an adaptation to the respective movements and loads that the shoulder experiences in reality. These are never symmetrical.

The legitimate question may arise as to whether all movement abnormalities are irrelevant and whether there are any relevant kinematic and biomechanical differences between patients and non-patients. Although differences were found, they are not as pronounced as often assumed. For example, a study showed that participants with shoulder pain had less mobility than participants without shoulder pain

(Roldán-Jiménez et al., 2022). This result was statistically significant and underlines the relevance of mobility examinations. However, it is a fallacy to deduce from this that the reduced mobility is the cause of the pain. Studies that demonstrate a correlation between such abnormalities and pain only show a statistical correlation and not causality. Thus, the conclusion that a premature elevation of the shoulder is the cause of the complaints is not permissible.

In addition to scapular dyskinesis, the glenohumeral internal rotation deficit (GIRD) is considered a risk factor for shoulder pain. When the mobility of shoulder rotation of swimmers, tennis players or handball players is measured, an increased external rotation and a decreased internal rotation is often found in the dominant arm compared to the other side (Torres & Gomes, 2009; Schmalzl et al., 2022). It is recommended to reduce the GIRD for the prevention of shoulder complaints in shoulder-dominant sports (Cools et al., 2015). Now the question arises whether this functional difference is a deficit or could possibly be interpreted as a positive adaptation to the sport-specific requirements. It should be discussed whether a GIRD is a risk factor for shoulder pain or merely an incidental finding in painful shoulders, the cause of which may not lie in the GIRD, but is nevertheless interpreted as such. If there is a correlation between shoulder problems and GIRD, it remains unclear whether it is a causal relationship. The literature on GIRD, pain and function provides some interesting insights. Studies show that handball players often have a GIRD (Fieseler et al., 2015). At the same time, it is known that handball players have an increased incidence of shoulder injuries (Vila et al., 2022). However, it is noteworthy that asymptomatic athletes without pain also have a GIRD (Torres & Gomes, 2009). Despite these observations, there is so far no scientific evidence that a GIRD directly leads to shoulder injuries. The coexistence of GIRD and an increased injury rate in handball players does not necessarily imply a causal relationship. Further research is needed to fully understand the complex interactions between GIRD, shoulder function and injury risk in handball players.

A study that only addressed biomechanics, but also examined strength in addition to mobility, showed that young performance handball players with a strength deficit in the external rotators have a higher probability of shoulder injuries (Achenbach et al., 2020). This was observed prospectively over 12 months. Thus, the statement that a strength deficit is a possible risk factor for shoulder injuries would be permissible. However, if a study examines handball players with and without shoulder pain and finds that handball players with shoulder pain have a greater GIRD than handball players without shoulder pain (Almeida et al., 2013), GIRD cannot be declared a risk factor, since firstly, asymptomatic athletes also have a GIRD and secondly, the observed greater mobility restriction in symptomatic athletes could also be a consequence of the pain. It cannot be presented as the cause of the pain. And if retrospective or cross-sectional studies without prospective observation are used for argumentation, meta-analyses should be favored. A meta-analysis of 2195 athletes with the question of whether shoulder mobility restrictions are a risk factor for shoulder injuries did not achieve significance (Keller et al., 2018). Perhaps the GIRD is not a deficit, but a biopositive adaptation to the demands of the sport. This thesis is supported by the fact that athletes with a GIRD show higher strength of the shoulder external rotators; in other words, higher GIRDs correlate with higher strength values (Vigolvino et al., 2020). The GIRD is of course not the cause of more strength, but both parameters are related and these observations are possibly adaptations to the stresses that the dominant arm experiences. In addition, pain-relieving therapy methods, consisting of special shoulder exercises, are not proof of the previously assumed cause of pain. Because the training neither centralizes the humeral head from ventralization, nor does it increase the space between the acromion and the supraspinatus tendon (Lin & Karduna, 2016). Rather, painful structures and movements are desensitized and their load capacity is increased.

In addition, there are indications that movements are classified as conspicuous and deficient when the therapist knows that the patient has pain. In the same study, therapists were allowed to visually analyze the posture and kinematics of the participants, but were told beforehand whether the patient had pain or not (Plummer et al., 2017). Scapula posture and kinematics were objectively the same in both groups, but interestingly, the subjective inspection by the therapists revealed more supposed posture and movement deficits and abnormalities in the symptomatic group than in the asymptomatic group. This underlines the influence of the therapist's bias and expectations on the examination results.

Another myth in medical practice is the supposedly unhealthy spinal curvature with poor lifting technique. A flexed posture when lifting (Fig. 4.7) is seen as a risk factor for pain or even disc herniation (Rialet-Micoulau et al., 2022), as it is associated with higher load.

Fig. 4.7 Lifting with a rounded back, own production

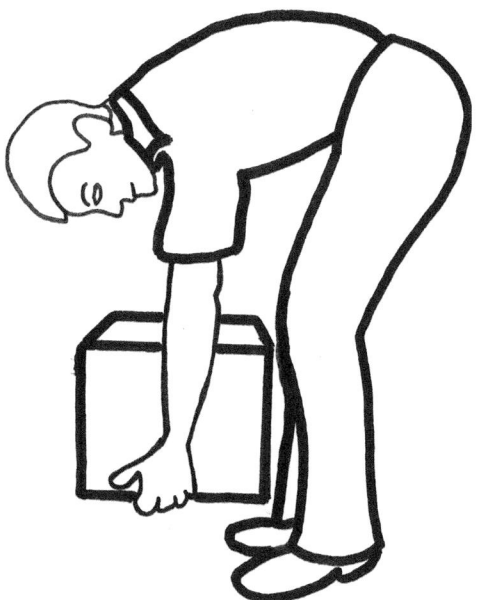

4.2 Movement Deficits

The pressure difference between lifting with a straight and rounded back is only 4% (Dreischarf et al., 2016). And even if it were at 40%, is more strain necessarily bad? Heavy loads are associated with the risk of more damage. For example, studies show that training loads increase the pressure on the intervertebral discs (Schäfer et al., 2023). However, whether an increase in pressure is a risk factor for pain cannot be answered by this, especially since intervertebral discs can highly adapt to the loads acting on them (Ruffilli et al., 2023). For example, intervertebral discs even become more robust and stronger the more load they experience, such as through a lot of running or cycling (Belavy et al., 2020), playing football or basketball (Owen et al., 2021) and strength training and lifting heavy weights (Granhed et al., 1987). Not the high load intensity, but rather the high load intensity coupled with high volume and high frequency and lack of recovery is a risk factor for degeneration and damage, but not high loads per se (Steele et al., 2015). Accordingly, there are indications that the risk of disc degeneration is increased with sudden increases in activity habits (Adams & Dolan, 1997). The implication for practice is thus load control, not load elimination or avoidance. Because too little load is also a risk factor for degeneration (Belavy et al., 2016). In addition to the load dose, the lifting technique plays a particularly large preventive and therapeutic role in medicine and patient education. However, the scientific data agree that lifting with a flexed lumbar spine neither increases the risk of pain nor injury (Saraceni et al., 2020; Washmuth et al., 2022); despite higher shear forces when lifting from the back with straight legs, than when lifting from the legs from a squat (von Arx et al., 2021). Especially since a back-friendly technique correction when lifting neither reduces pain nor prevents it (Clemes et al., 2010).

In one study, about three quarters of prospective physiotherapists stated that lifting with a rounded back should be avoided (Bassimtabar & Alfuth, 2024). This is transferred to the patients and can lead to fear of lifting with a rounded back, so that flexion is completely avoided and only lifted with a neutral lumbar spine. In fact, asymptomatic people who lift with a straight back have greater fear-avoidance behavior than people who lift with a rounder back (Knechtle et al., 2021). This is also consistent with other study results that have shown that people who advocate for the straight back as the better lifting technique have more negative beliefs about their back (Nolan et al., 2018) and greater kinesiophobia (Brox, 2018). In addition, the feeling of fragility is a strong indicator of a poor prognosis for back pain (Darlow et al., 2014), which is why avoidance strategies should not be recommended. Fear is not a favorable psychological prerequisite for a pain-free and movement-rich life. In addition, even an apparently neutral and extended lumbar spine bent upper body is still about 30° in vivo in the lumbar spine flexed (Arjmand & Shirazi-Adl, 2005; Holder, 2013). Thus, efforts for something of little relevance, which cannot even be avoided, should be reduced. In summary, a flexed lumbar spine when lifting is not a risk factor for the onset of pain. From a sports science perspective, in the search for the non-pain-related, optimal movement technique when lifting, data suggests that a round and flexed lifting technique seems to be more efficient than lifting with a straight back (Mawston et al., 2021).

In terms of the risk of pain onset, it does not seem particularly relevant how one moves. What is more important is whether and how much one moves. Symmetry is indeed beautiful and admirable to the eye (see architectural wonders), but it is man-made and not found in nature. Reality is asymmetrical.

Movement deficit? Movement abnormality? Movement diversity!

4.3 Structural Deficits

Presumably suboptimal postures and movement forms do not seem to be a risk factor for the development of pain. So where do the myths come from that, for example, knee valgus or varus are harmful? Possibly because studies show that axial deviations in certain areas of the knee joint can lead to higher loads (Werner et al., 2005) and their external correction, for example through orthoses, can reduce loads in certain areas (Shelburne et al., 2008). Key question: Why is high load equated with increased degeneration and structural damage risk and therefore avoided? Are higher loads automatically bad for the body? Higher loads are used purposefully in fitness training to strengthen muscle mass. There, high loads are not shied away from, but they are in relation to the joints. It may be assumed that passive tissue structures are not as adaptable as muscles and tendons. However, passive or non-consciously controllable structures such as bones, cartilage, and ligaments can adapt to loads and become stronger just like muscles. For example, the cartilage surfaces in the knee joint of professional weightlifters or the humerus of the throwing arm in baseball players are thicker and stronger than in untrained individuals (Grzelak et al., 2014; Warden et al., 2014). Increased mechanical load due to specific movement patterns does not necessarily imply an increased risk of injury. Rather, such loads can induce biopositive adaptation processes in the musculoskeletal system. These adaptations can potentially lead to improved resilience and performance of the affected structures. There is evidence that sport and the associated higher loads are not the cause of pain. For example, back pain occurs in professional overhead athletes (handball, volleyball, tennis), despite stronger biomechanical load on the lumbar spine, as frequently as in recreational athletes (Fett et al., 2019). In addition, athletes are more resistant compared to non-athletes and feel less pain with identical stimuli (Tesarz et al., 2012).

Assuming a structure changes due to lack of resilience and a degeneration, an injury or a structural deficit occurs: Is this the cause of pain? In people over 60, more structural degenerations can be detected, but they are less painful than those under 60. These are initial indications that pain does not necessarily correlate with the degree of degeneration (Andersson et al., 1993). The most common orthopedic reason for consulting a doctor is back pain (Finley et al., 2018), just as the most common diagnosis by German general practitioners and orthopedists (Müller-Schwefe, 2011). Changes in the intervertebral discs are often held responsible for this. Nakashima and colleagues examined 1211 people in Japan using MRI

4.3 Structural Deficits

and observed a clear disc herniation in 87.6% (2015). However, all were healthy and pain-free. In other studies, disc herniations were also observed in 30–50% of asymptomatic participants (Jensen et al., 1994; Maurer et al., 2011; Brinjikji et al., 2015). Although the prevalence increases with age, even pain-free 20–30 year olds showed a disc herniation in 30% of cases. One in four has an asymptomatic cervical spinal cord compression (Smith et al., 2021).

Asymptomatic structural deficits were also observed in the upper extremity. In one study, 72% of the 53 pain- and injury-free participants aged 45–60 years showed a SLAP lesion (Schwartzberg et al., 2016). In a larger study, 23% of the 411 asymptomatic shoulders showed a complete rotator cuff tear (Tempelhof et al., 1999). In 53% of 64 pain-free baseball players, an injury to the medial collateral ligament at the elbow was detected by MRI (Tanaka et al., 2017). The authors advocate for the term sport-specific adaptation, instead of structural deficit.

There is also ample scientific evidence for the lower extremity that tears or injuries do not always cause pain. 43 out of 44 asymptomatic participants showed meniscal damage, 27% even had 3-4 meniscal damages (Beattie et al., 2005). In another study with 115 pain-free participants, 97% of the knees showed a radiological abnormality. In 30% of the knees, meniscal tears were detected, in about 25% cartilage damage, and in 2% even tears in the anterior cruciate ligament (Horga et al., 2020). For example, 69% of 45 asymptomatic participants showed labrum tears in the hips (Register et al., 2012).

The prevalence of structural changes in the asymptomatic population raises the question of the clinical relevance of such findings. These observations primarily serve to critically question the often postulated direct causality between structural abnormalities and pain experience. A frequently cited counter-thesis is that structural abnormalities, which are asymptomatic at the time of examination, could possibly lead to complaints in the future. This argument is based on the assumption of a linear relationship from structural changes to symptomatic states. It is undisputed that pain is an integral part of human experience. However, the etiology of pain conditions is complex and multifactorial. The assumption that structural deficits inevitably represent the cause for future complaints neglects the complexity of pain genesis and perception. An analogy illustrates this: The claim that financial need is the primary cause of unhappiness could be refuted by empirical findings showing a similar incidence of sadness among financially different individuals. The conclusion that economic factors will inevitably lead to unhappiness in the future would be as speculative as the assumption that structural changes inevitably result in pain states. These considerations underline the need for a differentiated consideration of the relationships between structural findings, pain experience, and functional limitations in clinical practice and research. Whether structural abnormalities can predict future pain was investigated, for example, in a study from 2004 on 21 pain-free runners (Bergman et al., 2004). 43% (n = 9) showed a bony stress reaction of the tibia. None of the participants developed pain or other complaints in the following 12 and 48 months. This shows: abnormalities do not necessarily lead to pain. Asymptomatic abnormalities are not a risk factor for future pain.

That structural deficits in MRI and pain in most cases have no connection is already conclusively described in science. Nevertheless, MRIs have their raison d'être, especially in the case of acute injuries or traumas with loss of function, for medical examination of the integrity of structures. An MRI is always recommended in the case of red flags or severe acute injuries. However, imaging carries the risk that abnormalities (for example, a signal increase of the facets L3-5) are not postulated as a piece of the puzzle of the pain experience, but as the biomechanical main cause of pain, ignoring neurobiological processes and individual context factors, although many imaging findings, often interpreted as pathological, actually occur frequently in people without pain (Brinjikji et al., 2015). However, this should not imply that MRIs and imaging procedures cannot be helpful. Nevertheless, certain prerequisites should be given for an indication, such as sensory disturbances, radiating pain, muscle weaknesses, suspicion of fractures, progressive neurological pathologies, or complaints that persist for over 6 weeks. If these red flags are not present, an MRI is not indicated according to the German care guideline (BÄK et al., 2017). In addition, even MRI results, which are classified as far more reliable than, for example, clinical and manual tissue diagnostics, can also vary greatly depending on who evaluates them and what is being looked for (Herzog et al., 2017). Even MRIs do not seem to be objective. And even if they were, it is clear that structural deficits have no direct connection to non-traumatic pain.

Structural deficit? Structural abnormality? Structural diversity!

4.4 PSB Therapies

Therapies based on the PSB model assume that pain arises when PSB factors are impaired. Examples of this are postural weaknesses, movement deficits, or immobile muscle and joint structures. The therapy of these systems (posture training, muscle detoning, mobility improvement, and manual therapy of fasciae and joints) is intended to reverse impairments of the PSB system and reduce pain. The following will scientifically illuminate to what extent PSB therapies are effective and whether the propagated underlying treatment mechanisms are verifiable.

Where does the assumption come from that a theory or a hypothesis regarding a treatment mechanism could be correct? A sequence of 6 possible lines of thought could contribute to this assumption.

1. A fascial distortion is assumed to be a possible cause of pain.
2. A fascial distortion is diagnosed in the patient.
3. It is assumed that the elimination of the distortion will alleviate the pain.
4. Intensive pressure and traction techniques are applied.

4.4 PSB Therapies

5. After the treatment, the patient has less pain.
6. It is suspected that the fascia is now more supple, and therefore the pain relief occurred.

Point 6 is only correct if points 1, 2, 3, and 4 can be proven. The question arises whether point 1 is indeed a possible cause. If this is the case, point 2 must be demonstrably diagnosed. However, point 2 often cannot be objectively and reliably proven. Furthermore, it remains to be clarified whether the distortion has been eliminated by the therapy (point 4) (point 3). Often, the success of the treatment is used to prove the treatment mechanism. However, caution is advised here: A successful treatment (point 5) does not prove the correctness of the suspected treatment mechanism (point 6). The effectiveness of a therapy says nothing about the validity of the underlying theory. On the other hand, a pain-relieving therapy is not useless just because its suspected treatment mechanism cannot be proven. However, in education, no mechanisms should be conveyed as the reason for pain relief that cannot be proven.

Manual Therapy (MT) is the traditional cornerstone of physiotherapy. It is clear that manual therapy is currently in an identity crisis from which it is trying to reshape and reposition itself (Oostendorp, 2018). Long-held mechanisms of action seem increasingly not only scientifically unproven, but also refuted. Historically, MT is a very old discipline that had its place in many ancient cultures (Pettman, 2007). Possibly, MT gained importance through religious events like the healing hand of Jesus. It is possible that the current relevance of manual therapy has a religious and spiritual background. Nowadays, there is a great variety of schools of thought within MT, practiced by many different professions, including not only masseurs, physiotherapists, chiropractors or osteopaths. However, what all forms of manual therapy have in common is the touch of humans. Touch is an important part of human interaction and is used outside of medicine to underline communication or messages. It is not surprising that touch was used in the therapy of people who have pain. Many have recognized the power of touch and its influence on humans and developed new therapies. Touching people with pain has now evolved into special forms of physiotherapy, from simple massage to specific manual therapy or manipulation and everything in between. Pain relief does not occur due to a divine connection or healing spiritual power, but according to manual therapists traditionally through the correction of subluxated vertebrae, joint stiffness, adhesions or trigger points (Maitland, 1986; Henderson, 2012; Shah et al., 2015).

Here is a brief insight into the possible variables of touch or manual therapy: How can pressure or traction be applied?

The different variables of pressure application are visualized using our own designs (Figs. 4.8, 4.9, 4.10, 4.11, 4.12, 4.13 and 4.14). For simplicity, only pressure is shown, opposite arrow direction would mean tension.

Fig. 4.8 Angle of pressure

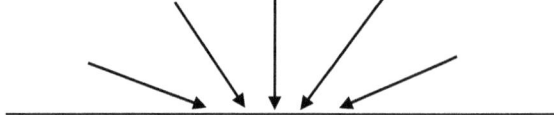

Fig. 4.9 Course of pressure

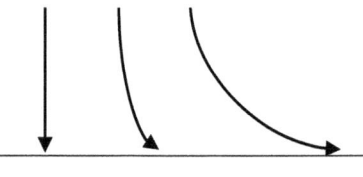

Fig. 4.10 Strength of pressure

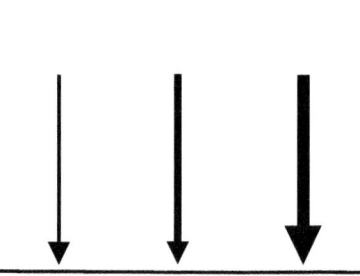

Fig. 4.11 Amplitude of pressure

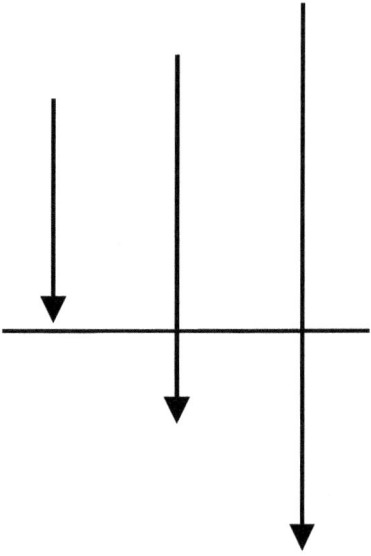

Fig. 4.12 Speed of pressure

Fig. 4.13 Frequency of pressure

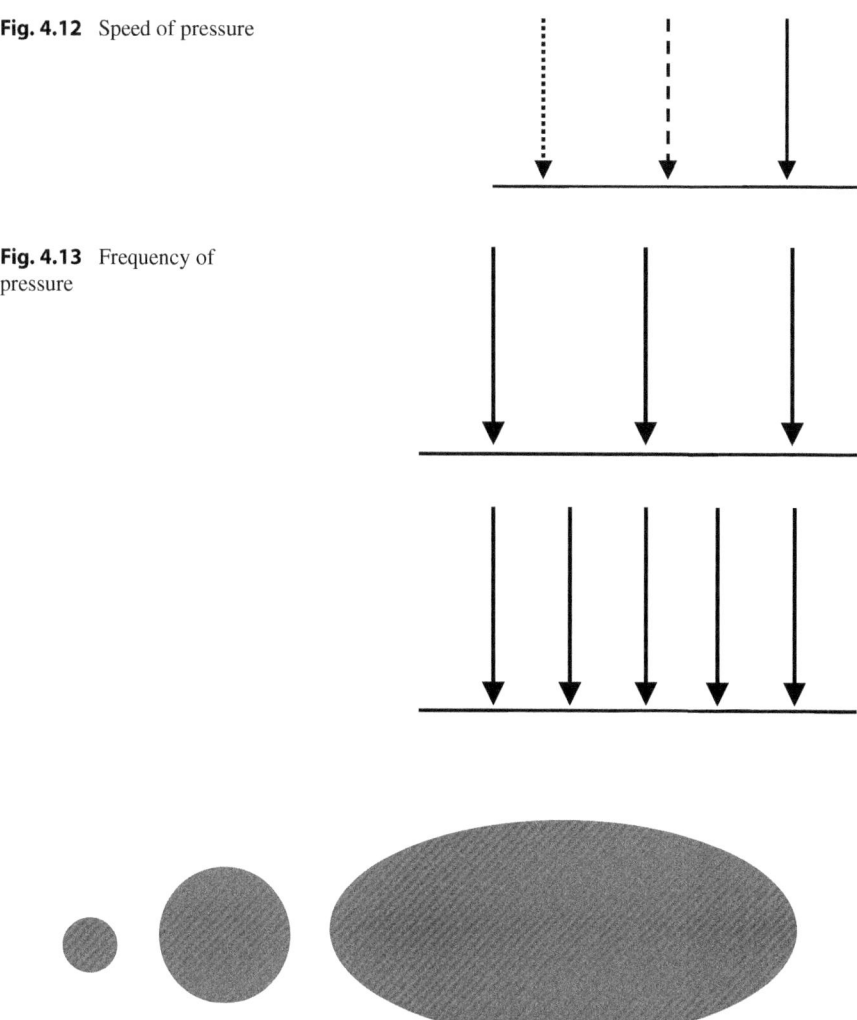

Fig. 4.14 Area of pressure

Now, using these variables, different techniques can be assembled and applied to the patient. However, the application of passive external force, such as pressure or tension, has no lasting influence on the biological structure (Vardiman et al., 2015; Konrad & Tilp, 2014). Thus, tissue structures do not adapt biopositively (as in training-induced adaptations) to manual techniques. They neither become longer, nor can adhesions or fasciae be morphologically changed.

> **Excursus**
> **Fascia Therapy**
> The fact that patients are more mobile after passive fascia therapy is not due to the fascia becoming longer, but to the fact that the tissue's tolerance threshold has been neurophysiologically modulated and increased for a short time (Langevin et al., 2018; Behm & Wilke, 2019). Although the tone of soft tissue (which is not soft, but quite stable) can be reduced by intensive stretching, pressure or traction application, this is not due to biological or morphological changes in the soft tissue, but to a vegetative sympathetic damping and central neurophysiological tone reflex reduction (Yoshimura et al., 2021). Fasciae are mechanically there to provide support to organs and muscles. It would not be beneficial if they could be lengthened or loosened by manual therapeutic force application. Moreover, the forces necessary to temporarily lengthen fasciae might not even be able to be applied by the therapist: To lengthen the Fascia Lata of the Tractus Iliotibialis by 1%, 9000 N of force are needed. Approximately 900 kg (Chaudhry et al., 2008). For the plantar fascia, 4500 N would be necessary. So about 450 kg, for 1%. The term *Myofascial Release* appears increasingly implausible (Thalhamer, 2018).

Some facts about Manual Therapy:

1. Manual therapeutic test procedures (passive ROM, end feel, pain provocation, static symmetries) are the basis for decision-making on which therapeutic techniques should be applied (Jull et al., 1994; Bialosky et al., 2012). However, these test procedures are not valid and not reliable (van Trijffel et al., 2005; van de Pol et al., 2010; van Trijffel et al., 2010).
2. MT cannot change the tissue in its morphology and structure (Bialosky et al., 2009; Zusman, 2011).
3. MT does not change the position of joints, and if it does, only temporarily and not sustainably (Tullberg et al., 1998; Colloca et al., 2003; Sato et al., 2014; Kardouni et al., 2015).
4. However, MT can relieve pain (Voogt et al., 2015). The treatment effect is thus proven. Therefore, it makes sense for therapists to use this effect to achieve the goal of pain relief in their patients. It is also logical for patients seeking pain relief to prefer a therapy that promises this effect. However, the question remains whether the only goal should be short-term pain relief and whether MT must be applied to this specific patient with his specific problems and by specific techniques to achieve the desired pain relief.
5. MT is not more effective in relieving pain in back and neck pain than other standard therapies, such as exercise therapy or oral analgesics (Rubinstein et al., 2011, 2012; Gross et al., 2015; Groeneweg et al., 2017). MT also does not seem to be more effective than *Wait and See,* where no therapy takes place

and only waiting is done (Artus et al., 2014). This can be explained by the natural healing course of the respective symptoms, which takes place regardless of the therapy.
6. Moreover, MT is not more effective than placebo or sham therapies (Ernst & Harkness, 2001; Bialosky et al., 2011, 2014; Guimarães et al., 2016; Aspinall et al., 2019). This means: If the patient is touched and it is implied that effective specific techniques are being performed, even though only an examination has taken place or techniques have been performed that are not meaningful in their direction, intensity, localization according to the textbook, the same pain relief is achieved as with the performance of specific techniques. The tactile contact alone, the touching per se, relieves pain through the release of inhibitory neurotransmitters and the activation of the endogenous pain control system by the brain (Dunbar, 2010; Geri et al., 2019). The specificity of the technique does not matter. Specific techniques in specific directions have no greater effect than non-specific techniques at non-specific locations in non-specific directions (Chiradejnant et al., 2003; Aquino et al., 2009; Kanlayanaphotporn et al., 2009; McCarthy et al., 2019).
7. MT, through the short-term modulation of the nervous system (inhibition of nociceptive afferents, reduction of central neurophysiological sensitivity and tolerance thresholds, vegetative inhibition of the sympathetic nervous system, activation of the endogenous pain control system, reduction of cortical activities such as those of the amygdala or insula) and the associated pain relief, has its justification in the use of physiotherapeutic measures, but should be used in the correct context. The mechanisms are based less on biomechanical correction, but on neurophysiological modulation (Oostendorp, 2007; Coronado et al., 2012; Sparks et al., 2013; Bialosky et al., 2017, 2018).

MT is not useless due to the facts mentioned above, just because the mechanisms assumed and propagated for centuries are not evident. MT has its justification in medicine due to its short-term pain-relieving effect, and should even be part of the therapy under certain circumstances. A nice quote on this is: "Manual therapy is always optional, but sometimes optimal." However, if manual therapy questions the justified movement variability, discourages movement and conveys a feeling of fragility and caution, this can unsettle the patient and lead to kinesiophobia. Data increasingly show that psychosocial factors are associated with chronicity and treatment failure. Outcomes are worse when patients exhibit kinesiophobia, fear avoidance, low self-efficacy expectation, and catastrophizing (Alhowimel et al., 2018). The demand to incorporate neurophysiological mechanisms of MT into the physiotherapy curriculum and to distance oneself from outdated biomechanical explanations is growing (Nijs et al., 2010; Bassimtabar & Alfuth, 2024).

In summary, increasing emphasis is being placed on not proceeding exclusively reductionistically or purely biomechanically. Instead, a broader context should be considered that includes psychosocial factors. Evidence-based practice is gaining importance over purely experience-based or technique-specific approaches. This allows for more flexible and individualized therapy. In addition, the active participation of the patient in the therapy process is recognized as a crucial factor for treatment success (Ferreira et al., 2013; Fuentes et al., 2014). Another important aspect is the consideration of patient perception. The goal is to avoid excessive fears of movement (kinesiophobia) or a feeling of fragility. Instead, the aim should be to strengthen patients' confidence in their own abilities.

These developments contribute to further developing MT as a modern, scientifically based, and patient-oriented therapy method. Considering the current evidence, MT can be used as an effective pain-relieving tool in the therapy of pain. However, after refuting structure-altering treatment mechanisms, it is important to emphasize that the effectiveness of a treatment does not depend solely on detectable structural changes. Functional improvements, pain reduction, and increased quality of life are equally important outcomes that show positive results in many MT studies (Falsiroli Maistrello et al., 2019; Zhu et al., 2024). Knowledge of its neurophysiological and psycho-social mechanisms of action is important in order not to attribute the effectiveness of MT exclusively to the supposed change of structures.

References

Achenbach, L., Laver, L., Walter, S. S., Zeman, F., Kuhr, M., & Krutsch, W. (2020). Decreased external rotation strength is a risk factor for overuse shoulder injury in youth elite handball athletes. *Knee surgery, sports traumatology, arthroscopy : Official journal of the ESSKA, 28*(4), 1202–1211. https://doi.org/10.1007/s00167-019-05493-4.

Adams, M. A., & Dolan, P. (1997). Could sudden increases in physical activity cause degeneration of intervertebral discs? *Lancet (London, England), 350*(9079), 734–735. https://doi.org/10.1016/S0140-6736(97)03021-3.

Alhowimel, A., AlOtaibi, M., Radford, K., & Coulson, N. (2018). Psychosocial factors associated with change in pain and disability outcomes in chronic low back pain patients treated by physiotherapist: A systematic review. *SAGE open medicine, 6*, 2050312118757387. https://doi.org/10.1177/2050312118757387.

Almeida, G. P., Silveira, P. F., Rosseto, N. P., Barbosa, G., Ejnisman, B., & Cohen, M. (2013). Glenohumeral range of motion in handball players with and without throwing-related shoulder pain. *Journal of shoulder and elbow surgery, 22*(5), 602–607. https://doi.org/10.1016/j.jse.2012.08.027.

Almeida, G. P., Silva, A. P., França, F. J., Magalhães, M. O., Burke, T. N., & Marques, A. P. (2016). Q-angle in patellofemoral pain: relationship with dynamic knee valgus, hip abductor torque, pain and function. Revista brasileira de ortopedia, 51(2), 181–186. https://doi.org/10.1016/j.rboe.2016.01.010.

Andersson, H. I., Ejlertsson, G., Leden, I., & Rosenberg, C. (1993). Chronic pain in a geographically defined general population: Studies of differences in age, gender, social class, and pain localization. *The Clinical journal of pain, 9*(3), 174–182. https://doi.org/10.1097/00002508-199309000-00004.

Aquino, R. L., Caires, P. M., Furtado, F. C., Loureiro, A. V., Ferreira, P. H., & Ferreira, M. L. (2009). Applying Joint Mobilization at Different Cervical Vertebral Levels does not Influence Immediate Pain Reduction in Patients with Chronic Neck Pain: A Randomized Clinical Trial. *The Journal of manual & manipulative therapy, 17*(2), 95–100. https://doi.org/10.1179/106698109790824686.

Arjmand, N., & Shirazi-Adl, A. (2005). Biomechanics of changes in lumbar posture in static lifting. *Spine, 30*(23), 2637–2648. https://doi.org/10.1097/01.brs.0000187907.02910.4f.

Artus, M., van der Windt, D., Jordan, K. P., & Croft, P. R. (2014). The clinical course of low back pain: A meta-analysis comparing outcomes in randomised clinical trials (RCTs) and observational studies. *BMC musculoskeletal disorders, 15,* 68. https://doi.org/10.1186/1471-2474-15-68.

Aspinall, S. L., Jacques, A., Leboeuf-Yde, C., Etherington, S. J., & Walker, B. F. (2019). No difference in pressure pain threshold and temporal summation after lumbar spinal manipulation compared to sham: A randomised controlled trial in adults with low back pain. *Musculoskeletal science & practice, 43,* 18–25. https://doi.org/10.1016/j.msksp.2019.05.011.

Bassimtabar, A., & Alfuth, M. (2024). Aktueller Wissensstand deutscher Physiotherapieschüler und -studenten über Schmerz und der Einfluss einer Lehrintervention [Current knowledge of German physiotherapy trainees and students on pain and the influence of a teaching intervention]. *Schmerz (Berlin, Germany),* https://doi.org/10.1007/s00482-024-00832-y. Advance online publication. https://doi.org/10.1007/s00482-024-00832-y.

Beattie, K. A., Boulos, P., Pui, M., O'Neill, J., Inglis, D., Webber, C. E., & Adachi, J. D. (2005). Abnormalities identified in the knees of asymptomatic volunteers using peripheral magnetic resonance imaging. *Osteoarthritis and cartilage, 13*(3), 181–186. https://doi.org/10.1016/j.joca.2004.11.001.

Behm, D. G., & Wilke, J. (2019). Do Self-Myofascial Release Devices Release Myofascia? Rolling Mechanisms: A Narrative Review. *Sports medicine (Auckland, N.Z.), 49*(8), 1173–1181. https://doi.org/10.1007/s40279-019-01149-y.

Belavy, D. L., Albracht, K., Bruggemann, G. P., Vergroesen, P. P., & van Dieën, J. H. (2016). Can Exercise Positively Influence the Intervertebral Disc?. *Sports medicine (Auckland, N.Z.), 46*(4), 473–485. https://doi.org/10.1007/s40279-015-0444-2.

Belavy, D. L., Brisby, H., Douglas, B., Hebelka, H., Quittner, M. J., Owen, P. J., Rantalainen, T., Trudel, G., & Lagerstrand, K. M. (2020). Characterization of intervertebral disc changes in asymptomatic individuals with distinct physical activity histories using three different quantitative MRI techniques. *Journal of clinical medicine, 9*(6), 1841. https://doi.org/10.3390/jcm9061841.

Bergman, A. G., Fredericson, M., Ho, C., & Matheson, G. O. (2004). Asymptomatic tibial stress reactions: MRI detection and clinical follow-up in distance runners. *AJR. American journal of roentgenology, 183*(3), 635–638. https://doi.org/10.2214/ajr.183.3.1830635.

Bialosky, J. E., Bishop, M. D., Price, D. D., Robinson, M. E., & George, S. Z. (2009). The mechanisms of manual therapy in the treatment of musculoskeletal pain: A comprehensive model. *Manual therapy, 14*(5), 531–538. https://doi.org/10.1016/j.math.2008.09.001.

Bialosky, J. E., Bishop, M. D., George, S. Z., & Robinson, M. E. (2011). Placebo response to manual therapy: Something out of nothing? *The Journal of manual & manipulative therapy, 19*(1), 11–19. https://doi.org/10.1179/2042618610Y.0000000001.

Bialosky, J. E., Simon, C. B., Bishop, M. D., & George, S. Z. (2012). Basis for spinal manipulative therapy: A physical therapist perspective. *Journal of electromyography and kinesiology: Official journal of the International Society of Electrophysiological Kinesiology, 22*(5), 643–647. https://doi.org/10.1016/j.jelekin.2011.11.014.

Bialosky, J. E., George, S. Z., Horn, M. E., Price, D. D., Staud, R., & Robinson, M. E. (2014). Spinal manipulative therapy-specific changes in pain sensitivity in individuals with low back pain (NCT01168999). *The journal of pain, 15*(2), 136–148. https://doi.org/10.1016/j.jpain.2013.10.005.

Bialosky, J. E., Bishop, M. D., & Penza, C. W. (2017). Placebo mechanisms of manual therapy: A sheep in wolf's clothing? *The Journal of orthopaedic and sports physical therapy, 47*(5), 301–304. https://doi.org/10.2519/jospt.2017.0604.

Bialosky, J. E., Beneciuk, J. M., Bishop, M. D., Coronado, R. A., Penza, C. W., Simon, C. B., & George, S. Z. (2018). Unraveling the mechanisms of manual therapy: Modeling an approach.

The Journal of orthopaedic and sports physical therapy, 48(1), 8–18. https://doi.org/10.2519/jospt.2018.7476.

Bontrup, C., Taylor, W. R., Fliesser, M., Visscher, R., Green, T., Wippert, P. M., & Zemp, R. (2019). Low back pain and its relationship with sitting behaviour among sedentary office workers. *Applied ergonomics, 81,* 102894. https://doi.org/10.1016/j.apergo.2019.102894.

Booth, F. W., Roberts, C. K., & Laye, M. J. (2012). Lack of exercise is a major cause of chronic diseases. *Comprehensive Physiology, 2*(2), 1143–1211. https://doi.org/10.1002/cphy.c110025.

Brinjikji, W., Luetmer, P. H., Comstock, B., Bresnahan, B. W., Chen, L. E., Deyo, R. A., Halabi, S., Turner, J. A., Avins, A. L., James, K., Wald, J. T., Kallmes, D. F., & Jarvik, J. G. (2015). Systematic literature review of imaging features of spinal degeneration in asymptomatic populations. *AJNR. American journal of neuroradiology, 36*(4), 811–816. https://doi.org/10.3174/ajnr.A4173.

Bundesärztekammer (BÄK), Kassenärztliche Bundesvereinigung (KBV), Arbeitsgemeinschaft der Wissenschaftlichen Medizinischen Fachgesellschaften (AWMF). (2017) Nationale Versorgungsleitlinie nicht-spezifischer Kreuzschmerz—Kurzfassung, 2. Auflage. Version 1. https://doi.org/10.6101/AZQ/000377. www.kreuzschmerz.versorgungsleitlinien.de. Zugegriffen: 9. Juni 2024.

Bunn, P. D. S., Lopes, T. J. A., Terra, B. S., Costa, H. F., Souza, M. P., Braga, R. M., Inoue, A., Ribeiro, F. M., Alves, D. S., & Bezerra da Silva, E. (2021). Association between movement patterns and risk of musculoskeletal injuries in navy cadets: A cohort study. *Physical therapy in sport: Official journal of the Association of Chartered Physiotherapists in Sports Medicine, 52,* 81–89. https://doi.org/10.1016/j.ptsp.2021.08.003.

Brox, J. I. (2018). Lifting with straight legs and bent spine is not bad for your back. *Scandinavian journal of pain, 18*(4), 563–564. https://doi.org/10.1515/sjpain-2018-0302.

Ceyssens, L., Vanelderen, R., Barton, C., Malliaras, P., & Dingenen, B. (2019). Biomechanical Risk Factors Associated with Running-Related Injuries: A Systematic Review. *Sports medicine (Auckland, N.Z.), 49*(7), 1095–1115. https://doi.org/10.1007/s40279-019-01110-z.

Chaudhry, H., Schleip, R., Ji, Z., Bukiet, B., Maney, M., & Findley, T. (2008). Three-dimensional mathematical model for deformation of human fasciae in manual therapy. *The Journal of the American Osteopathic Association, 108*(8), 379–390. https://doi.org/10.7556/jaoa.2008.108.8.379.

Chiradejnant, A., Maher, C. G., Latimer, J., & Stepkovitch, N. (2003). Efficacy of „therapist-selected" versus „randomly selected" mobilisation techniques for the treatment of low back pain: A randomised controlled trial. *The Australian journal of physiotherapy, 49*(4), 233–241. https://doi.org/10.1016/s0004-9514(14)60139-2.

Christensen, S. T., & Hartvigsen, J. (2008). Spinal curves and health: A systematic critical review of the epidemiological literature dealing with associations between sagittal spinal curves and health. *Journal of manipulative and physiological therapeutics, 31*(9), 690–714. https://doi.org/10.1016/j.jmpt.2008.10.004.

Chung, S. S., Lee, C. S., Kim, S. H., Chung, M. W., & Ahn, J. M. (2000). Effect of low back posture on the morphology of the spinal canal. *Skeletal radiology, 29*(4), 217–223. https://doi.org/10.1007/s002560050596.

Clemes, S. A., Haslam, C. O., & Haslam, R. A. (2010). What constitutes effective manual handling training? A systematic review. *Occupational medicine (Oxford, England), 60*(2), 101–107. https://doi.org/10.1093/occmed/kqp127.

Coenen, P., Gilson, N., Healy, G. N., Dunstan, D. W., & Straker, L. M. (2017). A qualitative review of existing national and international occupational safety and health policies relating to occupational sedentary behaviour. *Applied ergonomics, 60,* 320–333. https://doi.org/10.1016/j.apergo.2016.12.010.

Cools, A. M., Johansson, F. R., Borms, D., & Maenhout, A. (2015). Prevention of shoulder injuries in overhead athletes: A science-based approach. *Brazilian journal of physical therapy, 19*(5), 331–339. https://doi.org/10.1590/bjpt-rbf.2014.0109.

References

Colloca, C. J., Keller, T. S., & Gunzburg, R. (2003). Neuromechanical characterization of in vivo lumbar spinal manipulation. Part II. Neurophysiological response. *Journal of manipulative and physiological therapeutics, 26*(9), 579–591. https://doi.org/10.1016/j.jmpt.2003.08.004.

Coronado, R. A., Gay, C. W., Bialosky, J. E., Carnaby, G. D., Bishop, M. D., & George, S. Z. (2012). Changes in pain sensitivity following spinal manipulation: A systematic review and meta-analysis. *Journal of electromyography and kinesiology: Official journal of the International Society of Electrophysiological Kinesiology, 22*(5), 752–767. https://doi.org/10.1016/j.jelekin.2011.12.013.

Cronström, A., Creaby, M. W., & Ageberg, E. (2020). Do knee abduction kinematics and kinetics predict future anterior cruciate ligament injury risk? A systematic review and meta-analysis of prospective studies. *BMC musculoskeletal disorders, 21*(1), 563. https://doi.org/10.1186/s12891-020-03552-3.

Darlow, B., Perry, M., Stanley, J., Mathieson, F., Melloh, M., Baxter, G. D., & Dowell, A. (2014). Cross-sectional survey of attitudes and beliefs about back pain in New Zealand. *British Medical Journal Open, 4*(5), e004725. https://doi.org/10.1136/bmjopen-2013-004725.

Dillon, S., Burke, A., Whyte, E. F., O'Connor, S., Gore, S., & Moran, K. A. (2023). Running towards injury? A prospective investigation of factors associated with running injuries. *PLoS ONE, 18*(8), e0288814. https://doi.org/10.1371/journal.pone.0288814.

Dreischarf, M., Pries, E., Bashkuev, M., Putzier, M., & Schmidt, H. (2016). Differences between clinical „snap-shot" and „real-life" assessments of lumbar spine alignment and motion— What is the „real" lumbar lordosis of a human being? *Journal of biomechanics, 49*(5), 638–644. https://doi.org/10.1016/j.jbiomech.2016.01.032.

Driessen, M. T., Proper, K. I., van Tulder, M. W., Anema, J. R., Bongers, P. M., & van der Beek, A. J. (2010). The effectiveness of physical and organisational ergonomic interventions on low back pain and neck pain: A systematic review. *Occupational and environmental medicine, 67*(4), 277–285. https://doi.org/10.1136/oem.2009.047548.

Dunbar, R. I. (2010). The social role of touch in humans and primates: Behavioural function and neurobiological mechanisms. *Neuroscience and biobehavioral reviews, 34*(2), 260–268. https://doi.org/10.1016/j.neubiorev.2008.07.001.

Ernst, E., & Harkness, E. (2001). Spinal manipulation: A systematic review of sham-controlled, double-blind, randomized clinical trials. *Journal of pain and symptom management, 22*(4), 879–889. https://doi.org/10.1016/s0885-3924(01)00337-2.

Falsiroli Maistrello, L., Rafanelli, M., & Turolla, A. (2019). Manual therapy and quality of life in people with headache: Systematic review and meta-analysis of randomized controlled trials. *Current pain and headache reports, 23*(10), 78. https://doi.org/10.1007/s11916-019-0815-8.

Felson, D. T., Niu, J., Gross, K. D., Englund, M., Sharma, L., Cooke, T. D., Guermazi, A., Roemer, F. W., Segal, N., Goggins, J. M., Lewis, C. E., Eaton, C., & Nevitt, M. C. (2013). Valgus malalignment is a risk factor for lateral knee osteoarthritis incidence and progression: Findings from the Multicenter Osteoarthritis Study and the Osteoarthritis Initiative. *Arthritis and rheumatism, 65*(2), 355–362. https://doi.org/10.1002/art.37726.

Ferreira, P. H., Ferreira, M. L., Maher, C. G., Refshauge, K. M., Latimer, J., & Adams, R. D. (2013). The therapeutic alliance between clinicians and patients predicts outcome in chronic low back pain. *Physical therapy, 93*(4), 470–478. https://doi.org/10.2522/ptj.20120137.

Fett, D., Trompeter, K., & Platen, P. (2019). Prevalence of back pain in a group of elite athletes exposed to repetitive overhead activity. *PLoS ONE, 14*(1), e0210429. https://doi.org/10.1371/journal.pone.0210429.

Fieseler, G., Jungermann, P., Koke, A., Irlenbusch, L., Delank, K. S., & Schwesig, R. (2015). Glenohumeral range of motion (ROM) and isometric strength of professional team handball athletes, part III: Changes over the playing season. *Archives of orthopaedic and trauma surgery, 135*(12), 1691–1700. https://doi.org/10.1007/s00402-015-2308-5.

Finley, C. R., Chan, D. S., Garrison, S., Korownyk, C., Kolber, M. R., Campbell, S., Eurich, D. T., Lindblad, A. J., Vandermeer, B., & Allan, G. M. (2018). What are the most common conditions in primary care? Systematic review. *Canadian family physician Medecin de famille canadien, 64*(11), 832–840.

Foley, B., Engelen, L., Gale, J., Bauman, A., & Mackey, M. (2016). Sedentary behavior and musculoskeletal discomfort are reduced when office workers trial an activity-based work environment. *Journal of occupational and environmental medicine, 58*(9), 924–931. https://doi.org/10.1097/JOM.0000000000000828.

Fuentes, J., Armijo-Olivo, S., Funabashi, M., Miciak, M., Dick, B., Warren, S., Rashiq, S., Magee, D. J., & Gross, D. P. (2014). Enhanced therapeutic alliance modulates pain intensity and muscle pain sensitivity in patients with chronic low back pain: An experimental controlled study. *Physical therapy, 94*(4), 477–489. https://doi.org/10.2522/ptj.20130118.

Geri, T., Viceconti, A., Minacci, M., Testa, M., & Rossettini, G. (2019). Manual therapy: Exploiting the role of human touch. Musculoskeletal science & practice, 44, 102044. https://doi.org/10.1016/j.msksp.2019.07.008.

Ghamkhar, L., & Kahlaee, A. H. (2019). Is forward head posture relevant to cervical muscles performance and neck pain? A case-control study. *Brazilian journal of physical therapy, 23*(4), 346–354. https://doi.org/10.1016/j.bjpt.2018.08.007.

Goode, A., Hegedus, E. J., Sizer, P., Brismee, J. M., Linberg, A., & Cook, C. E. (2008). Three-dimensional movements of the sacroiliac joint: A systematic review of the literature and assessment of clinical utility. *The Journal of manual & manipulative therapy, 16*(1), 25–38. https://doi.org/10.1179/106698108790818639.

Gordon, R., & Bloxham, S. (2016). A Systematic Review of the Effects of Exercise and Physical Activity on Non-Specific Chronic Low Back Pain. *Healthcare (Basel, Switzerland), 4*(2), 22. https://doi.org/10.3390/healthcare4020022.

Granhed, H., Jonson, R., & Hansson, T. (1987). The loads on the lumbar spine during extreme weight lifting. *Spine, 12*(2), 146–149. https://doi.org/10.1097/00007632-198703000-00010.

Gregorić, P. (2005). Plato's and Aristotle's Explanation of Human Posture. *A Journal for Ancient Philosophy and Science, 2*, 183–196.

Groeneweg, R., van Assen, L., Kropman, H., Leopold, H., Mulder, J., Smits-Engelsman, B. C. M., Ostelo, R. W. J. G., Oostendorp, R. A. B., & van Tulder, M. W. (2017). Manual therapy compared with physical therapy in patients with non-specific neck pain: A randomized controlled trial. *Chiropractic & manual therapies, 25*, 12. https://doi.org/10.1186/s12998-017-0141-3.

Gross, A., Langevin, P., Burnie, S. J., Bédard-Brochu, M. S., Empey, B., Dugas, E., Faber-Dobrescu, M., Andres, C., Graham, N., Goldsmith, C. H., Brønfort, G., Hoving, J. L., & LeBlanc, F. (2015). Manipulation and mobilisation for neck pain contrasted against an inactive control or another active treatment. *The Cochrane database of systematic reviews, 2015*(9), CD004249. https://doi.org/10.1002/14651858.CD004249.pub4.

Grundy, P. F., & Roberts, C. J. (1984). Does unequal leg length cause back pain? A case-control study. *Lancet (London, England), 2*(8397), 256–258. https://doi.org/10.1016/s0140-6736(84)90300-3.

Grzelak, P., Domzalski, M., Majos, A., Podgórski, M., Stefanczyk, L., Krochmalski, M., & Polguj, M. (2014). Thickening of the knee joint cartilage in elite weightlifters as a potential adaptation mechanism. *Clinical anatomy (New York, N.Y.), 27*(6), 920–928. https://doi.org/10.1002/ca.22393.

Guimarães, J. F., Salvini, T. F., Siqueira, A. L., Jr., Ribeiro, I. L., Camargo, P. R., & Alburquerque- Sendín, F. (2016). Immediate Effects of Mobilization With Movement vs Sham Technique on Range of Motion, Strength, and Function in Patients With Shoulder Impingement Syndrome: Randomized Clinical Trial. *Journal of manipulative and physiological therapeutics, 39*(9), 605–615. https://doi.org/10.1016/j.jmpt.2016.08.001.

Hanna, F., Daas, R. N., El-Shareif, T. J., Al-Marridi, H. H., Al-Rojoub, Z. M., & Adegboye, O. A. (2019). The relationship between sedentary behavior, back pain, and psychosocial correlates among university employees. *Frontiers in public health, 7*, 80. https://doi.org/10.3389/fpubh.2019.00080.

Heino, J. G., Godges, J. J., & Carter, C. L. (1990). Relationship between Hip Extension Range of Motion and Postural Alignment. *The Journal of orthopaedic and sports physical therapy, 12*(6), 243–247. https://doi.org/10.2519/jospt.1990.12.6.243.

Henderson, C. N. (2012). The basis for spinal manipulation: Chiropractic perspective of indications and theory. *Journal of electromyography and kinesiology : Official journal of the International Society of Electrophysiological Kinesiology, 22*(5), 632–642. https://doi.org/10.1016/j.jelekin.2012.03.008.

Herrington, L. (2011). Assessment of the degree of pelvic tilt within a normal asymptomatic population. *Manual therapy, 16*(6), 646–648. https://doi.org/10.1016/j.math.2011.04.006.

Herzog, R., Elgort, D. R., Flanders, A. E., & Moley, P. J. (2017). Variability in diagnostic error rates of 10 MRI centers performing lumbar spine MRI examinations on the same patient within a 3-week period. *The spine journal : Official journal of the North American Spine Society, 17*(4), 554–561. https://doi.org/10.1016/j.spinee.2016.11.009.

Hodges, P. W. (2011). Pain and motor control: From the laboratory to rehabilitation. *Journal of electromyography and kinesiology: Official journal of the International Society of Electrophysiological Kinesiology, 21*(2), 220–228. https://doi.org/10.1016/j.jelekin.2011.01.002.

Hogan, C., Corbett, J. A., Ashton, S., Perraton, L., Frame, R., & Dakic, J. (2021). Scapular dyskinesis is not an isolated risk factor for shoulder injury in athletes: A systematic review and meta-analysis. *The American journal of sports medicine, 49*(10), 2843–2853. https://doi.org/10.1177/0363546520968508.

Holder, L. (2013). The effect of lumbar posture and pelvis fixation on back extensor torque and paravertebral muscle activation. https://openrepository.aut.ac.nz/server/api/core/bitstreams/d9496b7e-8373-4bee-90f1-8e4ed7a97efc/content. Zugegriffen: 25. Apr. 2024.

Holmgren, U., & Waling, K. (2008). Inter-examiner reliability of four static palpation tests used for assessing pelvic dysfunction. *Manual therapy, 13*(1), 50–56. https://doi.org/10.1016/j.math.2006.09.009.

Horga, L. M., Hirschmann, A. C., Henckel, J., Fotiadou, A., Di Laura, A., Torlasco, C., D'Silva, A., Sharma, S., Moon, J. C., & Hart, A. J. (2020). Prevalence of abnormal findings in 230 knees of asymptomatic adults using 3.0 T MRI. *Skeletal radiology, 49*(7), 1099–1107. https://doi.org/10.1007/s00256-020-03394-z.

Jafarian Tangrood, Z., Sole, G., & Cury Ribeiro, D. (2022). Association between changes in pain or function scores and changes in scapular rotations in patients with subacromial shoulder pain: A prospective cohort study. *Archives of physiotherapy, 12*(1), 18. https://doi.org/10.1186/s40945-022-00143-4.

Jensen, M. C., Brant-Zawadzki, M. N., Obuchowski, N., Modic, M. T., Malkasian, D., & Ross, J. S. (1994). Magnetic resonance imaging of the lumbar spine in people without back pain. *The New England journal of medicine, 331*(2), 69–73. https://doi.org/10.1056/NEJM199407143310201.

Johnson, C. D., Nijst, B. K. J. F., Eagle, S. R., Kessels, M. W. M., Lovalekar, M. T., Krajewski, K. T., Flanagan, S. D., Nindl, B. C., & Connaboy, C. (2019). Evaluation of shoulder strength and kinematics as risk factors for shoulder injury in United States special forces personnel. *Orthopaedic journal of sports medicine, 7*(3), 2325967119831272. https://doi.org/10.1177/2325967119831272.

Jull, G., Treleaven, J., & Versace, G. (1994). Manual examination: Is pain provocation a major cue for spinal dysfunction? *The Australian journal of physiotherapy, 40*(3), 159–165. https://doi.org/10.1016/S0004-9514(14)60574-2.

Kanlayanaphotporn, R., Chiradejnant, A., & Vachalathiti, R. (2009). The immediate effects of mobilization technique on pain and range of motion in patients presenting with unilateral neck pain: A randomized controlled trial. *Archives of physical medicine and rehabilitation, 90*(2), 187–192. https://doi.org/10.1016/j.apmr.2008.07.017.

Kantak, S. S., Johnson, T., & Zarzycki, R. (2022). Linking pain and motor control: Conceptualization of Movement Deficits in Patients with Painful Conditions. *Physical therapy, 102*(4), pzab289. https://doi.org/10.1093/ptj/pzab289.

Kardouni, J. R., Pidcoe, P. E., Shaffer, S. W., Finucane, S. D., Cheatham, S. A., Sousa, C. O., & Michener, L. A. (2015). Thoracic spine manipulation in individuals with subacromial impingement syndrome does not immediately alter thoracic spine kinematics, thoracic excursion, or scapular kinematics: A randomized controlled trial. *The Journal of orthopaedic and sports physical therapy, 45*(7), 527–538. https://doi.org/10.2519/jospt.2015.5647.

Keeve, J. P. (1967). „Fitness," „posture" and other selected school health myths. *The Journal of school health, 37*(1), 8–15. https://doi.org/10.1111/j.1746-1561.1967.tb07013.x.

Keller, R. A., De Giacomo, A. F., Neumann, J. A., Limpisvasti, O., & Tibone, J. E. (2018). Glenohumeral internal rotation deficit and risk of upper extremity injury in overhead athletes: A meta-analysis and systematic review. *Sports health, 10*(2), 125–132. https://doi.org/10.1177/1941738118756577.

Knechtle, D., Schmid, S., Suter, M., Riner, F., Moschini, G., Senteler, M., Schweinhardt, P., & Meier, M. L. (2021). Fear-avoidance beliefs are associated with reduced lumbar spine flexion during object lifting in pain-free adults. *Pain, 162*(6), 1621–1631. https://doi.org/10.1097/j.pain.0000000000002170.

Knutson G. A. (2005). Anatomic and functional leg-length inequality: A review and recommendation for clinical decision-making. Part I, anatomic leg-length inequality: Prevalence, magnitude, effects and clinical significance. *Chiropractic & osteopathy, 13,* 11. https://doi.org/10.1186/1746-1340-13-11.

Konrad, A., & Tilp, M. (2014). Increased range of motion after static stretching is not due to changes in muscle and tendon structures. *Clinical biomechanics (Bristol, Avon), 29*(6), 636–642. https://doi.org/10.1016/j.clinbiomech.2014.04.013.

Korakakis, V., O'Sullivan, K., O'Sullivan, P. B., Evagelinou, V., Sotiralis, Y., Sideris, A., Sakellariou, K., Karanasios, S., & Giakas, G. (2019). Physiotherapist perceptions of optimal sitting and standing posture. *Musculoskeletal science & practice, 39,* 24–31. https://doi.org/10.1016/j.msksp.2018.11.004.

Kudo, K., Nagura, T., Harato, K., Kobayashi, S., Niki, Y., Matsumoto, M., & Nakamura, M. (2020). Correlation between static limb alignment and peak knee adduction angle during gait is affected by subject pain in medial knee osteoarthritis. The Knee, 27(2), 348–355. https://doi.org/10.1016/j.knee.2019.11.008.

Laird, R. A., Gilbert, J., Kent, P., & Keating, J. L. (2014). Comparing lumbo-pelvic kinematics in people with and without back pain: A systematic review and meta-analysis. *BMC musculoskeletal disorders, 15,* 229. https://doi.org/10.1186/1471-2474-15-229.

Laird, R. A., Kent, P., & Keating, J. L. (2016). How consistent are lordosis, range of movement and lumbo-pelvic rhythm in people with and without back pain?. BMC musculoskeletal disorders, 17(1), 403. https://doi.org/10.1186/s12891-016-1250-1.

Langevin, H. M., Bishop, J., Maple, R., Badger, G. J., & Fox, J. R. (2018). Effect of stretching on thoracolumbar fascia injury and movement restriction in a porcine model. *American journal of physical medicine & rehabilitation, 97*(3), 187–191. https://doi.org/10.1097/PHM.0000000000000824.

Lederman, E. (2011). The fall of the postural-structural-biomechanical model in manual and physical therapies: Exemplified by lower back pain. *Journal of bodywork and movement therapies, 15*(2), 131–138. https://doi.org/10.1016/j.jbmt.2011.01.011.

Lin, Y. L., & Karduna, A. (2016). Exercises focusing on rotator cuff and scapular muscles do not improve shoulder joint position sense in healthy subjects. *Human movement science, 49,* 248–257. https://doi.org/10.1016/j.humov.2016.06.016.

Lund, J. P., Donga, R., Widmer, C. G., & Stohler, C. S. (1991). The pain-adaptation model: A discussion of the relationship between chronic musculoskeletal pain and motor activity. *Canadian journal of physiology and pharmacology, 69*(5), 683–694. https://doi.org/10.1139/y91-102.

Mahmoud, N. F., Hassan, K. A., Abdelmajeed, S. F., Moustafa, I. M., & Silva, A. G. (2019). The relationship between forward head posture and neck pain: A systematic review and meta-analysis. *Current reviews in musculoskeletal medicine, 12*(4), 562–577. https://doi.org/10.1007/s12178-019-09594-y.

Maitland G.D. (1986). *Vertebral Manipulation. Fifth Edition.* Butterworth-Heinemann. https://books.google.de/books?hl=de&lr=&id=HMM5EAAAQBAJ&oi=fnd&pg=PP&dq=matiland+1986+vertebral+manipulation&ots=M3hxvkXgVr&sig=l-WH1tRnhEhLxqdkjhCkTb1s

0U&redir_esc=y#v=onepage&q=matiland%201986%20vertebral%20manipulation&f=false. Zugegriffen: 22. März 2024.

Martinelli, N., Bergamini, A. N., Burssens, A., Toschi, F., Kerkhoffs, G. M. M. J., Victor, J., & Sansone, V. (2022). Does the foot and ankle alignment impact the patellofemoral pain syndrome? A systematic review and meta-analysis. *Journal of clinical medicine, 11*(8), 2245. https://doi.org/10.3390/jcm11082245.

Maurer, M., Soder, R. B., & Baldisserotto, M. (2011). Spine abnormalities depicted by magnetic resonance imaging in adolescent rowers. *The American journal of sports medicine, 39*(2), 392–397. https://doi.org/10.1177/0363546510381365.

Mawston, G., Holder, L., O'Sullivan, P., & Boocock, M. (2021). Flexed lumbar spine postures are associated with greater strength and efficiency than lordotic postures during a maximal lift in pain-free individuals. *Gait & posture, 86,* 245–250. https://doi.org/10.1016/j.gaitpost.2021.02.029.

McCarthy, C. J., Potter, L., & Oldham, J. A. (2019). Comparing targeted thrust manipulation with general thrust manipulation in patients with low back pain. A general approach is as effective as a specific one. A randomised controlled trial. *BMJ open sport & exercise medicine, 5*(1), e000514. https://doi.org/10.1136/bmjsem-2019-000514.

McGrath, M. C. (2006). Palpation of the sacroiliac joint: An anatomical and sensory challenge. *International Journal of Osteopathic Medicine, 9*(3), 103–107. https://doi.org/10.1016/j.ijosm.2006.03.001.

Müller-Schwefe, G. H. (2011). European survey of chronic pain patients: Results for Germany. *Current medical research and opinion, 27*(11), 2099–2106. https://doi.org/10.1185/03007995.2011.621935.

Nakashima, H., Yukawa, Y., Suda, K., Yamagata, M., Ueta, T., & Kato, F. (2015). Abnormal findings on magnetic resonance images of the cervical spines in 1211 asymptomatic subjects. *Spine, 40*(6), 392–398. https://doi.org/10.1097/BRS.0000000000000775.

Nolan, D., O'Sullivan, K., Stephenson, J., O'Sullivan, P., & Lucock, M. (2018). What do physiotherapists and manual handling advisors consider the safest lifting posture, and do back beliefs influence their choice? *Musculoskeletal science & practice, 33,* 35–40. https://doi.org/10.1016/j.msksp.2017.10.010.

Nourbakhsh, M. R., & Arab, A. M. (2002). Relationship between mechanical factors and incidence of low back pain. *The Journal of orthopaedic and sports physical therapy, 32*(9), 447–460. https://doi.org/10.2519/jospt.2002.32.9.447.

Nilstad, A., Petushek, E., Mok, K. M., Bahr, R., & Krosshaug, T. (2021). Kiss goodbye to the ‚kissing knees': No association between frontal plane inward knee motion and risk of future non-contact ACL injury in elite female athletes. *Sports biomechanics, 1–15.* Advance online publication. https://doi.org/10.1080/14763141.2021.1903541.

Nijs, J., Van Houdenhove, B., & Oostendorp, R. A. (2010). Recognition of central sensitization in patients with musculoskeletal pain: Application of pain neurophysiology in manual therapy practice. *Manual therapy, 15*(2), 135–141. https://doi.org/10.1016/j.math.2009.12.001.

Oostendorp, R. A. (2007). Manual physical therapy in the Netherlands: Reflecting on the past and planning for the future in an international perspective. *The Journal of manual & manipulative therapy, 15*(3), 133–141. https://doi.org/10.1179/106698107790819819.

Oostendorp, R. A. B. (2018). Credibility of manual therapy is at stake ‚Where do we go from here?' *The Journal of manual & manipulative therapy, 26*(4), 189–192. https://doi.org/10.1080/10669817.2018.1472948.

Owen, P. J., Hangai, M., Kaneoka, K., Rantalainen, T., & Belavy, D. L. (2021). Mechanical loading influences the lumbar intervertebral disc. A cross-sectional study in 308 athletes and 71 controls. *Journal of orthopaedic research: Official publication of the Orthopaedic Research Society, 39*(5), 989–997. https://doi.org/10.1002/jor.24809.

Palsson, T. S., Gibson, W., Darlow, B., Bunzli, S., Lehman, G., Rabey, M., Moloney, N., Vaegter, H. B., Bagg, M. K., & Travers, M. (2019). Changing the narrative in diagnosis and management of pain in the sacroiliac joint area. *Physical therapy, 99*(11), 1511–1519. https://doi.org/10.1093/ptj/pzz108.

Pettman, E. (2007). A history of manipulative therapy. *The Journal of manual & manipulative therapy, 15*(3), 165–174. https://doi.org/10.1179/106698107790819873.

Picavet, H. S., Vlaeyen, J. W., & Schouten, J. S. (2002). Pain catastrophizing and kinesiophobia: Predictors of chronic low back pain. *American journal of epidemiology, 156*(11), 1028–1034. https://doi.org/10.1093/aje/kwf136.

Plummer, H. A., Sum, J. C., Pozzi, F., Varghese, R., & Michener, L. A. (2017). Observational Scapular Dyskinesis: Known-groups validity in patients with and without shoulder pain. *The Journal of orthopaedic and sports physical therapy, 47*(8), 530–537. https://doi.org/10.2519/jospt.2017.7268.

Pope, M. H., Bevins, T., Wilder, D. G., & Frymoyer, J. W. (1985). The relationship between anthropometric, postural, muscular, and mobility characteristics of males ages 18–55. *Spine, 10*(7), 644–648. https://doi.org/10.1097/00007632-198509000-00009.

Preece, S. J., Willan, P., Nester, C. J., Graham-Smith, P., Herrington, L., & Bowker, P. (2008). Variation in pelvic morphology may prevent the identification of anterior pelvic tilt. *The Journal of manual & manipulative therapy, 16*(2), 113–117. https://doi.org/10.1179/106698108790818459.

Rabelo, N. D. D. A., & Lucareli, P. R. G. (2018). Do hip muscle weakness and dynamic knee valgus matter for the clinical evaluation and decision-making process in patients with patellofemoral pain? *Brazilian journal of physical therapy, 22*(2), 105–109. https://doi.org/10.1016/j.bjpt.2017.10.002.

Rees, D., Younis, A., & MacRae, S. (2019). Is there a correlation in frontal plane knee kinematics between running and performing a single leg squat in runners with patellofemoral pain syndrome and asymptomatic runners? *Clinical biomechanics (Bristol, Avon), 61*, 227–232. https://doi.org/10.1016/j.clinbiomech.2018.12.008.

Register, B., Pennock, A. T., Ho, C. P., Strickland, C. D., Lawand, A., & Philippon, M. J. (2012). Prevalence of abnormal hip findings in asymptomatic participants: A prospective, blinded study. *The American journal of sports medicine, 40*(12), 2720–2724. https://doi.org/10.1177/0363546512462124.

Rialet-Micoulau, J., Lucas, V., Demoulin, C., & Pitance, L. (2022). Misconceptions of physical therapists and medical doctors regarding the impact of lifting a light load on low back pain. *Brazilian journal of physical therapy, 26*(1), 100385. https://doi.org/10.1016/j.bjpt.2021.100385.

Richards, K. V., Beales, D. J., Smith, A. J., O'Sullivan, P. B., & Straker, L. M. (2016). Neck posture clusters and their association with biopsychosocial factors and neck pain in australian adolescents. *Physical therapy, 96*(10), 1576–1587. https://doi.org/10.2522/ptj.20150660.

Roffey, D. M., Wai, E. K., Bishop, P., Kwon, B. K., & Dagenais, S. (2010). Causal assessment of awkward occupational postures and low back pain: Results of a systematic review. *The spine journal : Official journal of the North American Spine Society, 10*(1), 89–99. https://doi.org/10.1016/j.spinee.2009.09.003.

Roldán-Jiménez, C., Cuesta-Vargas, A. I., & Martín-Martín, J. (2022). Three-dimensional kinematics during shoulder scaption in asymptomatic and symptomatic subjects by inertial sensors: A cross-sectional study. *Sensors (Basel, Switzerland), 22*(8), 3081. https://doi.org/10.3390/s22083081.

Rubinstein, S. M., van Middelkoop, M., Assendelft, W. J., de Boer, M. R., & van Tulder, M. W. (2011). Spinal manipulative therapy for chronic low-back pain. *The Cochrane database of systematic reviews*, (2), CD008112. https://doi.org/10.1002/14651858.CD008112.pub2.

Rubinstein, S. M., Terwee, C. B., Assendelft, W. J., de Boer, M. R., & van Tulder, M. W. (2012). Spinal manipulative therapy for acute low-back pain. *The Cochrane database of systematic reviews, 2012*(9), CD008880. https://doi.org/10.1002/14651858.CD008880.pub2.

Ruchholtz, S. & Wirtz, D. C. (2013). Orthopädie und Unfallchirurgie essentials. *Georg Thieme Verlag* (S. 537). https://doi.org/10.1055/b-002-35715.

Ruffilli, A., Viroli, G., Neri, S., Traversari, M., Barile, F., Manzetti, M., Assirelli, E., Ialuna, M., Vita, F., & Faldini, C. (2023). Mechanobiology of the human intervertebral disc: Systematic review of the literature and future perspectives. *International journal of molecular sciences, 24*(3), 2728. https://doi.org/10.3390/ijms24032728.

Sainz de Baranda, P., Andújar, P., Collazo-Diéguez, M., Pastor, A., Santonja-Renedo, F., Martínez-Romero, M. T., Aparicio-Sarmiento, A., Cejudo, A., Rodríguez-Ferrán, O., & Santonja-Medina, F. (2020). Sagittal standing spinal alignment and back pain in 8 to 12-year-old children from the region of Murcia, Spain: The ISQUIOS Program. *Journal of back and musculoskeletal rehabilitation, 33*(6), 1003–1014. https://doi.org/10.3233/BMR-191727.

Salamh, P. A., Hanney, W. J., Boles, T., Holmes, D., McMillan, A., Wagner, A., & Kolber, M. J. (2023). Is it time to normalize Scapular Dyskinesis? The incidence of Scapular Dyskinesis in those with and without Symptoms: A systematic review of the literature. *International journal of sports physical therapy, V18*(3), 558–576. https://doi.org/10.26603/001c.74388.

Sanchez, H. M., Sanchez, E. G., & Tavares, L. I. (2016). Association between Scapular Dyskinesia and shoulder pain in young adults. *Acta ortopedica brasileira, 24*(5), 243–248. https://doi.org/10.1590/1413-785220162405142225.

Saraceni, N., Kent, P., Ng, L., Campbell, A., Straker, L., & O'Sullivan, P. (2020). To flex or not to flex? Is there a relationship between Lumbar Spine Flexion during lifting and low back pain? A systematic review with meta-analysis. *The Journal of orthopaedic and sports physical therapy, 50*(3), 121–130. https://doi.org/10.2519/jospt.2020.9218.

Sato, T., Sato, N., Masui, K., & Hirano, Y. (2014). Immediate effects of manual traction on radiographically determined joint space width in the hip joint. *Journal of manipulative and physiological therapeutics, 37*(8), 580–585. https://doi.org/10.1016/j.jmpt.2014.08.002.

Schäfer, R., Trompeter, K., Fett, D., Heinrich, K., Funken, J., Willwacher, S., Brüggemann, G. P., & Platen, P. (2023). The mechanical loading of the spine in physical activities. *European spine journal: Official publication of the European Spine Society, the European Spinal Deformity Society, and the European Section of the Cervical Spine Research Society, 32*(9), 2991–3001. https://doi.org/10.1007/s00586-023-07733-1.

Schmalzl, J., Walter, H., Rothfischer, W., Blaich, S., Gerhardt, C., & Lehmann, L. J. (2022). GIRD syndrome in male handball and volleyball players: Is the decrease of total range of motion the turning point to pathology? *Journal of back and musculoskeletal rehabilitation, 35*(4), 755–762. https://doi.org/10.3233/BMR-191767.

Schmidt, H., Bashkuev, M., Weerts, J., Graichen, F., Altenscheidt, J., Maier, C., & Reitmaier, S. (2018). How do we stand? Variations during repeated standing phases of asymptomatic subjects and low back pain patients. *Journal of biomechanics, 70,* 67–76. https://doi.org/10.1016/j.jbiomech.2017.06.016.

Schwartzberg, R., Reuss, B. L., Burkhart, B. G., Butterfield, M., Wu, J. Y., & McLean, K. W. (2016). High prevalence of superior labral tears diagnosed by MRI in middle-aged patients with asymptomatic shoulders. *Orthopaedic journal of sports medicine, 4*(1), 2325967115623212. https://doi.org/10.1177/2325967115623212.

Shelburne, K. B., Torry, M. R., Steadman, J. R., & Pandy, M. G. (2008). Effects of foot orthoses and valgus bracing on the knee adduction moment and medial joint load during gait. *Clinical biomechanics (Bristol, Avon), 23*(6), 814–821. https://doi.org/10.1016/j.clinbiomech.2008.02.005.

Shah, J. P., Thaker, N., Heimur, J., Aredo, J. V., Sikdar, S., & Gerber, L. (2015). Myofascial trigger points then and now: A historical and scientific perspective. *PM & R: The journal of injury, function, and rehabilitation, 7*(7), 746–761. https://doi.org/10.1016/j.pmrj.2015.01.024.

Shumway-Cook, A., & Woollacott, M. (2006). Motor control: Translating research into clinical practice. *Osteoporos Int* (Bd. 18). https://doi.org/10.1007/s00198-007-0358-4.

Silverwood, V., Blagojevic-Bucknall, M., Jinks, C., Jordan, J. L., Protheroe, J., & Jordan, K. P. (2015). Current evidence on risk factors for knee osteoarthritis in older adults: A systematic review and meta-analysis. *Osteoarthritis and cartilage, 23*(4), 507–515. https://doi.org/10.1016/j.joca.2014.11.019.

Smith, S. S., Stewart, M. E., Davies, B. M., & Kotter, M. R. N. (2021). The prevalence of asymptomatic and symptomatic Spinal Cord compression on magnetic resonance imaging: A systematic review and meta-analysis. *Global spine journal, 11*(4), 597–607. https://doi.org/10.1177/2192568220934496.

Sparks, C., Cleland, J. A., Elliott, J. M., Zagardo, M., & Liu, W. C. (2013). Using functional magnetic resonance imaging to determine if cerebral hemodynamic responses to pain change following thoracic spine thrust manipulation in healthy individuals. *The Journal of orthopaedic and sports physical therapy, 43*(5), 340–348. https://doi.org/10.2519/jospt.2013.4631.

Steele, J., Bruce-Low, S., Smith, D., Osborne, N., & Thorkeldsen, A. (2015). Can specific loading through exercise impart healing or regeneration of the intervertebral disc? *The spine journal: Official journal of the North American Spine Society, 15*(10), 2117–2121. https://doi.org/10.1016/j.spinee.2014.08.446.

Su, D., Ai, Y., Zhu, G., Yang, Y., & Ma, P. (2023). Genetically predicted circulating levels of cytokines and the risk of osteoarthritis: A mendelian randomization study. *Frontiers in genetics, 14,* 1131198. https://doi.org/10.3389/fgene.2023.1131198.

Swain, C. T. V., Pan, F., Owen, P. J., Schmidt, H., & Belavy, D. L. (2020). No consensus on causality of spine postures or physical exposure and low back pain: A systematic review of systematic reviews. *Journal of biomechanics, 102,* 109312. https://doi.org/10.1016/j.jbiomech.2019.08.006.

Tanaka, K., Okamoto, Y., Makihara, T., Maehara, K., Yoshizawa, T., Minami, M., & Yamazaki, M. (2017). Clinical interpretation of asymptomatic medial collateral ligament injury observed on magnetic resonance imaging in adolescent baseball players. *Japanese journal of radiology, 35*(6), 319–326. https://doi.org/10.1007/s11604-017-0636-9.

Tanamas, S., Hanna, F. S., Cicuttini, F. M., Wluka, A. E., Berry, P., & Urquhart, D. M. (2009). Does knee malalignment increase the risk of development and progression of knee osteoarthritis? A systematic review. *Arthritis and rheumatism, 61*(4), 459–467. https://doi.org/10.1002/art.24336.

Tempelhof, S., Rupp, S., & Seil, R. (1999). Age-related prevalence of rotator cuff tears in asymptomatic shoulders. *Journal of shoulder and elbow surgery, 8*(4), 296–299. https://doi.org/10.1016/s1058-2746(99)90148-9.

Tesarz, J., Schuster, A. K., Hartmann, M., Gerhardt, A., & Eich, W. (2012). Pain perception in athletes compared to normally active controls: A systematic review with meta-analysis. *Pain, 153*(6), 1253–1262. https://doi.org/10.1016/j.pain.2012.03.005.

Thalhamer, C. (2018). A fundamental critique of the fascial distortion model and its application in clinical practice. *Journal of Bodywork and Movement Therapies, 22*(1), 112–117. https://doi.org/10.1016/j.jbmt.2017.07.009.

Tong, J. W., & Kong, P. W. (2013). Association between foot type and lower extremity injuries: Systematic literature review with meta-analysis. *The Journal of orthopaedic and sports physical therapy, 43*(10), 700–714. https://doi.org/10.2519/jospt.2013.4225.

Torres, R. R., & Gomes, J. L. (2009). Measurement of glenohumeral internal rotation in asymptomatic tennis players and swimmers. *The American journal of sports medicine, 37*(5), 1017–1023. https://doi.org/10.1177/0363546508329544.

Tullberg, T., Blomberg, S., Branth, B., & Johnsson, R. (1998). Manipulation does not alter the position of the sacroiliac joint. A roentgen stereophotogrammetric analysis. *Spine, 23*(10), 1124–1129. https://doi.org/10.1097/00007632-199805150-00010.

van de Pol, R. J., van Trijffel, E., & Lucas, C. (2010). Inter-rater reliability for measurement of passive physiological range of motion of upper extremity joints is better if instruments are used: A systematic review. *Journal of physiotherapy, 56*(1), 7–17. https://doi.org/10.1016/s1836-9553(10)70049-7.

Van Nieuwenhuyse, A., Crombez, G., Burdorf, A., Verbeke, G., Masschelein, R., Moens, G., Mairiaux, P., & BelCoBack Study Group. (2009). Physical characteristics of the back are not predictive of low back pain in healthy workers: A prospective study. *BMC musculoskeletal disorders, 10,* 2. https://doi.org/10.1186/1471-2474-10-2.

van Trijffel, E., Anderegg, Q., Bossuyt, P. M., & Lucas, C. (2005). Inter-examiner reliability of passive assessment of intervertebral motion in the cervical and lumbar spine: A systematic review. *Manual therapy, 10*(4), 256–269. https://doi.org/10.1016/j.math.2005.04.008.

van Trijffel, E., van de Pol, R. J., Oostendorp, R. A., & Lucas, C. (2010). Inter-rater reliability for measurement of passive physiological movements in lower extremity joints is generally low: A systematic review. *Journal of physiotherapy, 56*(4), 223–235. https://doi.org/10.1016/s1836-9553(10)70005-9.

Vardiman, J. P., Siedlik, J., Herda, T., Hawkins, W., Cooper, M., Graham, Z. A., Deckert, J., & Gallagher, P. (2015). Instrument-assisted soft tissue mobilization: Effects on the properties of human plantar flexors. *International journal of sports medicine, 36*(3), 197–203. https://doi.org/10.1055/s-0034-1384543.

Vigolvino, L. P., Barros, B. R. S., Medeiros, C. E. B., Pinheiro, S. M., & Sousa, C. O. (2020). Analysis of the presence and influence of Glenohumeral internal rotation deficit on posterior stiffness and isometric shoulder rotators strength ratio in recreational and amateur handball players. *Physical therapy in sport: Official journal of the Association of Chartered Physiotherapists in Sports Medicine, 42*, 1–8. https://doi.org/10.1016/j.ptsp.2019.12.004.

Vila, H., Barreiro, A., Ayán, C., Antúnez, A., & Ferragut, C. (2022). The most common handball injuries: A systematic review. *International journal of environmental research and public health, 19*(17), 10688. https://doi.org/10.3390/ijerph191710688.

von Arx, M., Liechti, M., Connolly, L., Bangerter, C., Meier, M. L., & Schmid, S. (2021). From stoop to squat: A comprehensive analysis of Lumbar loading among different lifting styles. *Frontiers in bioengineering and biotechnology, 9*, 769117. https://doi.org/10.3389/fbioe.2021.769117.

Voogt, L., de Vries, J., Meeus, M., Struyf, F., Meuffels, D., & Nijs, J. (2015). Analgesic effects of manual therapy in patients with musculoskeletal pain: A systematic review. *Manual therapy, 20*(2), 250–256. https://doi.org/10.1016/j.math.2014.09.001.

Walker, M. L., Rothstein, J. M., Finucane, S. D., & Lamb, R. L. (1987). Relationships between lumbar lordosis, pelvic tilt, and abdominal muscle performance. *Physical therapy, 67*(4), 512–516. https://doi.org/10.1093/ptj/67.4.512.

Warden, S. J., Mantila Roosa, S. M., Kersh, M. E., Hurd, A. L., Fleisig, G. S., Pandy, M. G., & Fuchs, R. K. (2014). Physical activity when young provides lifelong benefits to cortical bone size and strength in men. *Proceedings of the National Academy of Sciences of the United States of America, 111*(14), 5337–5342. https://doi.org/10.1073/pnas.1321605111.

Washmuth, N. B., McAfee, A. D., & Bickel, C. S. (2022). Lifting Techniques: Why are we not using evidence to optimize movement? *International journal of sports physical therapy, 17*(1), 104–110. https://doi.org/10.26603/001c.30023.

Werner, F. W., Ayers, D. C., Maletsky, L. P., & Rullkoetter, P. J. (2005). The effect of valgus/varus malalignment on load distribution in total knee replacements. *Journal of biomechanics, 38*(2), 349–355. https://doi.org/10.1016/j.jbiomech.2004.02.024.

Wilczyński, B., Zorena, K., & Ślęzak, D. (2020). Dynamic knee valgus in single-leg movement tasks. Potentially modifiable factors and exercise training options. A literature review. *International journal of environmental research and public health, 17*(21), 8208. https://doi.org/10.3390/ijerph17218208.

Wyndow, N., Collins, N. J., Vicenzino, B., Tucker, K., & Crossley, K. M. (2018). Foot and ankle characteristics and dynamic knee valgus in individuals with patellofemoral osteoarthritis. *Journal of foot and ankle research, 11*, 65. https://doi.org/10.1186/s13047-018-0310-1.

Xu, C., Wang, S., Ti, W., Yang, J., Yasen, Y., Memetsidiq, M., & Shi, S. Q. (2022). Role of dietary patterns and factors in determining the risk of knee osteoarthritis: A meta-analysis. *Modern rheumatology, 32*(4), 815–821. https://doi.org/10.1093/mr/roab059.

Yoshimura, A., Inami, T., Schleip, R., Mineta, S., Shudo, K., & Hirose, N. (2021). Effects of self-myofascial release using a foam roller on range of motion and morphological changes in muscle: A crossover study. *Journal of strength and conditioning research, 35*(9), 2444–2450. https://doi.org/10.1519/JSC.0000000000003196.

Zhu, B., Ba, H., Kong, L., Fu, Y., Ren, J., Zhu, Q., & Fang, M. (2024). The effects of manual therapy in pain and safety of patients with knee osteoarthritis: A systematic review and meta-analysis. *Systematic reviews, 13*(1), 91. https://doi.org/10.1186/s13643-024-02467-7.

Zusman, M. (2011). The modernisation of manipulative therapy. *International Journal of Clinical Medicine, 2*(5), 644–649. https://doi.org/10.4236/ijcm.2011.25110.

Examination and Treatment of Pain

5

Abstract

Pain medicine and therapy sciences have gained significant insights into the mechanisms of pain onset and relief over the past decades. These advances lead to concrete recommendations for clinical practice in the examination and treatment of pain patients. It is of high relevance to consider both the external evidence and the individual patient situation in the history taking, clinical examination, and therapy. The goal should be to comprehensively understand the affected person and their complaints, including relevant bio-psycho-social factors and drivers. Instead of focusing solely on the search for specific pain causes, it may be more advisable to precisely analyze the current state, include the context factors, and develop a therapy approach based on this, which does not necessarily have to derive from the identification of a specific cause.

When it comes to the comprehensive examination of a patient, many encounter a major problem: the discrepancy between the patient's perspective and that of the examiner regarding the causes of pain, drivers, or contextual factors. This discrepancy should be avoided as it poses an obstacle to a good patient-therapist alliance, which is absolutely necessary for successful treatment (Hall et al., 2010; Allen et al., 2017). When examining pain or painful restrictions, every examiner should first ask themselves: What is pain? And what is my purpose in the examination? An old definition of pain from 1968 by Margo McCaffery emphasizes that the patient should be at the forefront of the examination, not the examiner and what they think:

> "Pain is whatever the experiencing person says it is, existing whenever he/she says it does."

Pain is initially always a subjective and very personal experience. The way pain is described reveals different forms of evaluation, emotional involvement, and dealing with pain. Therefore, the therapist's opinion of why something hurts is secondary in the first place; not unimportant, but the patient and their version is the complete truth upon which the rest should be built. In the next step, an operationalization should and may take place, i.e., the attempt to capture this truth through questions and tests and to record numerical parameters. But how can tests and numerical parameters capture this subjective and personal truth? Clinical tests or questionnaires can hardly depict personal experiences, feelings, and beliefs of the patient, let alone define them. Nevertheless, they should be aimed at capturing the patient's version with all its facets and contextual factors (see Sect. 5.2). This collection should take place without influence and without manipulative conversation. Here, communication is of fundamental importance. Adequate communication can be simplified by a high degree of knowledge about pain. The therapist's knowledge about pain is crucial for how they best connect the topics of pain mechanisms, patient expression, examination, and therapy. Therefore, pain education plays a role not only in educating patients but also in training therapists and their narratives.

5.1 Pain Education

Therapists and doctors treat pain on a daily basis. How extensive is their knowledge about pain? Starting with a study in 2003, it was first revealed that healthcare personnel know too little about pain (Moseley, 2003). In this case, physiotherapists, doctors, occupational therapists, and psychologists only answered 55% of the questions correctly. The NPQ (Neurophysiology of Pain Questionnaire) was used as a measuring instrument. A possible explanation for the lack of knowledge could be that the competencies taught during training are still primarily based on biomechanical models and less on neurobiological and psychosocial models (Louw et al., 2016).

Physiotherapists often use the postural-structural-biomechanical (PSB) model to explain the symptom of pain with biomechanical deficits and are convinced that asymmetries and imbalances lead to pain (Lederman, 2011), thus neglecting the biopsychosocial model. A biomechanical deficit is, for example, poor posture, which is associated with a hyperkyphosis of the thoracic spine (T-spine) and a strong anteroposition of the cervical spine (C-spine), but contrary to popular belief, there is no causal relationship between supposedly poor posture and pain (Slater et al., 2019) (see Chap. 4). Despite the findings from neurobiology and pain science, physiotherapists continue to focus on biomechanical aspects and physical deficits in the examination and therapy of back pain patients and often neglect psychosocial drivers and contextual factors, possibly because they are not well enough informed or trained in this area (Synnott et al., 2015). This underscores the need to better and more holistically train healthcare personnel.

The knowledge of physiotherapists about the symptom of pain appears to be deficient. It is becoming increasingly known that physiotherapists know too little about pain and its adequate therapy, and that schools convey too little scientifically based content (Scudds et al., 2009; Clenzos et al., 2013). A recently

5.1 Pain Education

published nationwide study of approximately 300 prospective physiotherapists shows that the knowledge of physiotherapists about pain shortly before their professional entry is deficient and too PSB-oriented (Bassimtabar & Alfuth, 2024). Science demands better teaching and pain education for medical professionals (Vadivelu et al., 2012) and a content upgrade and scientific adaptation of the curricula (Hush et al., 2018). In therapy, the relevance of education for pain patients about the multifactoriality and neurobiology of pain using PNE (Pain Neuroscience Education) is increasing. PNE leads to improvements in pain knowledge for both patients (Moseley, 2003; Pate et al., 2019) and therapists (Moseley, 2003; Colleary et al., 2017; Cox et al., 2017). To close the knowledge gap between science and practice, the IASP (International Association of the study of pain) recommends not only educating patients in clinical practice, but also improving the training content of doctors and therapists (IASP, 2018).

Studies show that PNE can significantly increase therapists' knowledge of pain physiology (Fitzgerald et al., 2018; Maguire et al., 2019). The rNPQ (revised Neurophysiology of Pain Questionnaire) is often used as a measurement tool for knowledge about pain (Catley et al., 2013). For example, a 70-minute PNE lesson improved the rNPQ score from 48% to 75% among British physiotherapy students in their first and second year of training (Colleary et al., 2017). Marques and colleagues were able to record an improvement in the NPQ score from 62.5% to 90% among Brazilian physiotherapy students in their final year of training through twelve interactive PNE lessons (2016). Japanese physiotherapy students in their final year increased the NPQ score from 54% to 67.5% through an 80-minute PNE lesson. The improvement was still present after a one-month follow-up (Mine et al., 2017). In the USA, third-year physiotherapy doctoral students improved from 76.9% to 86% through a 2.5-week PNE teaching block (Bareiss et al., 2019). In the state of Missouri, physiotherapy doctoral students scored significantly worse in the pre-score of the NPQ with 41%, but reached a similar level with 87% correct answers after a three-hour lesson in the NPQ (Cox et al., 2017). In y, a single 4-hour online lesson led to an increase in the rNPQ score by 30% and in a newly designed questionnaire for recording PSB orientation, the EKPQ (Essential Knowledge of Pain Questionnaire), even by 71%; due to the low pre-test scores (Bassimtabar & Alfuth, 2023; Bassimtabar & Alfuth, 2024). Pain education not only leads to greater knowledge, but also to more confidence in dealing with chronic pain patients and to improving their clinical outcomes (Harris et al., 2008; Chelimsky et al., 2013).

The use of different terms by health professionals such as doctors, physiotherapists, osteopaths, and chiropractors, and the lack of a unified language, leads many patients to not understand the facts and explanations (Barker et al., 2009). This would be fatal in pain education. How do you explain to the patient why something hurts when the damage in the joint is not supposed to be the reason? When does it hurt? In the presence of noxious danger? At the risk of noxious danger? Or when the body has a need for protection? A need for protection presupposes an external noxious danger in nociceptive pain and implies this. However, in nociplastic pain, there is no external danger. Yet the patient perceives pain. The danger detectors of the nervous system have become autonomous. The mere realization that there is no danger, but that the danger detectors have become autonomous, can be a safety information and dampen the perception of pain; similar to an alarm, when it sounds, experts explore the situation, assess it, and possibly give the all-clear. The all-clear calms and should also be used as a therapeutic tool. Conversely, sometimes people feel no pain despite external dangers because there is no need for protection. Moseley and Butler, two leading pain researchers, recommend viewing pain as a need for protection, which arises when the danger information is greater than the safety information (Moseley & Butler, 2015). However, if the subjective feeling of being safe is greater than the subjective feeling of being in danger, pain is absent. The metaphor of the *Protectometer* is intended to illustrate the origin of pain (Fig. 5.1).

Pain arises when the body perceives itself to be more in danger and thus has a need for protection. From the reductionist biomedical perspective, it could now be illustrated why some noxious stimuli or pathologies do not result in a perception of pain (due to contextual and psycho-social damping) or conversely, in the absence of biological noxae or pathologies or supposedly non-pain-causing stimuli, pain still exists (due to contextual and psycho-social drivers). It should still be emphasized that psycho-social drivers are not a mental meta-phenomenon, but are biologically objectifiable (see Chap. 3). It only seems logical and consistent that additional danger information for patients, whose nervous system is already geared towards avoiding danger, is counterproductive. Danger information can be, for example, verbal suggestions made by therapists such as "The sleeping position is not good for you, it can cause damage." or "Stop that, it's not good for the joints." In medicine, such statements are called *Nocebos*.

Nocebos and Their Consequences
A nocebo is the opposite of a placebo and describes a harmful effect of an action or statement. The underlying mechanisms include the activation of stress and fear centers in the brain, such as the hippocampus and the amygdala, as well as the release of stress hormones like cortisol. The nocebo effect can be amplified by previous negative experiences or by negative information, such as negative verbal cues from the therapist (Cormack & Rossettini, 2023). Thus, words alone can

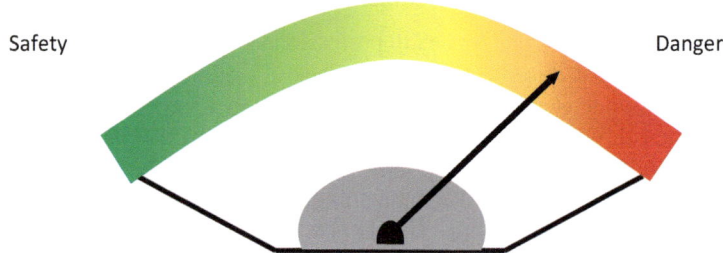

Fig. 5.1 Protectometer, own production

have a nocebo effect (Richter et al., 2010), suggesting that healthcare professionals should choose their words carefully when communicating with patients. The use of negative language by physiotherapists increases anxiety in patients and reinforces negative beliefs about their complaints (Fieke Linskens et al., 2023). Patients often have biomedical beliefs about their pain. There is evidence that these were caused by the therapists and their beliefs were shaped by the therapists' deficit-oriented attitudes and perspectives (Setchell et al., 2017). This highlights the susceptibility of patients to their therapists and shows that learning and adopting beliefs can have both positive (as in pain education) and negative (as in nocebos) effects.

Words create worlds: Nocebos lead to both increased pain experience (Blasini et al., 2017; Benedetti et al., 2020), and increased anxiety and catastrophizing (Darnall & Colloca, 2018). Anxiety and catastrophizing, in turn, are risk factors for chronic pain (Velly et al., 2011; Burns et al., 2015; Tan et al., 2020), higher opioid use (Martel et al., 2013) and other health problems, such as cardiovascular disorders (Leonard et al., 2013). False statements and nocebos negatively affect the psyche and can promote chronic pain (Chen et al., 2018).

Examples of false statements could be:

- "Lifting with a rounded back is dangerous."
- "You have pain because of your pelvic tilt."
- "Your poor posture is your problem."
- "Sport has damaged your intervertebral discs."
- "With your leg axis, pain is preprogrammed."

These are danger information, which, metaphorically speaking, can make the protectometer swing to red, increase the need for protection, and intensify the pain experience.

Example

In Tab. 5.1, some examples are discussed on how to rephrase and circumvent nocebos without altering their reality content. ◄

Nocebic Investigation?

Is the investigation itself, which seeks problems and deficits, a breeding ground for nocebos? Perhaps physiotherapists are trained to produce nocebos. Inspired by the well-known German physiotherapist Antje Hüter-Becker, criticism of the deficit-oriented approach in the examination and therapy of pain patients in physiotherapy is increasingly being confirmed. Physiotherapy is strongly characterized by a deficit-oriented perspective (Hüter-Becker, 2000; Synnott et al., 2015). Physiotherapists primarily focus on functional deficits and try to correct these using specific techniques. This deficit-oriented approach leads to physiotherapists losing themselves in a multitude of techniques and methods that are almost exclusively aimed at correcting functional deficits. In doing so, the holistic view of the patient is often neglected. The deficit-oriented action of physiotherapy is increasingly

Tab. 5.1 Paraphrasing of nocebos, own creation

Nocebo	Rephrasing	Comment
"Bone is pressing on bone in your knee."	"The X-ray shows a joint space narrowing."	Bone on bone does not exist, sometimes this sentence is used to explain something to patients more simply.
"According to the MRI, your discs have also degenerated."	"Your MRI shows normal adjustments to age and stress."	Asymptomatic incidental findings are very common, but that is no reason to put the image in the foreground.
"Your torso is totally unstable."	"The strength of your core muscles can be improved."	Exaggerations like *totally, very* or *massively* should be avoided. Moreover, it is worth not labeling conditions, but formulating the sentence as if the condition could be changed.
"Your left gluteus is not working at all." or "Your left hip is very stiff."	"The control is reduced" or better "The control of the left gluteal muscles should be trained." Or "The mobility of the left hip can be improved."	A muscle cannot not work. Except in cases of plegia. And if the examination results, such as strength, control, or mobility abnormalities, are directly coupled with solution-oriented verbs, not only the problem remains, but also a solution. It sounds banal, but it makes a big difference in the emotional world of (especially chronic) pain patients.
"Your pelvis is completely twisted."	–	This sentence cannot be saved by a rephrasing. Only by leaving it out.

failing to meet the complex realities of patients with chronic pain or disabilities. Deficit-oriented action in back pain therapy leads to negative beliefs and fears in patients (Darlow et al., 2015) and also increases the likelihood that the therapy will not only be unsuccessful, but may even cause harm and exacerbate problems (O'Sullivan et al., 2016). A reorientation of physiotherapy away from pure deficit orientation towards a more holistic and patient-centered approach therefore seems urgently necessary in order to meet the complex requirements of modern healthcare and to improve the effectiveness of physiotherapeutic interventions. The use of bio-psycho-social assessments coupled with neurobiological insights from pain research could accelerate this paradigm shift by reducing the relevance of postural-structural-biomechanical factors and highlighting the relevance of neurobiological processes and psycho-socio-economic and contextual drivers.

More and more experts, particularly due to the high proportion of manual therapy (MT) in physiotherapy training, are calling for the inclusion of neurobiological mechanisms of action of MT and distancing from outdated biomechanical explanations (Nijs et al., 2010). A special focus should also be placed on good communication between therapist and patient to prevent the creation of nocebos. Nocebos can lead to fears that impair the rehabilitation of musculoskeletal complaints (Fischerauer et al., 2018). Fear-avoidance behavior, in turn, is strongly associated with the onset and course of non-specific and chronic back pain (Fujii et al., 2019; Wertli et al., 2019), so this should be prevented. PNE can reduce fears

5.2 Investigation

and avoidance behavior in addition to the aforementioned effects of increasing knowledge about pain and relieving pain conditions (Fletcher et al., 2016). This can be useful both in the context of a patient's multimodal therapy and for the training of a physiotherapist. Because kinesiophobia and fear-avoidant attitudes of the therapist have a negative effect on patients, even reducing their strength and training abilities (Lakke et al., 2015). PNE can be used to avoid false beliefs and fear-avoidance behavior in therapists.

5.2 Investigation

The examination of a pain patient can be divided into anamnesis, clinical tests, and further assessments, such as questionnaires. The examination should be holistically oriented.

5.2.1 Medical History

The WHO recommends the ICF model (International Classification of Functioning, Disability and Health) for a bio-psycho-social and holistic recording of the patient's complaints. While ICDs (International Statistical Classification of Diseases and Related Health Problems) define pathologies and diseases, ICF stands for the consequences of diseases in relation to two sub-areas:

1. Functionality/Disability
2. Contextual Factors

Each of them includes two different components (Fig. 5.2):

1.1 Body Structure and Functions
1.2 Activity and Participation
2.2 Environmental Factors
2.2 Personal Factors.

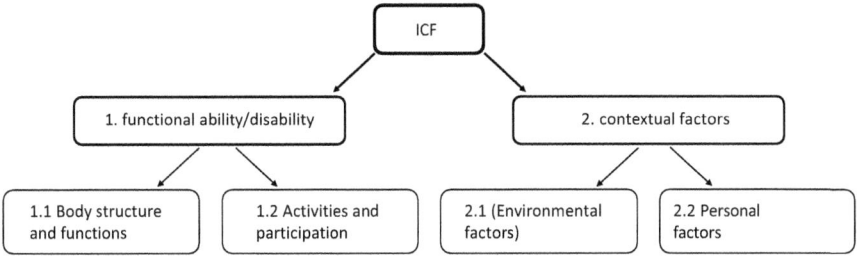

Fig. 5.2 ICF, own creation

However, supposed consequences of a diagnosis may also have been drivers or facilitating factors for the emergence of this diagnosis, so the reductionist view of psycho-social factors as an exclusive consequence is not recommended. When using the ICF model, the medical history comprehensively addresses the various areas of the person's life (Leonardi et al., 2022). This includes not only the medical aspects, but also the social, psychological, and environmental influences. Here come the entries for conspicuous flags, such as working conditions, the family environment, individual mental states, personality traits, expectations, and beliefs. Important: not only hindering, but also promoting factors should be considered. This helps in adequate therapy planning.

This holistic view can better understand how the health problem affects the person's daily life and what additional factors play a role. This allows for a more comprehensive and individual hypothesis to be formulated and a therapy to be planned that takes into account all relevant areas of the person's life. A checklist created by the WHO and freely available on the internet covers 8 pages. The fact that processing this checklist together with the patient not only appears utopian, but is also impossible in terms of time, is beyond question. However, it should at least serve as a suggestion to collect as many psycho-social and contextual factors as possible in addition to the structural and functional complaints. An exclusively PSB-oriented approach in the examination of pain patients could reduce compliance and result in poorer therapy outcomes (Nijs et al., 2013). Thus, the recording of factors that go beyond the physical structure is of elementary importance. And possibly the patient already directs to his most important drivers and factors. For this to happen, patients should be allowed to speak and be listened to. Patients wish to be involved in decision-making, to be listened to, and to receive explanations about interventions (Slade et al., 2009). If these wishes and expectations are not met, this can lead to frustration, which is known to be a driver for the chronification of pain. In addition to the need for multidimensional impressions of the patient, it is important to focus on the most important elements (dominant drivers) and to first capture these through tests for hypothesis and solution finding and in the further course by making them measurable for the course evaluation.

5.2.2 Clinical Tests

Inspection
Studies in which visual test results were checked with precise apparatus methods show that visual assessments in physiotherapy are often affected by significant subjective variability, are inaccurate and not reproducible, which questions their reliability and consistency (Goode et al., 2008; Holmgren and Waling, 2008; Gadotti et al., 2013; Wassinger et al., 2015; Paraskevopoulos et al., 2020; Fedorak et al., 2003).

Palpation

The purpose of palpation is to obtain information about the mechanical-thermal properties of the tissue through the fingertips. Here, in addition to checking for signs of inflammation such as heat, stiffness and tone are particularly tested. At this point, it should be critically mentioned that scientific skepticism is spreading about the ability to assess these parameters through palpation and the examiner should be aware of the limits of palpation skills. Overinterpretation of tactile perceptions could otherwise lead to erroneous conclusions and even false statements and nocebos ("The fascia is stuck."). Some therapists deceive themselves during palpation testing by believing they can perceive subtle changes or pathologies in the tissue that are beyond the limits of reliable tactile perception. This tendency may be facilitated by various factors, including ideological zeal or wishful thinking. There are some studies that prove the unreliability of such palpation findings, such as the inability of experienced examiners to correctly identify the painful side in back or neck pain solely through palpation (Maigne et al., 2012) or to determine trigger points or fascial restrictions (Myburgh et al., 2008; Lucas et al., 2009). Palpation findings may not be reliable and may not be based on a real existing evidence.

Despite this criticism, it should still be emphasized that palpation or touch alone establishes an interpersonal connection with the patient, builds trust, and can alleviate stress, negative affections, and even pain (Mancini et al., 2014; Erk et al., 2015; Goldstein et al., 2017; Fusaro et al., 2022) and is by no means illegitimate. On the contrary: Anatomical knowledge and palpation skills can indeed be valuable, but they should be used with the necessary humility and knowledge of the fallibility of human perception. Palpation may have primarily evolved for the examination of pain and its localization and drew further aspects, such as the assessment of swelling, temperature, and tissue condition, in its wake (Walker et al., 1990; Verghese & Horwitz, 2009).

Pain Assessment

Traditionally, questions about pain intensity and duration are very popular. In 1951, the first dolorimeter/algometer was invented to quantify pain. The device records the pressure applied to the tissue until the patient reports pain. This does not quantify the perception of pain, but the necessary stimulus intensity that leads to pain—the pain tolerance threshold (Haugen & Livingston, 1953). Dr. Beecher, a world-renowned doctor with significant contributions to modern pain science, did not find device-supported pain assessments useful; instead, he tried to capture individuality and subjectivity, including emotions. He did not try to objectify pain, but to quantify the subjective responses of patients by using simple numerical scales (McKeown & Warner, 2006). From the realization that clinical symptoms are a combination of physical, cognitive, and emotional components, he initiated various studies using simple numerical scales to quantify pain intensity from the patient's perspective, the predecessors of today's known VAS (Visual Analog

Scale) and NRPS (Numeric Rating Pain Scale). Later, Melzack and Warren developed five-level word-based scales and agreed on terminologies to describe pain intensities, such as *moderate* or *agonizing*. The goal was to create a language that all physicians could orient themselves by (Melzack, 1971). In 1975, Melzack finally developed a questionnaire, the McGill Pain Questionnaire (at McGill University in Canada), which proved to be an important tool and frequently used outcome in clinical studies (Melzack, 2005). This questionnaire captures both pain quality and intensity from the patient's perspective, as well as cognitive and emotional components of pain. Interestingly, the terms used in the MPQ to describe pain quality are almost completely identical to the terms of Avicenna, a significant polymath and physician of the 10th century (Tashani & Johnson, 2010). The MPQ certainly laid the foundation for the development of today's known questionnaires (see section 5.2.3). In parallel, based on the approaches of Hayes and Patterson 1921 (Delgado et al., 2018), two British psychiatrists, Bond and Pilowsky, designed the VAS in 1966. Another method used for pain assessment is the NRPS, which is based on a 10-cm long horizontal line (Bond & Pilowsky, 1966). This scale ranges from *no pain* (0) to *worst imaginable pain* (10) and is preferred in clinical practice due to its simplicity. However, the question arises whether such a simplified instrument can do justice to the multidimensionality of the pain experience. The reduction of complex pain perception to a one-dimensional scale carries the risk of overlooking important aspects of the pain phenomenon. The NRPS primarily captures the intensity of pain, but leaves out other relevant dimensions such as the affective component, functional impairment, or temporal dynamics. For a more comprehensive pain assessment, multidimensional assessment tools that consider various aspects of the pain experience could be considered. Nevertheless, due to its practicability, the NRPS remains an important screening tool in everyday clinical practice, but should be interpreted in the context of its limitations. Current guidelines recommend collecting more parameters than just numerical pain intensity, such as pain duration, the duration with which pain relief was associated, and functional tests such as ADLs, mobility, and strength.

Functional Tests
In physiotherapy, there are various active and passive functional tests that traditionally serve to evaluate the functionality of muscles, joints, and other structures. Generally, it can be said that basic motor skills (BMS) are tested at this point. They are traditionally divided into 5 BMS (Krug, 2022).

1. ROM/Mobility
2. Strength
3. Endurance
4. Coordination
5. Speed

In musculoskeletal medicine, mobility and strength are particularly in focus. These tests can be performed either with or without reference to pain.

The examination of BMS **without direct pain reference** aims to evaluate the performance of certain structures, such as the strength of a muscle, for example. Pain is not primarily in the foreground. These test methods are not limited to the actual pain area, but also include adjacent or more distant structures. This allows possible influences on the pain area to be identified—such as the mobility of the ankle joint in case of knee complaints or the strength of the shoulder external rotators in case of shoulder problems. Although these tests are related to pain, the focus during execution is not on the perception of pain itself. Rather, they serve to collect clues and formulate hypotheses about the cause of pain and the involvement of non-painful structures. However, it should be noted that there is a lack of solid studies and external evidence to fully substantiate this approach.

Despite the lack of scientific confirmation, the described approach should not be considered invalid. However, one should be cautious about hastily establishing causal relationships in order to minimize the risk of nocebo effects.

In contrast, the testing of **BMS with pain reference** aims to capture the extent of pain-related restrictions. Here, the precise question is of crucial importance. It would be a mistake to categorize movements merely as painful or non-painful. Supposedly specific tests often rely on this principle: If a patient experiences pain in 3 out of 5 tests, a high probability of structural damage (such as a labrum tear) is assumed. However, this simplified approach does not correspond to the actual purpose of functional tests. Instead of the dichotomous question "Is this movement painful?", which promotes black-and-white thinking and increases the risk of stigmatization, a more differentiated view is recommended: "From when and to what extent does a movement become painful?". The onset of pain can be related to the force exerted (load), the range of motion (ROM), or the number of repetitions. This more detailed view allows for a more precise assessment of the condition and avoids the pitfalls of dichotomous test results.

The collection and classification of problematic or painful movements into comfort and discomfort, related to specific motor characteristics (e.g., knee flexion from 70° ROM painful, NRPS 5), is of essential importance for several reasons:

1. Education: The patient can be precisely shown from which point a movement becomes problematic. Many patients often only perceive *that* a movement causes problems. Precise clarification ("You are pain-free up to this point.") provides security and can serve as motivation to maintain certain activities.
2. Training therapy planning: Knowing from when movements are restricted also implies up to which point they are not restricted. On this basis, exercises and movement sequences can be developed that carefully approach the border areas of the discomfort zone.
3. Progress evaluation: For an effective review of treatment success, the sole collection of dichotomous characteristics (hurts/does not hurt) is obstructive. Such a simplifying narrative would provoke the answer "It still hurts." when asked about the patient's current condition. Important details are overlooked: Has the pain intensity changed (e.g., from NRPS 5 to 3)? Has the pain trigger point shifted (e.g., from 70° to 100° ROM)? Has the duration of pain changed

(e.g., from 20 to 10 minutes)? A dichotomous view would not capture these improvements as such. Instead, the focus should be on positive changes and the respective expression of the parameters. Even with persistent complaints, improvements in other parameters can provide valuable safety information.

The collection of pain and its clinical characteristics should focus less on finding the cause of pain, but more on capturing the current state, its precise processing, education, and progress control.

5.2.3 Questionnaires

The quantification of impressions and factors or drivers deemed relevant by patients is particularly important for progress evaluation. Just as the severity of motor restrictions is determined by functional tests, questionnaires can be used to measure other factors that cannot be captured by functional tests, such as the impairment of quality of life, ADLs, or the severity of psychosocial abnormalities. It is recommended to have questionnaires filled out (or brought along already filled out) before the functional tests (or even before the anamnesis) so that information from these questionnaires can serve as reference points for the anamnesis or examination. Pain questionnaires can be oriented either towards motor-functional impairments in specific ADLs or towards psychosocial factors and mental states.

Pain Questionnaires for Motor-Functional Impairments
There are BMS or movements that cannot be tested in the therapeutic setting. These include many ADLs. In order to still be able to collect and quantify these restrictions, experts and researchers have created questionnaires for each body area that the patient can fill out themselves. Here too, dichotomous characteristics are not recorded, but rather the (categorical or numerical) severity of each restriction is recorded.

1. **General – PDI** (Pain Disability Index)
   Domains: Pain influence from family/social interaction and ADLs, such as profession or household work.
   Number of questions: 7
   Rating scale: The patient rates each question with 0–10 points (from no to maximum impairment)
   Score/Guidelines: The sum of the points results in a score between 0–70 points. A score of over 33 points can be assumed to indicate significant pain-related impairment (Soer et al., 2015). For a clinically relevant result, the score should have improved by at least 8.5 points.
2. **Head – HIT-6** (Headache Impact Test-6) (Bera et al., 2014; Houts, et al., 2021).
   Domains: Pain intensity, restrictions at work and in daily life, impairments of social activities, fatigue, irritability, and concentration difficulties.

Number of questions: 6
Rating scale: Each of the six questions has five answer options, which are rated as follows: never (6 points), rarely (8 points), sometimes (10 points), very often (11 points), always (13 points).
Score/Guidelines: The final result of the HIT-6 is calculated by summing the points of the six questions. The total score ranges from 36 to 78 points. Based on this total score, patients are divided into four categories: 36–49 points = little or no impairment, 50-55 points = moderate impairment, 56–59 points = substantial impairment, 60–78 points = severe impairment. For a clinically relevant result, the score should have improved by at least 5 points.

3. **Neck/Cervical Spine – NDI** (Neck Disability Index) (Jorritsma et al., 2012; Saltychev et al., 2024)
Domains: Pain intensity, ADLs, such as personal care, work, driving, sleeping, and concentration
Number of questions: 10
Rating scale: Each of the ten questions has six answer options, ranging from no restriction (0 points) to complete restriction (5 points).
Score/Guidelines: The final result of the NDI is calculated by summing the points of the ten questions. The total score ranges from 0 to 50 points. This total score is then converted into a percentage value to determine the severity of the restriction. The categorization is as follows: 0–4 points (0–8 %) = no disability, 5–14 points (10–28 %) = mild disability, 15–24 points (30–48 %) = moderate disability, 25–34 points (50–68 %) = severe disability, 35–50 points (70–100 %) = complete disability. For a clinically relevant result, the score should have improved by at least 8.4 points.

4.1. **LWS/BWS – ODI** (Oswestry Disability Index) (Mannion et al., 2006; Sheahan et al., 2015; Copay & Cher, 2016)
Domains: Pain and ADLs such as personal care, walking, sleeping, and social activities.
Number of questions: 10
Rating scale: Each of the ten questions has six possible answers, ranging from no limitation (0 points) to complete limitation (5 points).
Score/Guidelines: The final result of the ODI is calculated by summing the points of the ten questions. The total score ranges from 0 to 50 points. This total score is then converted into a percentage value (multiply by 2) to determine the severity of the disability. The categorization is as follows: 0-20% = minimal disability, 21–40% = moderate disability, 41–60% = significant disability, 61–80% = severe disability, 81–100% = complete disability. For a clinically relevant result, the score should have improved by at least 13%.

4.2. **LWS – RMDQ** (Roland Morris Disability Questionnaire) (Chiarotto et al., 2016)
Domains: Pain, ADLs and also emotional well-being.
Number of statements: 24

Rating scale: The patient should mark each statement as *true* or *not true* depending on their current situation. Each statement marked as *true* receives one point.

Score/Guidelines: The total score ranges from 0 to 24 points. The categorization is as follows: 0–9 points = minor disability, 10–15 points = moderate disability, >16 points = major disability. For a clinically relevant result, the score should have improved by 2–8 points.

Further questionnaires depending on the body region:

5. **Hip – HOOS** (Hip disability and Osteoarthritis Outcome Score).
6. **Knee – KOOS** (Knee injury and Osteoarthritis Outcome Score).
7. **Foot/Ankle – FAOS** (Foot and Ankle Outcome Score).
8. **Upper Extremity – DASH** (Disabilities of arm, shoulder, hand).
9. **Shoulder – CMS** (Constant-Murley Score).
10. **Elbow – ESAS** (Elbow Self-Assessment Score).
11. **Hand – MHQ** (Michigan Hand Outcomes Questionnaire).

Pain questionnaires for mental and psycho-social drivers

As already explained in section 5.2.1, the holistic and multidimensional examination of the patient plays a central role in modern medicine. This includes environmental and personal factors. The classic flag system is taken into account here. The suspicion of the presence of yellow, blue or black flags can arise from certain statements or behaviors of the patient. However, this suspicion should be checked. To identify classic risk factors of chronicity or low treatment success, such as fear, kinesiophobia or catastrophizing, early on, different questionnaires have been developed.

1. **Kinesiophobia – TSK-11** (Tampa Scale of Kinesiophobia-11) (Hapidou et al., 2012; Dupuis et al., 2023)

    Domains: pain-related movement fear
    Number of statements: 11
    Rating scale: Each statement is rated on a 4-point Likert scale from 1 (I completely disagree) to 4 points (I completely agree).
    Score/Guidelines: The points for each question are added up to obtain a total score. The total score ranges from 11 to 44, with higher scores indicating a stronger kinesiophobia.

2. **Catastrophizing – PCS** (Pain Catastrophizing Scale) (Meyer et al., 2008)

    Domains: Pain-related catastrophizing (helplessness, magnification, rumination)
    Number of statements: 13
    Rating scale: Each statement is rated on a 5-point Likert scale from 0 (not at all) to 4 points (always).
    Score/Guidelines: The points for each question are added up to obtain a total score. The total score ranges from 0–52: low catastrophizing = 0–20 points,

moderate catastrophizing = 21–30 points, high catastrophizing = 31–52 points. For a clinically relevant result, the score should have improved by at least 13%.

3. **Fear-Avoidance – FAB-Q** (Fear Avoidance Belief-Questionnaire) (George et al., 2010; Pagels et al., 2023)

Domains: pain-related fear and avoidance behavior; a scale for physical activity (PA) and a scale for work (W)
   Number of statements: 16 (FAB-PA = 5 and FAB-W = 11)
   Rating scale: Each statement will be rated on a 7-point Likert scale, from 0 points (completely disagree) to 6 points (completely agree).
   Score/Guidelines: The points for each question are added up to obtain a total score. The total score for the FAB-PA is composed only of statements 2,3,4,5 (without the 1) for better psychometric properties and ranges from 0–24 points and for the FAB-W from statements 6, 7, 9, 10, 11, 12, 15 (without 8, 13 and 14) and ranges from 0–42 points. An increased risk of chronicity exists at >15 points (FAB-PA) and >34 points (FAB-W). For clinically relevant results, the scores should have improved by 5.4 (FAB-PA) and 6.8 (FAB-W) points respectively.

Attention: The guidelines of these questionnaires should not be used to instruct the patient ("It's not that bad, says the following study."), nor to induce nocebo fear ("Your score puts you in a critical range."), but initially for baseline testing for the evaluation of progress and the exploration of potential drivers.
   In addition, there are some questionnaires that can simplify the highlighting of a specific pain mechanism (neuropathic, nociplastic). Since the measurability of sensitization processes is not possible in clinical practice, certain key symptoms are recorded using questionnaires such as the **Central Sensitisation Inventory (CSI)**, (Mayer et al., 2012). Its domains include musculoskeletal pain, sleep disorders, cognitive problems, urogenital and gastrointestinal problems, mood swings and states of exhaustion (Nebelt et al., 2013). A pathology associated with sensitization and nociplastic processes is, for example, fibromyalgia. Here, the use of the **FibroDetectÒ**questionnaire can be useful to support the hypothesis (Baron et al., 2014). Questionnaires with a neuropathic focus are the **painDETECT** (Cappelleri et al., 2016; Foadi et al., 2024), the **S-LANSS**(selfreported Leeds Assessment of Neuropathic Symptoms and Signs) (Bennett et al., 2005) or the **DN4** (Bouhassira et al., 2005), which ask for and quantify neuropathic symptoms, such as special pain qualities (electrifying, burning,..) localizations (diffuse, radiating,..) and neurological symptoms (sensory and motor), and can indicate neural and somatosensory damage. In the case of neuropathic components, a careful neurological examination should take place. For the evaluation of progress, the drawing of pain areas or sensory deficient skin areas is useful, to allow for image progression control through photography (Bonezzi et al., 2020).
   These questionnaires do not replace a careful medical history, they serve as a supplement. The evaluation, localization, sensitivity, and movement dependence of the pain and a thorough examination are crucial to obtain clues about the nature

of the pain. By systematically collecting information about the pain symptoms and the underlying medical history, important hypothetical conclusions can be drawn.

5.2.4 Documentation and Illustration

Although a patient's subjective pain experience cannot be objectified, quantifying this experience and converting it into numerical parameters for illustration and especially for progress control is of great benefit. This conversion is not intended to explain the subjective pain experience, but rather to create a measurable basis for the documentation and analysis of changes in pain perception. Therefore, the collection of such parameters is highly recommended. Experience shows that the documentation of these parameters, whether written or digital, is in line form. Precise data processing is not guaranteed with this. Possible parameters that can be collected include pain intensity on the NRPS during certain movements or ADLs, questionnaire scores in points, and BMS in degrees, kilograms, centimeters, or other units.

Example
Patient Z.n. Weber C re. 12 months post OP, NRPS 2 at rest, NRPS 4 when walking, NRPS 7 when jogging, NRPS 6 pressure tenderness distal third of fibula, ROM Knee to Wall re. 2 cm, li. 8 cm, Plantarflexion re. 10° li. 25°, Strength Eversion re. 9 kg, li. 25 kg, FAOS 35%.

Tabular Documentation
The time points (TP) at which the measurements were taken are shown the first line, in column 1 the respective parameters and from column 2 the respective values per parameter and time point. When entering new values a few weeks later, the data is clearly arranged (Tab. 5.2).

Graphical Documentation:
Simple pre-programmed Excel files can convert these data directly into a graph. This way, trends and developments can be visualized (Fig. 5.3). It is

Tab. 5.2 Table with clinical examination results, own production

Parameter	Time point 1	Time point 2
Pain (Rest)	2	1
Pain (Walking)	4	2
Pain (Jogging)	7	5
Pressure pain	6	3
KTW	25% (re. 2, li. 8)	63% (re. 5, li. 8)
Strength Eversion	36% (re. 9, li. 25)	52% (re. 14, li. 27)
FAOS	45%	70%

Fig. 5.3 Graph with clinical pain reports. (Own creation)

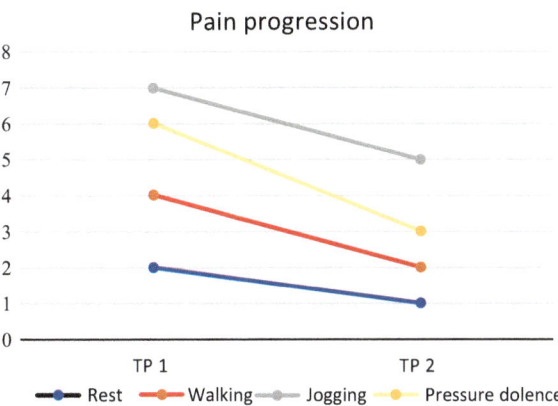

recommended to create a graph for each of the pain reports, mobility, strength, and questionnaire score. An exemplary graph for the pain reports would look like the following based on the data from the above example:

Discussion on Pain Assessment

Does the parameterization of pain really measure pain perception? How valid are subjective pain reports? Do patients really report what they perceive? Or what they want to disclose? Does the number 7 indicate pain intensity? Or does the number 7 embody the patient's coping and dealing with his pain? Pain signals a kind of need for protection and help. Wouldn't a decrease from 7 to 3 signal that one no longer needs help/therapy/care? Could patients persist in pain because the need for protection and help seems greater and more tangible than the state of painlessness and independence? Perhaps it does not help to see pain as the primary parameter for treatment success in chronic pain patients, but other factors such as activity level? Thus, the effectiveness of a therapy can also be measured by an increase in activity level, if the pain does not increase at the same time. Same pain despite increased activity is an improvement.

In clinical practice, the numerical rating scale from 0 to 10 has established itself as a common tool for pain assessment. This seemingly simple method suggests an objective measurability of pain, which can be deceptive upon closer inspection. The parameterization of pain using a numerical scale offers both opportunities and risks for patient care and medical research. Pain is, as already postulated by the renowned nursing scientist Margo McCaffery, a deeply subjective experience. McCaffery's famous definition "Pain is whatever a person says it is and exists whenever a person perceives it." emphasizes the inviolability of individual pain experience. This definition puts the patient's perspective in the foreground and simultaneously deprives pain of any external validation or objectification. Unlike other physical sensations or symptoms, pain cannot be verified or falsified by simple tests. While the feeling of stiffness can be objectified by mobility tests or the feeling of muscle weakness by strength measurements, pain remains an intangible, inner experience of the individual. The numerical pain scale attempts to bring this subjective experience into a seemingly objective form, which can lead to various problems and misunderstandings.

The indication of a number on the pain scale is far more complex than it may appear at first glance. It can be influenced by various factors:

1. Individual pain tolerance and experience: Each person has a different pain threshold and different experiences with pain that influence his or her rating.
2. Cultural and social background: The way pain is expressed and communicated can be strongly shaped by cultural norms and social expectations.
3. Emotional state: Fear, depression, or stress can significantly influence pain perception and rating.
4. Cognitive factors: Understanding of the scale, ability for self-reflection, and current cognitive performance play a role.
5. Contextual factors: The environment in which the pain assessment takes place, as well as the relationship to the asking therapist, can significantly influence the response.

The question of the validity of subjective pain reports is of central importance for clinical practice and pain research. Patients could exaggerate or downplay their pain intensity for various reasons:

- Fear of stigmatization or disregard of their complaints
- Desire to maintain a sick role or avoid responsibility
- Unconscious psychological processes that distort pain perception
- Difficulty differentiating between pain intensity and emotional distress caused by pain

The number on the pain scale can thus reflect more than just the pure pain intensity. It can express the total suffering, coping strategies, or the need for support and care. The evolutionary function of pain as a warning and protective signal must not be overlooked. Pain not only signals physical danger, but also the need for social support and care. In this context, the persistence of pain in chronic pain patients can also be understood as an expression of a deeply rooted need for protection and help. The reduction of pain from a 7 to a 3 could be perceived unconsciously as a threat—as a signal that the needed support and attention could be lost. This could possibly explain in some cases why some patients report no improvement in their pain despite therapy, or even report a worsening. At the same time, these assumptions should in no way result in an insinuation of alleged exaggeration or a trivialization of the patient's expression of pain.

Given the complexity and potential unreliability of numerical pain recording, especially in chronic pain patients, it seems sensible to use alternative or supplementary parameters to evaluate treatment success. Some possible approaches could be:

1. Activity level: The patient's ability to perform everyday activities or participate in social interactions can be a meaningful indicator of quality of life and treatment success.
2. Functional improvement: The regaining of specific physical functions or the expansion of the range of motion can be objectively measured.
3. Quality of life: Standardized questionnaires for assessing general quality of life can provide a more comprehensive picture of the patient's situation.
4. Medication consumption: A reduction in pain medication with improved or stable functionality can be seen as a positive sign.
5. Coping strategies: The development and application of effective pain management strategies can be an important indicator of treatment success.
6. Work ability: Returning to work or increasing work ability can be a significant marker for improvement and treatment success.

The parameterization of pain through a simple numerical scale is undoubtedly a useful tool in clinical practice, but it carries the risk of oversimplifying a highly complex phenomenon and a reductionist approach. It is important that therapists and doctors are aware of the limits and potential pitfalls of this method.

A multidimensional approach that considers functional, psychological, and social aspects in addition to pain intensity promises a more comprehensive and meaningful picture of the patient's situation, as also proposed in the ICF model. The numerical data collection is to be considered as a helpful supplement, but should never serve as the sole basis for clinical reasoning, education, or therapy. Especially in chronic pain patients, the focus should be on improving quality of life, beliefs, and physical functions, with pain reduction being an important, but not the only goal.

The challenge for the future will be to develop individualized methods for pain assessment that do justice to the complexity of the pain experience and are at the same time practical for everyday clinical use. Until then, critical reflection and sensitive handling of pain reports remain a central task for all professionals involved in pain therapy.

5.3 Therapy

Pain therapy has undergone a special transformation over the last centuries. From spiritual and religious actions to surgeries, to medicinal, physical, or psycho-social therapies, almost nothing has been left untried in pain therapy to alleviate pain. And even today, all possibilities are still available and no type of attempt to alleviate pain seems to have become extinct. The fame and attention for each therapy may vary, but they all exist simultaneously. However, in the therapy of (especially chronic) pain, the aim should not only be to directly alleviate pain through the execution of a specific intervention. Instead, the mechanism of pain should be reversed. And this is not achievable with long-standing problems, where central sensitization, top-down processes, and other emotional and cognitive aspects are involved, through a single treatment or other *quick fixes*. The mechanistic reversal can only take place when the dominant mechanism with its drivers could be identified through a thorough examination.

5.3.1 General Recommendations for Pain Therapy

Due to the high prevalence of back and lower back pain, most studies and guidelines refer to the therapy of these body areas. The most recent European guidelines provide four different recommendations for **acute nonspecific back pain** (after exclusion of red flags) (van Tulder et al., 2006):

1. The patient should be encouraged through education to minimize uncertainties and worry.
2. Bed rest should be avoided.
3. The patient should remain as active as possible at his highest possible load capacity, capable of sports and work.
4. No specific active or passive measures are recommended.

Acute back pain usually heals by itself (Apkarian et al., 2009). Therefore, and due to the effectiveness of *Wait and See*, a specific intervention, such as a stretching exercise program, may be effective but not efficient. A thorough examination, by excluding red flags followed by education, seems to be the best therapy for acute back pain according to guidelines.

Chronic back pain is a widespread health problem that has significant impacts on the quality of life of those affected. The weak correlation between structural anomalies and pain has led to the suggestion that factors other than just structural pathologies are predictors for clinical outcomes. These factors include psycho-social factors. These psycho-social factors include, among other things, the extent of depression, anxiety, pain catastrophizing, fear and/or helplessness, job satisfaction, and environmental influences such as compensation and litigation. Given these findings, it is crucial that approaches to the therapy of chronic back pain not only consider biomechanical aspects but also address the psycho-social drivers. A holistic therapy approach that integrates both physical and psychological components could therefore be more effective in improving the quality of life of back pain patients and supporting pain management. Conservative or surgical measures for pain relief that directly target the back often show no effect. Although these patients exhibit various biomechanical anomalies, therapies to normalize these supposed anomalies hardly lead to an improvement. Moreover, there is no correlation between therapy outcomes and changes in biomechanical parameters. This suggests that even biomechanically oriented therapies lead to pain relief through mechanisms other than the actual change in biomechanics (Wand & O´Connell, 2008).

The European guidelines for **chronic nonspecific back pain** provide different recommendations (Airaksinen et al., 2006):

1. Supervised exercise therapy with modifiable and patient-adaptable exercises without great effort or machines. A specific form of exercise is not recommended as they all seem to be equally effective (patient preference should be considered here).
2. Short education strategies
3. a bio-psycho-social approach
4. Cognition-based therapies

Drug therapies are only recommended for short-term use and in case of failure of other therapies. Classic quick-fix interventions, such as heat/laser/shock wave/ electro or massage therapies, are not recommended. Manual therapeutic measures are not recommended as primary therapy, but can be used for a short time (Airaksinen et al., 2006).

> **Excursus**
> **Dealing with Pain**
> The interpretation and evaluation of pain experiences play a central role in pain perception and processing. Cognitive evaluation processes significantly influence the emotional and behavior-related reaction to pain. Negative associations, such as attributing pain to structural damage and a resulting feeling of fragility, can lead to maladaptive coping strategies and an intensification of pain perception (Vlaeyen & Linton, 2000). In contrast, reinterpreting pain as a normal physiological adaptation reaction can contribute to a reduction in pain intensity and improved functionality (Moseley & Butler, 2015). This reinterpretation is in line with the bio-psycho-social pain model (Gatchel et al., 2007) and promotes adaptive coping strategies. Pain processing includes various strategies, including acceptance, adaptation, avoidance, and active intervention. Research results show that acceptance-based approaches, such as Acceptance and Commitment Therapy (ACT), can effectively contribute to improving the quality of life in chronic pain (McCracken & Vowles, 2014). It is important to emphasize that many nonspecific pain conditions are self-limiting (Artus et al., 2014). Excessive interventions or a focus on the pain problem can paradoxically contribute to chronicity (Hasenbring et al., 2001). Instead, appropriate education about the benign course of many pain conditions, combined with encouragement to normal activity, can often be sufficient to promote adaptive coping strategies and maintain functionality (O'Sullivan et al., 2016).

5.3.2 Specific Recommendations for Pain Therapy

The relief of nociceptive pain, after excluding red flags and serious pathologies, may be less complex than the relief of nociplastic pain. The effectiveness of many different therapies for nociceptive pain may be due to the fact that the nociceptive input often subsides on its own through the natural healing process, and thus the pain also subsides. Accompanying this process, providing explanatory care, reducing functional decline, controlling disturbing factors, and restoring optimal fitness is still a challenge that requires trained health experts. More challenging is the therapy of nociplastic pain, which is not based on regression to the mean or a natural healing process. To set up targeted therapies for nociplastic pain, an analysis is needed to determine which components make up the nociplastic pain and which contributing factors and drivers people with nociplastic pain have. In addition to the clinical pain and movement patterns to be collected in section 5.2, nociplastic pain, unlike nociceptive pain, is accompanied by many affective and psycho-social abnormalities, which are associated with neuroplastic cortical restructurings. These include (Jackson et al., 2014; Manchikanti et al., 2014; Yang & Chang, 2019):

- Stress
- Depression
- Anxiety/Kinesiophobia
- low self-efficacy expectation
- Catastrophizing

Based on these findings, it is logical to identify the most important drivers for the patient and to include these in the goal formulation, in addition to pain relief. The therapy of nociplastic pain should aim at the mechanistic reversal of the reversibility of neuroplastic changes and the reduction of negative top-down processes. And this is not possible with purely biomedical and biomechanical approaches. Bio-psycho-social therapies that can reverse neuroplastic changes, alleviate pain, and improve functions will now be summarized.

Pain Education/PNE
Pain education or PNE (Pain Neuroscience Education) is an essential component of multimodal pain therapy for patients with chronic pain. It aims to improve patients' understanding of their pain, to educate about the multifactorial nature and neurobiological mechanisms, and to provide them with tools for better coping (Moseley & Butler, 2015).

Pain education typically covers the following topics:

1. Neurobiology of pain
2. Bio-psycho-social model of chronic pain
3. Central sensitization and pain chronification

4. Influence of thoughts, emotions, and behaviors on pain
5. Pain coping strategies and self-management techniques

PNE can take place in various settings that can be adapted to the individual needs and circumstances of the patients. Individual sessions offer the possibility of personalized care, while group programs promote exchange between those affected. Inpatient rehabilitation programs provide intensive, holistic care, and online courses as well as telemedical offers ensure flexibility and accessibility, especially for patients with limited mobility or in remote areas.

Education and PNE can contribute to pain relief in addition to increasing knowledge. A multimodal therapy, which included PNE, achieved better results in terms of pain relief compared to standard therapy (Wälti et al., 2015). PNE alleviates pain, fears, false beliefs, catastrophizing, and kinesiophobia, and improves motor functions (Moseley, 2002; Moseley et al., 2004; Meeus et al., 2010; van Oosterwijck et al., 2013; Bodes Pardo et al., 2018; Watson et al., 2019; Wood & Hendrick, 2019). In addition, PNE can reduce the use of the healthcare system and thus be cost-effective (Louw et al., 2014). Wood and Hendrick summarized in a meta-analysis in 2019 that the addition of PNE to usual physiotherapy seems to be more effective in the short term for patients with chronic back pain than standalone physiotherapy without education. However, this statement could not yet be confirmed for long-term effects due to a lack of studies. Education for pain patients has also been included in European and German guidelines (Airaksinen et al., 2006; Arnold et al., 2014), but there is still a lack of sufficiently extensive and meaningful studies to recommend PNE as a standalone therapy (Geneen et al., 2015).

Whether neuroplastic changes at the cortical level can be reversed through pain education cannot be conclusively proven, as research in this area is still relatively young and the evidence is limited. Many studies have small sample sizes and long-term studies are lacking. However, there are some indications that pain education can indeed influence neuroplastic changes: Moseley (2005) showed in a study with fMRI that a single session of pain education led to a change in brain activity that was associated with a reduction in pain perception. Further theoretical cortical overlap mechanisms between chronic pain and education suggest that pain education can modulate activity in pain-processing brain regions (Zimney et al., 2023). The exact mechanisms by which pain education influences neuroplastic changes are not yet fully understood. It is suspected that the change in beliefs and behaviors regarding pain leads to a reorganization of neuronal networks (Nijs et al., 2014).

Pain education should be understood as a partnership, empathetic process that respects and includes the individual experiences and perceptions of the patient. Instead of merely explaining the patient's symptoms in a factual and possibly condescending manner, the approach should be reassuring, enlightening, and motivating.

An effective education approach does not tell the patient what he perceives, but helps him understand which factors can influence his perception—both positively and negatively. This promotes a deeper understanding of the complexity of the pain experience and enables the patient to actively participate in his recovery.

Therapists should develop a fine sense for when and to what extent education is appropriate. It's about finding a balance between information and interaction, so that the sessions do not become one-sided lectures. The connection of theoretical knowledge with practical experiences is crucial in this context.

A constructive approach could be, for example: "Let's look together at why this movement is not an immediate threat from various perspectives. We will proceed cautiously and work with targeted measures to bring about positive changes and establish new behavior patterns."

In contrast, statements like "Studies show that these movements are absolutely harmless. What you were told is nonsense. Just keep going." should be avoided. Such formulations can be perceived as derogatory and burden the patient-therapist alliance. Patient-centered pain education should aim to create a trusting atmosphere in which the patient feels understood and taken seriously. It should leave room for questions and concerns and encourage the patient to actively participate in the therapy process. This respectful and cooperative approach can strengthen the therapeutic alliance and increase the effectiveness of pain education. Ultimately, it's about empowering the patient to better understand and manage his pain experience, without negating or devaluing his individual perspective. A sensitive and individualized pain education can thus become an important part of successful therapy.

Training

Active training is more effective for pain relief in chronic pain patients than passive hands-on therapies, such as manual therapy, osteopathy, or chiropractic (Owen et al., 2020). Current European guidelines recommend the use of physical exercises and strength training in the therapy of chronic nonspecific back pain (Airaksinen et al., 2006). Strength training can reduce pain intensity in various chronic pain conditions and simultaneously improve functions, such as ADLs and logically strength (Jackson et al., 2011; Geneen et al., 2017; Cortell-Tormo et al., 2018). Often, the question or uncertainty about the safe intensity and load is a hurdle for the progression of strength exercises, which is why exercises that initially go down well with the patient are not or only marginally increased. However, progressive strength training with successively increasing intensities shows positive effects on pain relief (Calatayud et al., 2020; Syroyid Syroyid et al., 2022). The intensity of the training seems to play a role in pain relief. Intensive strength training is low-risk and has a greater pain-relieving effect compared to moderate strength training (Verbrugghe et al., 2019). A meta-analysis favors the use of strength and stability training over cardio-pulmonary/aerobic exercises (Searle et al., 2015). Other studies show that aerobic exercises with low mechanical load have a similar pain-relieving effect as intensive strength training (Wewege et al., 2018). Another meta-analysis showed that Pilates was slightly superior compared to other forms of training, but all forms of training including core stability, strength, aqua, stretching or yoga training show pain-relieving effects (Owen et al., 2020). The type of training does not necessarily have a specific effect on pain relief and no form of training is clearly superior to others (Oesch et al., 2010; de Zoete et al., 2020). This can be taken as an opportunity to include the preferences of the patients and adapt the active plan to their wishes. However, when it comes to strength training, as described above, higher intensities show greater pain-relieving effects. Strength training could be considered one of the best forms of training due to its far-reaching positive effects on comorbidities, which go beyond relieving chronic pain, such as risk minimization for diabetes, heart attacks, high blood pressure, obesity, osteoporosis, and depression (Westcott, 2012; Callow et al., 2020; Maestroni et al., 2020).

The pain-relieving effects of strength training, however, seem not only to be attributable to the primarily propagated mechanisms of physical resilience enhancement, which now better protects and stabilizes the painful tissue, but also to the descending pain inhibition of the brainstem, which is neurobiologically activated by strength training (Sluka et al., 2018; Song et al., 2022). The descending pain-inhibiting system and the release activity of endogenous opioids is higher in physically active people than in less active people (Naugle et al., 2017). Another study showed the involvement of non-opioid systems, in which strength training led to the activation of the endocannabinoid system, and thus to the release of endocannabinoids, which correlated with the degree of increase in the pain tolerance threshold (Koltyn et al., 2014). Further studies highlight other non-physical or tissue-specific mechanisms of strength training. Strength training reduces pro-inflammatory cytokines, such as interleukin 6, TNF-α and C-reactive protein, and minimizes their new formation (Calle & Fernandez, 2010; Macêdo Santiago et al., 2018; Zheng et al., 2024). These markers are drivers for central sensitization and pain chronification (Fang et al., 2023).

In summary, three different mechanisms are attributed to the training-induced relief of chronic pain (Jiang et al., 2023):

1. Activation of the descending pain-inhibiting system by the release of endogenous opioids, such as beta-endorphins
2. Activation of the endocannabinoid system by the release of endogenous cannabis-like endocannabinoids
3. Release of anti-inflammatory myokines to reduce pro-inflammatory cytokines

Furthermore, although strength training does not primarily aim at cognition, it also positively influences cognitive and psycho-social factors in chronic pain patients. Studies show that strength training not only increases physical performance, but also leads to a reduction of catastrophizing thoughts and an increase in self-efficacy expectation in chronic pain patients (Smeets et al., 2006; Vincent et al., 2014; Shinohara et al., 2022; Gilanyi et al., 2023). These improvements in psychological yellow flags—i.e., unfavorable beliefs and attitudes towards pain—are discussed as an important additional factor contributing to long-term pain relief and improvement of pain coping. These pain-relieving mechanisms, which are not specifically attributable to the increase in the morphological resilience of the painful body area, are supported by study results. These show that training of peripheral, non-painful body regions can alleviate the pain in the primarily affected, painful areas just as much, if not more, than direct training and loading of the painful areas themselves (Vincent et al., 2014; Atalay et al., 2017).

This phenomenon suggests that strength training exerts its pain-relieving effect at least partially through central and systemic mechanisms that go beyond a mere increase in tissue resilience. In addition, studies show the training-induced influence on brain activities, which are associated with pain relief. On the one hand, the activity of the reward center, which is disturbed in chronic pain patients, is normalized through the release of dopamine, on the other hand, the activity of glutamatergic neurons in the hippocampus, which project to the amygdala and are responsible for the encoding of fear and avoidance, is reduced (Kami et al., 2022).

A few studies have examined the effect of strength training on neuroplastic changes in chronic pain patients. These suggest a cortical reorganization, which is discussed as a possible mechanism of pain relief (de Zoete et al., 2023; Zou & Hao, 2024).

Graded Activity and Graded Exposure
The Graded Activity (GA) approach, also known as Graded Exercise Therapy, translates to: gradual or step-by-step activity. In the therapy of chronic pain, this concept is based on the principles of operant conditioning and cognitive-behavioral therapy (CBT), which was first introduced by Fordyce and colleagues in the 1970s. The basic idea is that chronic pain often goes hand in hand with avoidance behavior and a decrease in physical activity. This can lead to a vicious cycle of pain, rest, deconditioning, and further intensification of pain (Vlaeyen & Linton, 2000). Through GA, the patient is gradually guided to increased physical activity and resilience, regardless of the pain (Vlaeyen et al., 1995; Macedo et al., 2010). The promotion of healthy behavior is the focus here, less the direct confrontation with or reduction of fear, which is primarily treated in Graded Exposure. In GA, a problematic action is selected, for example, prolonged jogging. Then a baseline is determined, i.e., when which symptoms occur how strongly. Subsequently, a comfortable or feasible tolerable training range is set, which is then gradually increased.

The central aspects here are:

1. Setting realistic, patient-specific activity goals, such as being able to walk a certain distance again.
2. Slow, gradual approach to these goals, initially regardless of the pain.
3. Setbacks are accepted as normal and possibly met with a training adjustment, but not with excessive rest or protection.
4. Positive reinforcement and promotion of self-management.

Studies have shown that this approach can lead to improvements in pain, functionality, anxiety, and depression in patients with chronic pain (Macedo et al., 2010; Kuss et al., 2016; Magalhães et al., 2018).

5.3 Therapy

The Graded Exposure (GE) approach translates to gradual or step-by-step exposure. In the therapy of chronic pain, GE is based on the fear-avoidance model and aims to reduce pain-associated fears and avoidance behavior. GE addresses the kinesiophobia present in many chronic pain patients, which leads to avoidance behavior and ultimately to an intensification of the pain symptoms (Leeuw et al., 2007).

The core elements of GE are:

1. Identification of feared activities or movements
2. Hierarchical arrangement of these activities according to the degree of triggered fear
3. Step-by-step exposure to these activities in vivo, starting with the least feared.
4. Cognitive restructuring to correct obstructive beliefs about pain and movement, which is achieved through educative and physically implemented exposure.

The goal is to reduce the fear of movement through repeated exposure and to enable positive experiences with physical activity (de Jong et al., 2005). Studies have proven the effectiveness of this approach in various chronic pain syndromes, especially in chronic back pain and CRPS (Leeuw et al., 2008; den Hollander et al., 2016).

GA and GE are therapeutic approaches to the treatment of chronic pain, which are firmly rooted in CBT. They are based on the principles of behavior change and the modification of thoughts and beliefs, which are central elements of CBT. Although they have some similarities, there are important differences in their theoretical foundations and practical applications.

1. Objective:
   - GA: aims to reinforce healthy behavior and focuses on the gradual increase of general physical activity.
   - GE: aims to reduce pain-associated fears and focuses on confronting specific fear-laden movements.
2. Implementation:
   - GA: The increase in activity is time-based, regardless of the pain.
   - GE: The exposure is fear- and experience-based, with pain also being accepted as part of the experience.

Commonalities:

1. Both approaches use a gradual, structured approach.
2. Both require active participation of the patient and promote self-management.
3. Both can lead to a reduction of pain and disability.

Both concepts aim to break maladaptive associations between specific movements and pain experiences that have been learned and manifested in the nervous system over time. These learned links often stem from past pain experiences and lead to certain movements continuing to be perceived as threatening and triggering pain, even when there is no longer any acute tissue damage or threat. At the neurobiological level, the goal is to reduce the hypersensitivity of central pain networks and promote new adaptive neuronal connections. Through repeated and controlled exposure to movements perceived as threatening, habituation is to be achieved. This allows the brain to reassess the perception of threat and learn that the movement can be performed safely. The goal is to break, unlearn, and replace the learned association *movement* = *pain* and the resulting belief *pain* = *danger* with new positive movement experiences. This restructuring can be brought about by GA and GE and other measures within the framework of CBT, such as education, stress management, and relaxation techniques (Ehde et al., 2014). The effectiveness of CBT in terms of pain relief may be explained by its ability to reverse neuroplastic changes. Seminowicz and colleagues (2013) observed structural changes in the brain after CBT in chronic pain patients, suggesting the reversibility of some neuroplastic changes. CBT is a broadly applicable therapeutic approach that was originally developed for the treatment of psychiatric disorders (Urits et al., 2019). When applied to chronic pain, CBT aims to identify and change maladaptive behaviors, thought patterns, and situations that can contribute to the maintenance or exacerbation of the pain experience. The approach includes various techniques such as relaxation exercises, breathing exercises, cognitive restructuring, and problem-solving activities. Patients learn to develop new, more adaptive behaviors to improve their psychological functioning and better cope with pain. Graded Activity and Graded Exposure can be incorporated into a CBT, as well as into a CFT (cognitive functional therapy). CFT is a newer approach and, unlike CBT, was specifically developed by physiotherapists for the treatment of chronic back pain (O'Sullivan et al., 2018). It is a behavior-oriented approach that aims to identify modifiable risk factors, change behaviors and maladaptive thought patterns to regain functionality and improve pain management. CFT follows a three-step process: cognitive training, functional movement training with exposure and control, and physical activity and lifestyle changes (Urits et al., 2019; Hadley & Novic, 2021). Both forms of therapy aim to change maladaptive thinking and behavior patterns and take into account psychological factors in pain perception and coping. They strive to improve functionality and quality of life and promote self-management and active patient participation. The main difference between the two approaches lies in their focus and structure. While CBT is primarily oriented towards psychological aspects and is used for a broader range of conditions, CFT consciously integrates physical movement and functionality and was specifically developed for back pain. CFT has a more specific structure with the aim of transitioning to functional activity changes. Both forms of therapy have proven effective in the treatment of chronic pain. The choice between CBT and CFT often depends on the specific situation of the patient, the type of pain, and the available resources. In many cases, elements of both approaches can be combined to ensure comprehensive and individualized therapy, with CFT specifically targeting patients with chronic musculoskeletal complaints. Due to large similarities, the practical boundaries between the two approaches are anyway fluid.

Acceptance-Commitment Therapy

ACT is a form of behavioral therapy aimed at increasing psychological flexibility. ACT was developed in the 1980s by Steven Hayes and colleagues and adapted in the context of pain therapy to specifically address the challenges of chronic pain patients (Vowles et al., 2014).

In chronic pain, ACT does not primarily focus on pain reduction, but on the acceptance of pain. It supports patients in leading a fulfilling life despite chronic pain by changing patients' expectations from complete pain relief to the best possible life despite chronic pain. The primary goal is to teach patients a non-judgmental attitude towards pain experiences. An increased acceptance of pain and the execution of activities despite pain correlate positively with improved quality of life and lead to pain relief; presumably through improved coping and a re-evaluation of sensations, which reduces the threat and thus pain perception (Johnston et al., 2010; Wetherell et al., 2011; Veehof et al., 2016; Hughes et al., 2017). ACT promotes openness to emotions, thoughts, and physical sensations. The prefrontal cortex, which is mainly involved in cognitive control, plays a central role here. ACT modulates activity in this area, which can lead to improved regulation of emotions and pain perception (Jensen et al., 2012). After ACT treatment, increased activation was observed in areas of the ventrolateral prefrontal and lateral orbitofrontal cortex (vlPFC/lOFC). These regions are important for emotion regulation and re-evaluation of situations. The increased activation in these areas could explain why patients are better able to cope with pain and negative emotions after ACT. The changes in brain activity also correlate with a reduction in anxiety symptoms. In addition, after ACT, increased connectivity between vlPFC and the thalamus is observed: This is significant because the thalamus plays an important role in the transmission and modulation of sensory information, including nociception. An enhanced connection between vlPFC and thalamus could indicate improved top-down control of nociceptive afferents. Another study also documented the influence of ACT on pain-relevant brain activities (Smallwood et al., 2016). After the ACT intervention, patients showed a significant decrease in activation in several brain regions, such as the insula and the anterior cingulate cortex. This reduced activation suggests that ACT reduces the brain's affective-emotional reactivity to painful stimuli. It also leads to a decreased connectivity between pain-processing areas and the Default Mode Network (DMN). The DMN is a network of brain regions that is active when one is not focused on the outside world and is in a resting state.

Sensory Discrimination Training

Patients with chronic back pain have a reduced ability to discriminate sensory stimuli compared to asymptomatic individuals. For example, they cannot accurately locate sensory stimuli applied to the back or distinguish between two points in close proximity, for which cortical somatotopic restructuring is considered the cause. For instance, after amputations, the intensity of phantom pain is strongly associated with the degree of cortical restructuring (the extent of the cortical representation of the amputated limb) (Flor et al., 1995). Sensory Discrimination

Training (SDT) aims to improve sensory perception and normalize the cortical representation of the affected body part. In addition, several studies have shown that SDT led to significant pain reduction and functional improvement in patients with phantom pain (Flor et al., 2001), fibromyalgia (Mhalla et al., 2010), and CRPS (Pleger et al., 2005; Moseley et al., 2008), as well as in patients with chronic back pain (Wand et al., 2011; Louw et al., 2015). The pain reduction was accompanied by a decrease in neuroplastic changes, specifically cortical reorganization and normalization of somatotopy. These studies demonstrate the increasing evidence for the effectiveness of SDT in various chronic pain syndromes. Imaging studies attribute similar mechanisms and effects to Graded Motor Imagery, in which both pain can be alleviated and the activation of various brain areas involved in pain processing can be normalized (Diers et al., 2010).

Graded Motor Imagery
Graded Motor Imagery (GMI) is a therapeutic approach developed in the context of chronic pain therapy, particularly for complex pain syndromes such as CRPS or phantom pain. GMI was significantly developed by Lorimer Moseley, based on neuroscientific findings about the plasticity of the brain and the role of cortical representation in chronic pain (Moseley, 2004, 2006). GMI is based on the idea that in chronic pain, there is often a disturbance in the processing and representation of movements in the brain. Through a gradual and controlled activation of motor imagination, a reorganization of these cortical representations is to be achieved. GMI typically consists of three consecutive phases:

1. Laterality training: Patients practice quickly recognizing whether a shown body part (e.g., a hand) is on the left or right side.
2. Explicit motor imagery: Patients imagine performing certain movements without actually carrying them out.
3. Mirror therapy: Patients observe movements of the unaffected body part in a mirror, creating the illusion that the affected body part is moving painlessly.

Several studies have investigated the effectiveness of GMI in various chronic pain syndromes:

- A systematic review by Bowering and colleagues (2013) found moderate evidence for the effectiveness of GMI in CRPS and phantom pain.
- A meta-analysis by Lakatos and colleagues (2016) showed that GMI was significantly more effective in pain reduction than conventional physiotherapy with manual and exercise therapy in patients with CRPS.
- Furthermore, GMI can also be used to reduce pain in patients with chronic back pain (Wand et al., 2012).

GMI is often used as part of a more comprehensive treatment plan. The therapy is carried out step by step and is individually adapted, with each phase typically lasting 2–4 weeks. Patients practice daily, often with the help of special picture cards or digital applications. The evidence for the use of GMI in chronic back pain is still limited. The application often relies on the transfer of findings from other chronic pain syndromes and the theoretical basis that changes in cortical representation of the back could also play a role in chronic back pain.

Mindfulness-Based Stress Reduction
The **mindfulness-based stress reduction** (MBSR) was developed in 1979 by Jon Kabat-Zinn in the USA, who wanted to create a secular, scientifically based approach to help chronic pain patients (Kabat-Zinn, 2005). MBSR is understood as a western counterpart to meditation. Relaxation caused by mindfulness of one's own body leads to stress reduction, which can alleviate chronic pain and associated fears (Reich et al., 2017; Liu et al., 2019; Schell et al., 2019; Burrowes et al., 2022; Soundararajan et al., 2022). A central component of MBSR is the body scan, in which a body journey is made from the feet to the head while lying on the back and with closed eyes. Patients should describe their sensations without evaluating them. This trains a non-judgmental attitude towards sensations, aiming for emotion regulation. Non-sensations, i.e., pain-free body areas, should also be consciously perceived. Other contents of MBSR include seated meditation, active yoga exercises, and educational content on the effects of stress with experience exchange. MBSR shows similar pain-relieving effects as CBT (Cherkin et al., 2016) and can lead to cortical reorganization and reverse pain-related neuroplastic changes (Hölzel et al., 2011; Zeidan et al., 2011; Tang et al., 2015; Wielgosz et al., 2022).

Sleep and Nutrition
The combination of multimodal, i.e., differently targeted, and patient-tailored therapy is recommended as the most promising treatment for chronic pain (Nijs et al., 2024). This includes, in addition to the already mentioned movement and stress management, other lifestyle factors, such as sleep and nutrition. There is a bidirectional relationship between sleep deprivation and chronic pain (Finan et al., 2013). The treatment of sleep disorders can positively influence chronic pain (Jungquist et al., 2010; Whale & Gooberman-Hill, 2022). Mechanisms include improved descending pain inhibition, reduced inflammation markers, improved mood, and better coping. An integrative therapy that addresses both sleep disorders (if present) and chronic pain is considered a very effective approach. Nutrition therapy also has a growing influence on the treatment of chronic pain, as some studies show. Nutritional interventions can reduce inflammation, improve antioxidant capacity, positively influence the gut microbiome, and support neurotransmitter modulation, which contributes to pain relief (Rondanelli et al., 2018; Brain et al., 2019; Kaushik et al., 2020). The dietary recommendations include basics, such as daily consumption of enough water, whole grains (whole grain bread, whole grain pasta, rice, quinoa), vegetables (green leafy vegetables, broccoli, cabbage), fruit (berries and color-intensive fruits), as well as anti-inflammatory herbs and spices (turmeric, ginger, rosemary, thyme). Legumes (beans, lentils, chickpeas), nuts and seeds (walnuts, almonds, flax seeds, chia seeds), olive oil, and fish (salmon, mackerel, sardines) should be consumed several times a week to benefit from their

omega-3 fatty acids and other nutrients. Lean meat, eggs, and fermented dairy products are allowed in moderation, while red meat, processed products, and sugar should only be eaten rarely. The nutrition pyramid by Rondanelli and colleagues for chronic pain patients emphasizes the importance of omega-3 fatty acids, vitamin D, magnesium, and other micronutrients to reduce inflammation and thus maintain central sensitization processes.

All these therapeutic approaches (PNE, training, GA, GE, CBT, CFT, ACT, SDT, GMI, and MBSR) recognize the multidimensionality of chronic pain and give hope for promising results for often seemingly hopeless pain patients. These therapies focus not only on the pain, which can be seen as a symptom of nociplastic changes, but also on their bio-psycho-social drivers. Simple derivations can be made for practice:

1. Education about pain mechanisms and drivers
2. Promotion of progressive movement, activity, and participation
3. Reduction of fears by promoting positive thoughts, statements, and beliefs
4. Training of self-efficacy and non-judgmental handling of sensations
5. Cognitive relaxation techniques
6. Lifestyle changes such as sleep and nutrition optimization

Complex mechanisms, like those of chronic pain, do not require complicated approaches. On the other hand, reductionist and oversimplified approaches do not do justice to its complexity. Nevertheless, take-aways for patients should be tangible. Possibly, a good mix of basics, such as brief education and adapted movement exercises, is enough to start with. Individually relevant lifestyle changes, systematic training plans, and behavioral therapeutic approaches can be added gradually so that the patient is not overwhelmed at the beginning.

5.3.3 Change Management

In this philosophical-logical subchapter, change and what is necessary for it are discussed. In pain therapy, change is at the center. Whether it is the relief of pain or the application of a new therapy method—the goal is always a change in the existing state. However, change is a complex process that brings challenges for both patients and therapists, as well as the health system as a whole. This chapter illuminates the various aspects of change management in pain therapy and shows ways in which changes can be successfully initiated and implemented.

1. The therapeutic perspective: To bring about changes in pain therapy, it is first crucial to consider the perspective of the therapists. Therapists play a key role in implementing new approaches and influencing the patient perspective. Here, not only the *what* is important, but above all the *how*. The way therapists communicate and implement changes has a direct impact on their success. A crucial aspect is the conviction of the therapists themselves. Only if they are

convinced of the necessity and benefit of a change, such as their own level of knowledge, can they process it and then credibly convey it to the patients. This often requires a process of self-reflection and continuous further education. Therapists must be willing to critically question their own beliefs and practices and adjust them if necessary. Collaboration and exchange with colleagues also play an important role. Through professional discourse, new ideas can emerge and be disseminated. At the same time, this can also lead to resistance when established practices are questioned. It is therefore important to promote a culture of open dialogue and constructive criticism.
2. Systemic perspective: When considering changes in pain therapy, it is essential to also consider the systemic aspects. The handling of pain is often shaped by deeply rooted cultural and societal patterns, depending on the population group. These can hinder or favor changes. A significant system error lies in the often too one-sided focus on the purely physical dimension of pain. This often leads to an overemphasis on imaging procedures and drug therapies, while psycho-social and contextual factors are neglected. To correct this system error, a holistic approach is required that takes into account the bio-psycho-social nature of pain. Structural obstacles such as the specifications of statutory health insurance, limited time resources in practices, or standardized anamnesis questionnaires can also hinder changes. These structures must be made more flexible to enable innovative approaches in pain therapy.
3. The patient perspective: Ultimately, it is the patients in whom a change is to take place. Their perspective and willingness to change are crucial for the success of any therapy. It should be noted that patients often come into therapy with entrenched beliefs and expectations. Many patients expect a quick, passive solution for their pain, often in the form of medication, surgical interventions, or miraculous manual techniques. The switch to a more active, self-responsible approach can initially meet with resistance. Here it is important to gently introduce patients to new concepts and convey the benefits of a holistic approach. A crucial aspect is the education of the patients. Only if they understand how pain arises and what factors influence it, can they actively participate in their recovery. This requires time and patience on the part of the therapists, but pays off in the long run.
4. Implementation of changes: The implementation of changes in pain therapy is often associated with challenges. Psychologically speaking, people find it difficult to give up tried and tested things and to embrace new ones. The comfort of the familiar and various cognitive biases can hinder the change process.

To overcome these obstacles, a strategic approach is required. This can include the following steps:

a) Problem recognition: The first step is to clearly identify and communicate the problem. This often requires a detailed analysis of the current state.
b) Status quo report: An accurate measurement and documentation of the current situation is important in order to evaluate progress later on.

c) Acceptance: Both therapists and patients must accept the current situation. Only through acceptance of the current state can changes be brought about to a desired state.
d) Change of thoughts and actions: Based on acceptance, concrete steps for change can now be initiated. This includes both cognitive restructuring and behavior-oriented measures.
e) Reevaluation: After a set period of time, the status quo should be measured again and the problem reanalyzed. This allows for an evaluation of progress and, if necessary, an adjustment of the strategy.

The question of how best to motivate people to change is complex. Should one present an opposing extreme to move people to the middle? Or is it more effective to directly aim for the regulated middle? In practice, it often turns out that the path to the middle leads through experiencing extremes. People tend to switch from one extreme to another before they find a balanced position. In pain therapy, this could mean that the path from a purely biomedical view to a balanced bio-psycho-social approach leads through a phase in which psycho-social factors are overrated. The challenge is to design this process in such a way that it does not lead to new problems. To bring about changes, it is crucial to convince people. This applies to both therapists who are supposed to implement new approaches and patients who need to change their attitude towards pain and therapy.

Effective persuasion is based on several factors:

- Sympathy: People are more willing to accept ideas from someone they like. A trusting, empathetic relationship between therapist and patient is therefore of great importance.
- Consistency: The message must be coherent. Contradictory statements undermine credibility and make it harder to accept new ideas.
- Evidence: Scientific evidence for the effectiveness of new approaches can help convince skeptics.
- Adaptation: The way of communication should be adapted to the respective recipient. What works with a colleague may not necessarily be effective with a patient.

The question of whether to fully adapt to the goal of change or to find a compromise depends on the specific situation. In some cases, it may be sensible to proceed step by step and initially make a stopover to make the actual goal more attractive. In pain therapy, this could mean that patients are first made familiar with less radical changes before more comprehensive approaches are introduced. For example, one could start with simple relaxation techniques before introducing more complex behavioral therapeutic interventions.

Change management in pain therapy is a complex process that requires patience, empathy, and strategic thinking. It is about finding a balance between the need for change and the maintenance of proven practices. It encourages a continuous process of reflection and adjustment, both on an individual and systemic level.

Fig. 5.4 Correction to the middle, own creation

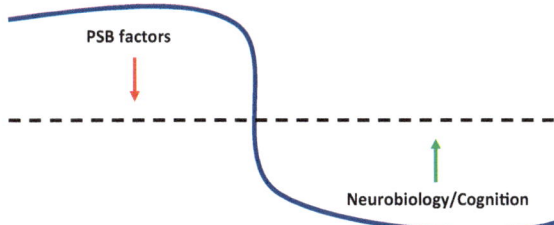

> **Excursus**
> Both in the teaching and knowledge expansion of health professionals, as well as in patient education, the motto is: **The correction to the middle** (Fig. 5.4) – Education for regulation, not elimination. Not everything old is wrong, and not everything new is right. It is about reducing and relativizing overrepresented, possibly less effective views/interventions/beliefs and underlining and recruiting underrepresented, possibly more relevant views.
> In this way, beliefs are brought into a homeostasis, which can coexist, interact with each other and even complement each other, without creating a gap between supposedly good and supposedly bad.

References

Allen, M. L., Cook, B. L., Carson, N., Interian, A., La Roche, M., & Alegría, M. (2017). Patient-provider therapeutic alliance contributes to patient activation in community mental health clinics. *Administration and policy in mental health, 44*(4), 431–440. https://doi.org/10.1007/s10488-015-0655-8.

Airaksinen, O., Brox, J. I., Cedraschi, C., Hildebrandt, J., Klaber-Moffett, J., Kovacs, F., Mannion, A. F., Reis, S., Staal, J. B., Ursin, H., Zanoli, G., & COST B13 Working Group on Guidelines for Chronic Low Back Pain (2006). Chapter 4. European guidelines for the management of chronic nonspecific low back pain. *European spine Journal : Official publication of the European Spine Society, the European Spinal Deformity Society, and the European Section of the Cervical Spine Research Society, 15 Suppl 2*(Suppl 2), S192–S300. https://doi.org/10.1007/s00586-006-1072-1.

Apkarian, A. V., Baliki, M. N., & Geha, P. Y. (2009). Towards a theory of chronic pain. *Progress in neurobiology, 87*(2), 81–97. https://doi.org/10.1016/j.pneurobio.2008.09.018.

Arnold, B., Brinkschmidt, T., Casser, H.-R., Diezemann, A., Gralow, I., Irnich, D., Kaiser, U., Klasen, B., Klimczyk, K., Lutz, J., Nagel, B., Pfingsten, M., Sabatowski, R., Schesser, R., Schesser, R., Schiltenwolf, M., Seeger, D., & Söllner, W. (2014). Multimodale Schmerztherapie für die Behandlung chronischer Schmerzsyndrome. *Der Schmerz, 28*(5), 459–472. https://doi.org/10.1007/s00482-014-1471-x.

Artus, M., van der Windt, D., Jordan, K. P., & Croft, P. R. (2014). The clinical course of low back pain: A meta-analysis comparing outcomes in randomised clinical trials (RCTs) and observational studies. *BMC musculoskeletal disorders, 15,* 68. https://doi.org/10.1186/1471-2474-15-68.

Atalay, E., Akova, B., Gür, H., & Sekir, U. (2017). Effect of upper-extremity strengthening exercises on the lumbar strength, disability and pain of patients with chronic low back pain: A randomized controlled study. *Journal of sports science & medicine, 16*(4), 595–603.

Bareiss, S. K., Nare, L., & McBee, K. (2019). Evaluation of pain knowledge and attitudes and beliefs from a pre-licensure physical therapy curriculum and a stand-alone pain elective. *BMC Medical Education, 19*(1), 375. https://doi.org/10.1186/s12909-019-1820-7.

Barker, K. L., Reid, M., & Minns Lowe, C. J. (2009). Divided by a lack of common language? A qualitative study exploring the use of language by health professionals treating back pain. *BMC musculoskeletal disorders, 10*, 123. https://doi.org/10.1186/1471-2474-10-123.

Baron, R., Perrot, S., Guillemin, I., Alegre, C., Dias-Barbosa, C., Choy, E., Gilet, H., Cruccu, G., Desmeules, J., Margaux, J., Richards, S., Serra, E., Spaeth, M., & Arnould, B. (2014). Improving the primary care physicians' decision making for fibromyalgia in clinical practice: Development and validation of the Fibromyalgia Detection (FibroDetect®) screening tool. *Health and quality of life outcomes, 12*, 128. https://doi.org/10.1186/s12955-014-0128-x.

Bassimtabar, A., & Alfuth, M. (2023). Entwicklung und Validierung eines Fragebogens zur Erfassung postural-strukturell-biomechanisch orientierter Überzeugungen von Physiotherapeut: Innen zu Schmerzen [Development and validation of a questionnaire to assess physiotherapists' postural-structural-biomechanical-oriented beliefs about pain]. *Schmerz (Berlin, Germany),* https://doi.org/10.1007/s00482-023-00757-y. Advance online publication. https://doi.org/10.1007/s00482-023-00757-y.

Bassimtabar, A., & Alfuth, M. (2024). Aktueller Wissensstand deutscher Physiotherapieschüler und -studenten über Schmerz und der Einfluss einer Lehrintervention [Current knowledge of German physiotherapy trainees and students on pain and the influence of a teaching intervention]. *Schmerz (Berlin, Germany),* https://doi.org/10.1007/s00482-024-00832-y. Advance online publication. https://doi.org/10.1007/s00482-024-00832-y.

Benedetti, F., Frisaldi, E., Barbiani, D., Camerone, E., & Shaibani, A. (2020). Nocebo and the contribution of psychosocial factors to the generation of pain. *Journal of neural transmission (Vienna, Austria: 1996), 127*(4), 687–696. https://doi.org/10.1007/s00702-019-02104-x.

Bennett, M. I., Smith, B. H., Torrance, N., & Potter, J. (2005). The S-LANSS score for identifying pain of predominantly neuropathic origin: Validation for use in clinical and postal research. *The Journal of pain, 6*(3), 149–158. https://doi.org/10.1016/j.jpain.2004.11.007.

Bera, S. C., Khandelwal, S. K., Sood, M., & Goyal, V. (2014). A comparative study of psychiatric comorbidity, quality of life and disability in patients with migraine and tension type headache. *Neurology India, 62*(5), 516–520. https://doi.org/10.4103/0028-3886.144445.

Blasini, M., Corsi, N., Klinger, R., & Colloca, L. (2017). Nocebo and pain: An overview of the psychoneurobiological mechanisms. *Pain reports, 2*(2), e585. https://doi.org/10.1097/PR9.0000000000000585.

Bodes Pardo, G., Lluch Girbés, E., Roussel, N. A., Gallego Izquierdo, T., Jiménez Penick, V., & Pecos Martín, D. (2018). Pain Neurophysiology education and therapeutic exercise for patients with chronic low back pain: A single-blind randomized controlled trial. *Archives of physical medicine and rehabilitation, 99*(2), 338–347. https://doi.org/10.1016/j.apmr.2017.10.016.

Bond, M. R., & Pilowsky, I. (1966). Subjective assessment of pain and its relationship to the administration of analgesics in patients with advanced cancer. *Journal of psychosomatic research, 10*(2), 203–208. https://doi.org/10.1016/0022-3999(66)90064-x.

Bonezzi, C., Fornasari, D., Cricelli, C., Magni, A., & Ventriglia, G. (2020). Not all pain is created equal: Basic definitions and diagnostic work-up. *Pain and therapy, 9*(Suppl 1), 1–15. https://doi.org/10.1007/s40122-020-00217-w.

Bouhassira, D., Attal, N., Alchaar, H., Boureau, F., Brochet, B., Bruxelle, J., Cunin, G., Fermanian, J., Ginies, P., Grun-Overdyking, A., Jafari-Schluep, H., Lantéri-Minet, M., Laurent, B., Mick, G., Serrie, A., Valade, D., & Vicaut, E. (2005). Comparison of pain syndromes associated with nervous or somatic lesions and development of a new neuropathic pain diagnostic questionnaire (DN4). *Pain, 114*(1–2), 29–36. https://doi.org/10.1016/j.pain.2004.12.010.

References

Bowering, K. J., O'Connell, N. E., Tabor, A., Catley, M. J., Leake, H. B., Moseley, G. L., & Stanton, T. R. (2013). The effects of graded motor imagery and its components on chronic pain: A systematic review and meta-analysis. *The Journal of pain, 14*(1), 3–13. https://doi.org/10.1016/j.jpain.2012.09.007.

Brain, K., Burrows, T. L., Rollo, M. E., Chai, L. K., Clarke, E. D., Hayes, C., Hodson, F. J., & Collins, C. E. (2019). A systematic review and meta-analysis of nutrition interventions for chronic noncancer pain. *Journal of human nutrition and dietetics: The official Journal of the British Dietetic Association, 32*(2), 198–225. https://doi.org/10.1111/jhn.12601.

Burns, L. C., Ritvo, S. E., Ferguson, M. K., Clarke, H., Seltzer, Z., & Katz, J. (2015). Pain catastrophizing as a risk factor for chronic pain after total knee arthroplasty: A systematic review. *Journal of pain research, 8,* 21–32. https://doi.org/10.2147/JPR.S64730.

Burrowes, S. A. B., Goloubeva, O., Stafford, K., McArdle, P. F., Goyal, M., Peterlin, B. L., Haythornthwaite, J. A., & Seminowicz, D. A. (2022). Enhanced mindfulness-based stress reduction in episodic migraine-effects on sleep quality, anxiety, stress, and depression: A secondary analysis of a randomized clinical trial. *Pain, 163*(3), 436–444. https://doi.org/10.1097/j.pain.0000000000002372.

Calatayud, J., Guzmán-González, B., Andersen, L. L., Cruz-Montecinos, C., Morell, M. T., Roldán, R., Ezzatvar, Y., & Casaña, J. (2020). Effectiveness of a group-based progressive strength training in primary care to improve the recurrence of low back pain exacerbations and function: A randomised trial. *International Journal of environmental research and public health, 17*(22), 8326. https://doi.org/10.3390/ijerph17228326.

Calle, M. C., & Fernandez, M. L. (2010). Effects of resistance training on the inflammatory response. *Nutrition research and practice, 4*(4), 259–269. https://doi.org/10.4162/nrp.2010.4.4.259.

Callow, D. D., Arnold-Nedimala, N. A., Jordan, L. S., Pena, G. S., Won, J., Woodard, J. L., & Smith, J. C. (2020). The mental health benefits of physical activity in older adults survive the COVID-19 pandemic. *The American Journal of geriatric psychiatry: Official Journal of the American Association for Geriatric Psychiatry, 28*(10), 1046–1057. https://doi.org/10.1016/j.jagp.2020.06.024.

Cappelleri, J. C., Koduru, V., Bienen, E. J., & Sadosky, A. (2016). Characterizing neuropathic pain profiles: Enriching interpretation of painDETECT. *Patient related outcome measures, 7,* 93–99. https://doi.org/10.2147/PROM.S101892.

Catley, M. J., O'Connell, N. E., & Moseley, G. L. (2013). How good is the neurophysiology of pain questionnaire? A rasch analysis of psychometric properties. *The Journal of pain: Official Journal of the American Pain Society, 14*(8), 818–827. https://doi.org/10.1016/j.jpain.2013.02.008.

Chelimsky, T. C., Fischer, R. L., Levin, J. B., Cheren, M. I., Marsh, S. K., & Janata, J. W. (2013). The primary practice physician program for chronic pain (© 4PCP): Outcomes of a primary physician-pain specialist collaboration for community-based training and support. *The Clinical Journal of pain, 29*(12), 1036–1043. https://doi.org/10.1097/AJP.0b013e3182851584.

Chen, Y., Campbell, P., Strauss, V. Y., Foster, N. E., Jordan, K. P., & Dunn, K. M. (2018). Trajectories and predictors of the long-term course of low back pain: Cohort study with 5-year follow-up. *Pain, 159*(2), 252–260. https://doi.org/10.1097/j.pain.0000000000001097.

Chiarotto, A., Maxwell, L. J., Terwee, C. B., Wells, G. A., Tugwell, P., & Ostelo, R. W. (2016). Roland-morris disability questionnaire and oswestry disability index: Which has better measurement properties for measuring physical functioning in nonspecific low back pain? Systematic review and meta-analysis. *Physical therapy, 96*(10), 1620–1637. https://doi.org/10.2522/ptj.20150420.

Clenzos, N., Naidoo, N., & Parker, R. (2013). Physiotherapists' knowledge of pain: A cross-sectional correlational study of members of the South African Sports and Orthopaedic Manipulative Special Interest Groups. *South African Journal of Sports Medicine, 25,* 95. https://doi.org/10.17159/2078-516X/2013/v25i4a337.

Colleary, G., O'Sullivan, K., Griffin, D., Ryan, C. G., & Martin, D. J. (2017). Effect of pain neurophysiology education on physiotherapy students' understanding of chronic pain, clinical recommendations and attitudes towards people with chronic pain: A randomised controlled trial. *Physiotherapy, 103*(4), 423–429. https://doi.org/10.1016/j.physio.2017.01.006.

Copay, A. G., & Cher, D. J. (2016). Is the Oswestry disability Index a valid measure of response to sacroiliac joint treatment? *Quality of life research: An international Journal of quality of life aspects of treatment, care and rehabilitation, 25*(2), 283–292. https://doi.org/10.1007/s11136-015-1095-3.

Cormack, B., & Rossettini, G. (2023). Are patients picking up what we are putting down? Considering nocebo effects in exercise for musculoskeletal pain. *Frontiers in psychology, 14,* 1291770. https://doi.org/10.3389/fpsyg.2023.1291770.

Cortell-Tormo, J. M., Sánchez, P. T., Chulvi-Medrano, I., Tortosa-Martínez, J., Manchado-López, C., Llana-Belloch, S., & Pérez-Soriano, P. (2018). Effects of functional resistance training on fitness and quality of life in females with chronic nonspecific low-back pain. *Journal of back and musculoskeletal rehabilitation, 31*(1), 95–105. https://doi.org/10.3233/BMR-169684.

Cox, T., Louw, A., & Puentedura, E. J. (2017). An abbreviated therapeutic neuroscience education session improves pain knowledge in first-year physical therapy students but does not change attitudes or beliefs. *The Journal of manual & manipulative therapy, 25*(1), 11–21. https://doi.org/10.1080/10669817.2015.1122308.

Darlow, B., Dean, S., Perry, M., Mathieson, F., Baxter, G. D., & Dowell, A. (2015). Easy to harm, hard to heal: patient views about the back. *Spine, 40*(11), 842–850. https://doi.org/10.1097/BRS.0000000000000901.

Darnall, B. D., & Colloca, L. (2018). Optimizing placebo and minimizing nocebo to reduce pain, catastrophizing, and opioid use: a review of the science and an evidence-informed clinical toolkit. *International review of neurobiology, 139,* 129–157. https://doi.org/10.1016/bs.irn.2018.07.022.

de Jong, J. R., Vlaeyen, J. W. S., Onghena, P., Cuypers, C., den Hollander, M., & Ruijgrok, J. (2005). Reduction of pain-related fear in complex regional pain syndrome type I: The application of graded exposure in vivo. *Pain, 116*(3), 264–275. https://doi.org/10.1016/j.pain.2005.04.019.

den Hollander, M., Goossens, M., de Jong, J., Ruijgrok, J., Oosterhof, J., Onghena, P., Smeets, R., & Vlaeyen, J. W. S. (2016). Expose or protect? A randomized controlled trial of exposure in vivo vs pain-contingent treatment as usual in patients with complex regional pain syndrome type 1. *Pain, 157*(10), 2318–2329. https://doi.org/10.1097/j.pain.0000000000000651.

Delgado, D. A., Lambert, B. S., Boutris, N., McCulloch, P. C., Robbins, A. B., Moreno, M. R., & Harris, J. D. (2018). Validation of digital visual analog scale pain scoring with a traditional paper-based visual analog scale in adults. *Journal of the American Academy of Orthopaedic Surgeons. Global research & reviews, 2*(3), e088. https://doi.org/10.5435/JAAOSGlobal-D-17-00088.

de Zoete, R. M., Armfield, N. R., McAuley, J. H., Chen, K., & Sterling, M. (2020). Comparative effectiveness of physical exercise interventions for chronic non-specific neck pain: A systematic review with network meta-analysis of 40 randomised controlled trials. *British Journal of sports medicine,* bjsports-2020-102664. Advance online publication. https://doi.org/10.1136/bjsports-2020-102664.

de Zoete, R. M. J., Berryman, C. F., Nijs, J., Walls, A., & Jenkinson, M. (2023). Differential structural brain changes between responders and nonresponders after physical exercise therapy for chronic nonspecific neck pain. *The Clinical Journal of pain, 39*(6), 270–277. https://doi.org/10.1097/AJP.0000000000001115.

Diers, M., Christmann, C., Koeppe, C., Ruf, M., & Flor, H. (2010). Mirrored, imagined and executed movements differentially activate sensorimotor cortex in amputees with and without phantom limb pain. *Pain, 149*(2), 296–304. https://doi.org/10.1016/j.pain.2010.02.020.

Dupuis, F., Cherif, A., Batcho, C., Massé-Alarie, H., & Roy, J. S. (2023). The Tampa scale of Kinesiophobia: A systematic review of its psychometric properties in people with musculoskeletal pain. *The clinical Journal of pain, 39*(5), 236–247. https://doi.org/10.1097/AJP.0000000000001104.

Ehde, D. M., Dillworth, T. M., & Turner, J. A. (2014). Cognitive-behavioral therapy for individuals with chronic pain: Efficacy, innovations, and directions for research. *The American psychologist, 69*(2), 153–166. https://doi.org/10.1037/a0035747.

Erk, S. M., Toet, A., & Van Erp, J. B. (2015). Effects of mediated social touch on affective experiences and trust. *PeerJ, 3,* e1297. https://doi.org/10.7717/peerj.1297.

Fang, X. X., Zhai, M. N., Zhu, M., He, C., Wang, H., Wang, J., & Zhang, Z. J. (2023). Inflammation in pathogenesis of chronic pain: Foe and friend. *Molecular pain, 19,* 17448069231178176. https://doi.org/10.1177/17448069231178176.

Fedorak, C., Ashworth, N., Marshall, J., & Paull, H. (2003). Reliability of the visual assessment of cervical and lumbar lordosis: How good are we? *Spine, 28*(16), 1857–1859. https://doi.org/10.1097/01.BRS.0000083281.48923.BD.

Fieke Linskens, F. G., van der Scheer, E. S., Stortenbeker, I., Das, E., Staal, J. B., & van Lankveld, W. (2023). Negative language use of the physiotherapist in low back pain education impacts anxiety and illness beliefs: A randomised controlled trial in healthy respondents. *Patient education and counseling, 110,* 107649. https://doi.org/10.1016/j.pec.2023.107649.

Finan, P. H., Goodin, B. R., & Smith, M. T. (2013). The association of sleep and pain: An update and a path forward. *The Journal of pain, 14*(12), 1539–1552. https://doi.org/10.1016/j.jpain.2013.08.007.

Fischerauer, S. F., Talaei-Khoei, M., Bexkens, R., Ring, D. C., Oh, L. S., & Vranceanu, A. M. (2018). What is the relationship of fear avoidance to physical function and pain intensity in injured athletes? *Clinical orthopaedics and related research, 476*(4), 754–763. https://doi.org/10.1007/s11999.0000000000000085.

Fitzgerald, K., Fleischmann, M., Vaughan, B., de Waal, K., Slater, S., & Harbis, J. (2018). Changes in pain knowledge, attitudes and beliefs of osteopathy students after completing a clinically focused pain education module. *Chiropractic & manual therapies, 26,* 42. https://doi.org/10.1186/s12998-018-0212-0.

Fletcher, C., Bradnam, L., & Barr, C. (2016). The relationship between knowledge of pain neurophysiology and fear avoidance in people with chronic pain: A point in time, observational study. *Physiotherapy theory and practice, 32*(4), 271–276. https://doi.org/10.3109/09593985.2015.1138010.

Flor, H., Elbert, T., Knecht, S., Wienbruch, C., Pantev, C., Birbaumer, N., Larbig, W., & Taub, E. (1995). Phantom-limb pain as a perceptual correlate of cortical reorganization following arm amputation. *Nature, 375*(6531), 482–484. https://doi.org/10.1038/375482a0.

Foadi, N., Winkelmann, I., Rhein, M., et al. (2024). Retrospektive Auswertung elektronisch erhobener Patientenfragebögen einer universitären Schmerzambulanz mit dem painDETECT®-Fragebogen. *Schmerz, 38,* 205–215. https://doi.org/10.1007/s00482-022-00677-3.

Fujii, T., Oka, H., Takano, K., Asada, F., Nomura, T., Kawamata, K., Okazaki, H., Tanaka, S., & Matsudaira, K. (2019). Association between high fear-avoidance beliefs about physical activity and chronic disabling low back pain in nurses in Japan. *BMC musculoskeletal disorders, 20*(1), 572. https://doi.org/10.1186/s12891-019-2965-6.

Fusaro, M., Bufacchi, R. J., Nicolardi, V., & Provenzano, L. (2022). The analgesic power of pleasant touch in individuals with chronic pain: Recent findings and new insights. *Frontiers in integrative neuroscience, 16,* 956510. https://doi.org/10.3389/fnint.2022.956510.

Gadotti, I. C., Armijo-Olivo, S., Silveira, A., & Magee, D. (2013). Reliability of the craniocervical posture assessment: Visual and angular measurements using photographs and radiographs. *Journal of manipulative and physiological therapeutics, 36*(9), 619–625. https://doi.org/10.1016/j.jmpt.2013.09.002.

Gatchel, R. J., Peng, Y. B., Peters, M. L., Fuchs, P. N., & Turk, D. C. (2007). The biopsychosocial approach to chronic pain: Scientific advances and future directions. *Psychological bulletin, 133*(4), 581–624. https://doi.org/10.1037/0033-2909.133.4.581.

Geneen, L. J., Martin, D. J., Adams, N., Clarke, C., Dunbar, M., Jones, D., McNamee, P., Schofield, P., & Smith, B. H. (2015). Effects of education to facilitate knowledge about

chronic pain for adults: A systematic review with meta-analysis. *Systematic reviews, 4,* 132. https://doi.org/10.1186/s13643-015-0120-5.
Geneen, L. J., Moore, R. A., Clarke, C., Martin, D., Colvin, L. A., & Smith, B. H. (2017). Physical activity and exercise for chronic pain in adults: An overview of Cochrane Reviews. *The Cochrane database of systematic reviews, 4*(4), CD011279. https://doi.org/10.1002/14651858.CD011279.pub3.
George, S. Z., Valencia, C., & Beneciuk, J. M. (2010). A psychometric investigation of fear-avoidance model measures in patients with chronic low back pain. *The Journal of orthopaedic and sports physical therapy, 40*(4), 197–205. https://doi.org/10.2519/jospt.2010.3298.
Gilanyi, Y. L., Wewege, M. A., Shah, B., Cashin, A. G., Williams, C. M., Davidson, S. R. E., McAuley, J. H., & Jones, M. D. (2023). Exercise increases pain self-efficacy in adults with nonspecific chronic low back pain: A systematic review and meta-analysis. *The Journal of orthopaedic and sports physical therapy, 53*(6), 335–342. https://doi.org/10.2519/jospt.2023.1162.
Goldstein, P., Weissman-Fogel, I., & Shamay-Tsoory, S. G. (2017). The role of touch in regulating inter-partner physiological coupling during empathy for pain. *Scientific reports, 7*(1), 3252. https://doi.org/10.1038/s41598-017-03627-7.
Goode, A., Hegedus, E. J., Sizer, P., Brismee, J. M., Linberg, A., & Cook, C. E. (2008). Three-dimensional movements of the sacroiliac joint: A systematic review of the literature and assessment of clinical utility. *The Journal of manual & manipulative therapy, 16*(1), 25–38. https://doi.org/10.1179/106698108790818639.
Hadley, G., & Novitch, M. B. (2021). CBT and CFT for chronic pain. *Current pain and headache reports, 25*(5), 35. https://doi.org/10.1007/s11916-021-00948-1.
Hall, A. M., Ferreira, P. H., Maher, C. G., Latimer, J., & Ferreira, M. L. (2010). The influence of the therapist-patient relationship on treatment outcome in physical rehabilitation: A systematic review. *Physical therapy, 90*(8), 1099–1110. https://doi.org/10.2522/ptj.20090245.
Hapidou, E. G., O'Brien, M. A., Pierrynowski, M. R., de Las Heras, E., Patel, M., & Patla, T. (2012). Fear and avoidance of movement in people with chronic pain: Psychometric properties of the 11-Item Tampa Scale for Kinesiophobia (TSK-11). *Physiotherapy Canada. Physiotherapie Canada, 64*(3), 235–241. https://doi.org/10.3138/ptc.2011-10.
Harris, J. M., Jr, Elliott, T. E., Davis, B. E., Chabal, C., Fulginiti, J. V., & Fine, P. G. (2008). Educating generalist physicians about chronic pain: Live experts and online education can provide durable benefits. *Pain medicine (Malden, Mass.), 9*(5), 555–563. https://doi.org/10.1111/j.1526-4637.2007.00399.x.
Hasenbring, M., Hallner, D., & Klasen, B. (2001). Psychologische Mechanismen im Prozess der Schmerzchronifizierung. *Der Schmerz, 15,* 442–447.
Haugen, F. P., & Livingston, W. K. (1953). Experiences with the Hardy-Wolff-Goodell dolorimeter. *Anesthesiology, 14*(2), 109–116. https://doi.org/10.1097/00000542-195303000-00001.
Holmgren, U., & Waling, K. (2008). Inter-examiner reliability of four static palpation tests used for assessing pelvic dysfunction. *Manual therapy, 13*(1), 50–56. https://doi.org/10.1016/j.math.2006.09.009.
Hölzel, B. K., Carmody, J., Vangel, M., Congleton, C., Yerramsetti, S. M., Gard, T., & Lazar, S. W. (2011). Mindfulness practice leads to increases in regional brain gray matter density. *Psychiatry research, 191*(1), 36–43. https://doi.org/10.1016/j.pscychresns.2010.08.006.
Houts, C. R., McGinley, J. S., Wirth, R. J., Cady, R., & Lipton, R. B. (2021). Reliability and validity of the 6-item headache impact test in chronic migraine from the PROMISE-2 study. *Quality of life research: An international Journal of quality of life aspects of treatment, care and rehabilitation, 30*(3), 931–943. https://doi.org/10.1007/s11136-020-02668-2.
Hughes, L. S., Clark, J., Colclough, J. A., Dale, E., & McMillan, D. (2017). Acceptance and Commitment Therapy (ACT) for chronic pain: A systematic review and meta-analyses. *The clinical Journal of pain, 33*(6), 552–568. https://doi.org/10.1097/AJP.0000000000000425.
Hush, J. M., Nicholas, M., & Dean, C. M. (2018). Embedding the IASP pain curriculum into a 3-year pre-licensure physical therapy program: Redesigning pain education for future clinicians. *Pain reports, 3*(2), e645. https://doi.org/10.1097/PR9.0000000000000645.

Hüter-Becker, A. (2000). Der Paradigmenwechsel in der Physiotherapie und das Bobath-Konzept. *Krankengymnastik, 52*(2), 277–282.

International Association for the Study of Pain (IASP). IASP Curriculum outline on pain for physical therapy (2018). Abgerufen 07.07.2024 von https://www.iasp-pain.org/Education/CurriculumDetail.aspx?ItemNumber=2055.

Jackson, J. K., Shepherd, T. R., & Kell, R. T. (2011). The influence of periodized resistance training on recreationally active males with chronic nonspecific low back pain. *Journal of strength and conditioning research, 25*(1), 242–251. https://doi.org/10.1519/JSC.0b013e3181b2c83d.

Jackson, T., Wang, Y., Wang, Y., & Fan, H. (2014). Self-efficacy and chronic pain outcomes: A meta-analytic review. *The Journal of pain, 15*(8), 800–814. https://doi.org/10.1016/j.jpain.2014.05.002.

Jensen, K. B., Kosek, E., Wicksell, R., Kemani, M., Olsson, G., Merle, J. V., Kadetoff, D., & Ingvar, M. (2012). Cognitive behavioral therapy increases pain-evoked activation of the prefrontal cortex in patients with fibromyalgia. *Pain, 153*(7), 1495–1503. https://doi.org/10.1016/j.pain.2012.04.010.

Jiang, Y., Angeletti, P. C., & Hoffman, A. J. (2023). Investigating the physiological mechanisms between resistance training and pain relief in the cancer population: A literature review. *Journal of cancer therapy, 14*(2), 80–101. https://doi.org/10.4236/jct.2023.142008.

Johnston, M., Foster, M., Shennan, J., Starkey, N. J., & Johnson, A. (2010). The effectiveness of an acceptance and commitment therapy self-help intervention for chronic pain. *The clinical Journal of pain, 26*(5), 393–402. https://doi.org/10.1097/AJP.0b013e3181cf59ce.

Jorritsma, W., Dijkstra, P. U., de Vries, G. E., Geertzen, J. H., & Reneman, M. F. (2012). Detecting relevant changes and responsiveness of neck pain and disability scale and neck disability index. *European spine Journal: Official publication of the European Spine Society, the European Spinal Deformity Society, and the European Section of the Cervical Spine Research Society, 21*(12), 2550–2557. https://doi.org/10.1007/s00586-012-2407-8.

Jungquist, C. R., O'Brien, C., Matteson-Rusby, S., Smith, M. T., Pigeon, W. R., Xia, Y., Lu, N., & Perlis, M. L. (2010). The efficacy of cognitive-behavioral therapy for insomnia in patients with chronic pain. *Sleep medicine, 11*(3), 302–309. https://doi.org/10.1016/j.sleep.2009.05.018.

Kabat-Zinn, J. (2005). Full catastrophe living: using the wisdom of your body and mind to face stress, pain, and illness. *Random House*. https://books.google.de/books?hl=de&lr=&id=TVsrK0sjGiUC&oi=fnd&pg=PR13&ots=eHm4d0jn00&sig=mLgIysnSpXAQseewyHzNlxHF9VM&redir_esc=y#v=onepage&q&f=false. Zugegriffen: 22. Aug. 2024.

Kami, K., Tajima, F., & Senba, E. (2022). Brain mechanisms of exercise-induced Hypoalgesia: To find a way out from "Fear-Avoidance Belief". *International Journal of molecular sciences, 23*(5), 2886. https://doi.org/10.3390/ijms23052886.

Kaushik, A. S., Strath, L. J., & Sorge, R. E. (2020). Dietary interventions for treatment of chronic pain: oxidative stress and inflammation. *Pain and therapy, 9*(2), 487–498. https://doi.org/10.1007/s40122-020-00200-5.

Koltyn, K. F., Brellenthin, A. G., Cook, D. B., Sehgal, N., & Hillard, C. (2014). Mechanisms of exercise-induced hypoalgesia. *The Journal of pain, 15*(12), 1294–1304. https://doi.org/10.1016/j.jpain.2014.09.006.

Krug, J. (2022). Motorische Fähigkeiten: Konzept, Entwicklungen, Theorienvergleiche. In Güllich, A., & Krüger, M. (Eds) Bewegung, Training, Leistung und Gesundheit. Springer, Berlin, Heidelberg. https://doi.org/10.1007/978-3-662-53386-4_40-2.

Kuss, K., Leonhardt, C., Quint, S., Seeger, D., Pfingsten, M., Wolf Pt, U., Basler, H. D., & Becker, A. (2016). Graded activity for older adults with chronic low back pain: Program development and mixed methods feasibility cohort study. *Pain medicine (Malden, Mass.), 17*(12), 2218–2229. https://doi.org/10.1093/pm/pnw062.

Lakke, S. E., Soer, R., Krijnen, W. P., van der Schans, C. P., Reneman, M. F., & Geertzen, J. H. (2015). Influence of physical therapists' Kinesiophobic beliefs on lifting capacity in healthy adults. *Physical therapy, 95*(9), 1224–1233. https://doi.org/10.2522/ptj.20130194.

Lederman, E. (2011). The fall of the postural-structural-biomechanical model in manual and physical therapies: Exemplified by lower back pain. *Journal of bodywork and movement therapies, 15*(2), 131–138. https://doi.org/10.1016/j.jbmt.2011.01.011.

Leeuw, M., Goossens, M. E., Linton, S. J., Crombez, G., Boersma, K., & Vlaeyen, J. W. (2007). The fear-avoidance model of musculoskeletal pain: Current state of scientific evidence. *Journal of behavioral medicine, 30*(1), 77–94. https://doi.org/10.1007/s10865-006-9085-0.

Leeuw, M., Goossens, M. E. J. B., van Breukelen, G. J. P., de Jong, J. R., Heuts, P. H. T. G., Smeets, R. J. E. M., Köke, A. J. A., & Vlaeyen, J. W. S. (2008). Exposure in vivo versus operant graded activity in chronic low back pain patients: Results of a randomized controlled trial. *Pain, 138*(1), 192–207. https://doi.org/10.1016/j.pain.2007.12.009.

Leonard, M. T., Chatkoff, D. K., & Gallaway, M. (2013). Association between pain catastrophizing, spouse responses to pain, and blood pressure in chronic pain patients: A pathway to potential comorbidity. *International Journal of behavioral medicine, 20*(4), 590–598. https://doi.org/10.1007/s12529-012-9262-1.

Leonardi, M., Lee, H., Kostanjsek, N., Fornari, A., Raggi, A., Martinuzzi, A., Yáñez, M., Almborg, A. H., Fresk, M., Besstrashnova, Y., Shoshmin, A., Castro, S. S., Cordeiro, E. S., Cuenot, M., Haas, C., Maart, S., Maribo, T., Miller, J., Mukaino, M., ... Kraus de Camargo, O. (2022). 20 Years of ICF-International Classification of Functioning, disability and health: Uses and applications around the world. *International Journal of environmental research and public health, 19*(18), 11321. https://doi.org/10.3390/ijerph191811321.

Limakatso, K., Madden, V. J., Manie, S., & Parker, R. (2020). The effectiveness of graded motor imagery for reducing phantom limb pain in amputees: A randomised controlled trial. *Physiotherapy, 109,* 65–74. https://doi.org/10.1016/j.physio.2019.06.009.

Liu, H., Gao, X., & Hou, Y. (2019). Effects of mindfulness-based stress reduction combined with music therapy on pain, anxiety, and sleep quality in patients with osteosarcoma. *Revista brasileira de psiquiatria (Sao Paulo, Brazil: 1999), 41*(6), 540–545. https://doi.org/10.1590/1516-4446-2018-0346.

Louw, A., Diener, I., Landers, M. R., & Puentedura, E. J. (2014). Preoperative pain neuroscience education for lumbar radiculopathy: A multicenter randomized controlled trial with 1-year follow-up. *Spine, 39*(18), 1449–1457. https://doi.org/10.1097/BRS.0000000000000444.

Louw, A., Farrell, K., Wettach, L., Uhl, J., Majkowski, K., & Welding, M. (2015). Immediate effects of sensory discrimination for chronic low back pain: A case series. *The New Zealand Journal of physiotherapy, 43.* https://doi.org/10.15619/NZJP/43.2.06.

Louw, A., Puentedura, E. J., Zimney, K., & Schmidt, S. (2016). Know pain, know gain? A perspective on pain neuroscience education in physical therapy. *The Journal of orthopaedic and sports physical therapy, 46*(3), 131–134. https://doi.org/10.2519/jospt.2016.0602.

Lucas, N., Macaskill, P., Irwig, L., Moran, R., & Bogduk, N. (2009). Reliability of physical examination for diagnosis of myofascial trigger points: A systematic review of the literature. *The clinical Journal of pain, 25*(1), 80–89. https://doi.org/10.1097/AJP.0b013e31817e13b6.

Macedo, L. G., Smeets, R. J., Maher, C. G., Latimer, J., & McAuley, J. H. (2010). Graded activity and graded exposure for persistent nonspecific low back pain: A systematic review. *Physical therapy, 90*(6), 860–879. https://doi.org/10.2522/ptj.20090303.

Macêdo Santiago, L. Â., Neto, L. G. L., Borges Pereira, G., Leite, R. D., Mostarda, C. T., de Oliveira Brito Monzani, J., Sousa, W. R., Rodrigues Pinheiro, A. J. M., & Navarro, F. (2018). Effects of resistance training on immunoinflammatory response, TNF-Alpha gene expression, and body composition in elderly women. *Journal of aging research, 2018,* 1467025. https://doi.org/10.1155/2018/1467025.

Maestroni, L., Read, P., Bishop, C., Papadopoulos, K., Suchomel, T. J., Comfort, P., & Turner, A. (2020). The benefits of strength training on musculoskeletal system health: practical applications for interdisciplinary care. *Sports medicine (Auckland, N.Z.), 50*(8), 1431–1450. https://doi.org/10.1007/s40279-020-01309-5.

Magalhães, M. O., Comachio, J., Ferreira, P. H., Pappas, E., & Marques, A. P. (2018). Effectiveness of graded activity versus physiotherapy in patients with chronic nonspecific low back pain: Midterm follow up results of a randomized controlled trial. *Brazilian Journal of physical therapy, 22*(1), 82–91. https://doi.org/10.1016/j.bjpt.2017.07.002.

Maguire, N., Chesterton, P., & Ryan, C. (2019). The effect of pain neuroscience education on sports therapy and rehabilitation students' knowledge, attitudes, and clinical recommendations toward athletes with chronic pain. *Journal of sport rehabilitation, 28*(5), 438–443. https://doi.org/10.1123/jsr.2017-0212.

Maigne, J. Y., Cornelis, P., & Chatellier, G. (2012). Lower back pain and neck pain: Is it possible to identify the painful side by palpation only? *Annals of physical and rehabilitation medicine, 55*(2), 103–111. https://doi.org/10.1016/j.rehab.2012.01.001.

Manchikanti, L., Singh, V., Falco, F. J., Benyamin, R. M., & Hirsch, J. A. (2014). Epidemiology of low back pain in adults. *Neuromodulation: Journal of the International Neuromodulation Society, 17*(Suppl 2), 3–10. https://doi.org/10.1111/ner.12018.

Mancini, F., Nash, T., Iannetti, G. D., & Haggard, P. (2014). Pain relief by touch: A quantitative approach. *Pain, 155*(3), 635–642. https://doi.org/10.1016/j.pain.2013.12.024.

Mannion, A. F., Junge, A., Fairbank, J. C., Dvorak, J., & Grob, D. (2006). Development of a German version of the Oswestry disability index. Part 1: Cross-cultural adaptation, reliability, and validity. *European spine Journal: Official publication of the European Spine Society, the European Spinal Deformity Society, and the European Section of the Cervical Spine Research Society, 15*(1), 55–65. https://doi.org/10.1007/s00586-004-0815-0.

Marques, E., Xarles, T., Antunes, T., da Silva, K. K., Reis, F., Oliveira, L., & Nogueira, L. (2016). Evaluation of physiologic pain knowledge by physiotherapy students. *Revista Dor, 17.* https://doi.org/10.5935/1806-0013.20160008.

Martel, M. O., Wasan, A. D., Jamison, R. N., & Edwards, R. R. (2013). Catastrophic thinking and increased risk for prescription opioid misuse in patients with chronic pain. *Drug and alcohol dependence, 132*(1–2), 335–341. https://doi.org/10.1016/j.drugalcdep.2013.02.034.

Mayer, T. G., Neblett, R., Cohen, H., Howard, K. J., Choi, Y. H., Williams, M. J., Perez, Y., & Gatchel, R. J. (2012). The development and psychometric validation of the central sensitization inventory. *Pain practice: The official Journal of World Institute of Pain, 12*(4), 276–285. https://doi.org/10.1111/j.1533-2500.2011.00493.x.

McCracken, L. M., & Vowles, K. E. (2014). Acceptance and commitment therapy and mindfulness for chronic pain: Model, process, and progress. *The American psychologist, 69*(2), 178–187. https://doi.org/10.1037/a0035623.

Meeus, M., Nijs, J., Van Oosterwijck, J., Van Alsenoy, V., & Truijen, S. (2010). Pain physiology education improves pain beliefs in patients with chronic fatigue syndrome compared with pacing and self-management education: A double-blind randomized controlled trial. *Archives of physical medicine and rehabilitation, 91*(8), 1153–1159. https://doi.org/10.1016/j.apmr.2010.04.020.

Melzack, R., & Torgerson, W. S. (1971). On the language of pain. *Anesthesiology, 34*(1), 50–59. https://doi.org/10.1097/00000542-197101000-00017.

Melzack, R. (2005). The McGill pain questionnaire: From description to measurement. *Anesthesiology, 103*(1), 199–202. https://doi.org/10.1097/00000542-200507000-00028.

Meyer, K., Sprott, H., & Mannion, A. F. (2008). Cross-cultural adaptation, reliability, and validity of the German version of the pain catastrophizing scale. *Journal of psychosomatic research, 64*(5), 469–478. https://doi.org/10.1016/j.jpsychores.2007.12.004.

Mhalla, A., de Andrade, D. C., Baudic, S., Perrot, S., & Bouhassira, D. (2010). Alteration of cortical excitability in patients with fibromyalgia. *Pain, 149*(3), 495–500. https://doi.org/10.1016/j.pain.2010.03.009.

Mine, K., Gilbert, S., Tsuchiya, J., & Nakayama, T. (2017). The Short-Term Effects of a Single Lecture on Undergraduate Physiotherapy Students' Understanding Regarding Pain Neurophysiology: A Prospective Case Series. *Journal of Musculoskeletal Disorders and Treatment, 3.* https://doi.org/10.23937/2572-3243.1510041.

Moseley, L. (2002). Combined physiotherapy and education is efficacious for chronic low back pain. *The Australian Journal of physiotherapy, 48*(4), 297–302. https://doi.org/10.1016/s0004-9514(14)60169-0.

Moseley, L. (2003). Unraveling the barriers to reconceptualization of the problem in chronic pain: The actual and perceived ability of patients and health professionals to understand the neurophysiology. *The Journal of pain, 4*(4), 184–189. https://doi.org/10.1016/s1526-5900(03)00488-7.

Moseley, G. L. (2004). Graded motor imagery is effective for long-standing complex regional pain syndrome: A randomised controlled trial. *Pain, 108*(1–2), 192–198. https://doi.org/10.1016/j.pain.2004.01.006.

Moseley, G. L., Nicholas, M. K., & Hodges, P. W. (2004). A randomized controlled trial of intensive neurophysiology education in chronic low back pain. *The clinical Journal of pain, 20*(5), 324–330. https://doi.org/10.1097/00002508-200409000-00007.

Moseley, G. L. (2005). Widespread brain activity during an abdominal task markedly reduced after pain physiology education: FMRI evaluation of a single patient with chronic low back pain. *The Australian Journal of physiotherapy, 51*(1), 49–52. https://doi.org/10.1016/s0004-9514(05)70053-2.

Moseley, G. L. (2006). Graded motor imagery for pathologic pain: A randomized controlled trial. *Neurology, 67*(12), 2129–2134. https://doi.org/10.1212/01.wnl.0000249112.56935.32.

Moseley, L. G., Zalucki, N. M., & Wiech, K. (2008). Tactile discrimination, but not tactile stimulation alone, reduces chronic limb pain. *Pain, 137*(3), 600–608. https://doi.org/10.1016/j.pain.2007.10.021.

Moseley, G. L., & Butler, D. S. (2015). Fifteen years of explaining pain: The past, present, and future. *The Journal of Pain, 16*(9), 807–813. https://doi.org/10.1016/j.jpain.2015.05.005.

McKeown, J. L., & Warner, M. A. (2009). Enduring contributions of Henry K. Beecher to medicine, science, and society. *Anesthesiology 45*(4), 110–952. https://doi.org/10.1097/ALN.0b013e31819c49ac.

Myburgh, C., Larsen, A. H., & Hartvigsen, J. (2008). A systematic, critical review of manual palpation for identifying myofascial trigger points: Evidence and clinical significance. *Archives of physical medicine and rehabilitation, 89*(6), 1169–1176. https://doi.org/10.1016/j.apmr.2007.12.033.

Naugle, K. M., Ohlman, T., Naugle, K. E., Riley, Z. A., & Keith, N. R. (2017). Physical activity behavior predicts endogenous pain modulation in older adults. *Pain, 158*(3), 383–390. https://doi.org/10.1097/j.pain.0000000000000769.

Neblett, R., Cohen, H., Choi, Y., Hartzell, M. M., Williams, M., Mayer, T. G., & Gatchel, R. J. (2013). The Central Sensitization Inventory (CSI): Establishing clinically significant values for identifying central sensitivity syndromes in an outpatient chronic pain sample. *The Journal of pain, 14*(5), 438–445. https://doi.org/10.1016/j.jpain.2012.11.012.

Nijs, J., Van Houdenhove, B., & Oostendorp, R. A. (2010). Recognition of central sensitization in patients with musculoskeletal pain: Application of pain neurophysiology in manual therapy practice. *Manual therapy, 15*(2), 135–141. https://doi.org/10.1016/j.math.2009.12.001.

Nijs, J., Roussel, N., Paul van Wilgen, C., Köke, A., & Smeets, R. (2013). Thinking beyond muscles and joints: Therapists' and patients' attitudes and beliefs regarding chronic musculoskeletal pain are key to applying effective treatment. *Manual therapy, 18*(2), 96–102. https://doi.org/10.1016/j.math.2012.11.001.

Nijs, J., Meeus, M., Cagnie, B., Roussel, N. A., Dolphens, M., Van Oosterwijck, J., & Danneels, L. (2014). A modern neuroscience approach to chronic spinal pain: Combining pain neuroscience education with cognition-targeted motor control training. *Physical therapy, 94*(5), 730–738. https://doi.org/10.2522/ptj.20130258.

Nijs, J., Malfliet, A., Roose, E., Lahousse, A., Van Bogaert, W., Johansson, E., Runge, N., Goossens, Z., Labie, C., Bilterys, T., Van Campenhout, J., Polli, A., Wyns, A., Hendrix, J., Xiong, H. Y., Ahmed, I., De Baets, L., & Huysmans, E. (2024). Personalized multimodal lifestyle intervention as the best-evidenced treatment for chronic pain: State-of-the-art clinical perspective. *Journal of clinical medicine, 13*(3), 644. https://doi.org/10.3390/jcm13030644.

Oesch, P., Kool, J., Hagen, K. B., & Bachmann, S. (2010). Effectiveness of exercise on work disability in patients with non-acute non-specific low back pain: Systematic review and meta-analysis of randomised controlled trials. *Journal of rehabilitation medicine, 42*(3), 193–205. https://doi.org/10.2340/16501977-0524.

O'Sullivan, P., Caneiro, J. P., O'Keeffe, M., & O'Sullivan, K. (2016). Unraveling the complexity of low back pain. *The Journal of orthopaedic and sports physical therapy, 46*(11), 932–937. https://doi.org/10.2519/jospt.2016.0609.

O'Sullivan, P. B., Caneiro, J. P., O'Keeffe, M., Smith, A., Dankaerts, W., Fersum, K., & O'Sullivan, K. (2018). Cognitive functional therapy: An integrated behavioral approach for the targeted management of disabling low back pain. *Physical therapy, 98*(5), 408–423. https://doi.org/10.1093/ptj/pzy022.

Owen, P. J., Miller, C. T., Mundell, N. L., Verswijveren, S. J. J. M., Tagliaferri, S. D., Brisby, H., Bowe, S. J., & Belavy, D. L. (2020). Which specific modes of exercise training are most effective for treating low back pain? Network meta-analysis. *British Journal of sports medicine, 54*(21), 1279–1287. https://doi.org/10.1136/bjsports-2019-100886.

Paraskevopoulos, E., Papandreou, M., & Gliatis, J. (2020). Reliability of assessment methods for scapular dyskinesis in asymptomatic subjects: A systematic review. *Acta orthopaedica et traumatologica turcica, 54*(5), 546–556. https://doi.org/10.5152/j.aott.2020.19088.

Pate, J. W., Veage, S., Lee, S., Hancock, M. J., Hush, J. M., & Pacey, V. (2019). Which patients with chronic pain are more likely to improve pain biology knowledge following education? *Pain practice: The official Journal of World Institute of Pain, 19*(4), 363–369. https://doi.org/10.1111/papr.12748.

Pleger, B., Tegenthoff, M., Ragert, P., Förster, A. F., Dinse, H. R., Schwenkreis, P., Nicolas, V., & Maier, C. (2005). Sensorimotor retuning [corrected] in complex regional pain syndrome parallels pain reduction. *Annals of neurology, 57*(3), 425–429. https://doi.org/10.1002/ana.20394.

Reich, R. R., Lengacher, C. A., Alinat, C. B., Kip, K. E., Paterson, C., Ramesar, S., Han, H. S., Ismail-Khan, R., Johnson-Mallard, V., Moscoso, M., Budhrani-Shani, P., Shivers, S., Cox, C. E., Goodman, M., & Park, J. (2017). Mindfulness-based stress reduction in post-treatment breast cancer patients: Immediate and sustained effects across multiple symptom clusters. *Journal of pain and symptom management, 53*(1), 85–95. https://doi.org/10.1016/j.jpainsymman.2016.08.005.

Richter, M., Eck, J., Straube, T., Miltner, W., & Weiss, T. (2010). Do words hurt? Brain activation during the processing of pain-related words. *Pain, 148*(2), 198–205. https://doi.org/10.1016/j.pain.2009.08.009.

Rondanelli, M., Faliva, M. A., Miccono, A., Naso, M., Nichetti, M., Riva, A., Guerriero, F., De Gregori, M., Peroni, G., & Perna, S. (2018). Food pyramid for subjects with chronic pain: Foods and dietary constituents as anti-inflammatory and antioxidant agents. *Nutrition research reviews, 31*(1), 131–151. https://doi.org/10.1017/S0954422417000270.

Saltychev, M., Pylkäs, K., Karklins, A., & Juhola, J. (2024). Psychometric properties of neck disability index—A systematic review and meta-analysis. *Disability and rehabilitation,* 1–17. Advance online publication. https://doi.org/10.1080/09638288.2024.2304644.

Schell, L. K., Monsef, I., Wöckel, A., & Skoetz, N. (2019). Mindfulness-based stress reduction for women diagnosed with breast cancer. *The Cochrane database of systematic reviews, 3*(3), CD011518. https://doi.org/10.1002/14651858.CD011518.pub2.

Scudds, R., Scudds, R., & Simmonds, M. (2009). Pain in the physical therapy (PT) curriculum: A faculty survey. *Physiotherapy Theory and Practice, 17,* 239–256. https://doi.org/10.1080/095939801753385744.

Seminowicz, D. A., Shpaner, M., Keaser, M. L., Krauthamer, G. M., Mantegna, J., Dumas, J. A., Newhouse, P. A., Filippi, C. G., Keefe, F. J., & Naylor, M. R. (2013). Cognitive-behavioral therapy increases prefrontal cortex gray matter in patients with chronic pain. *The Journal of pain, 14*(12), 1573–1584. https://doi.org/10.1016/j.jpain.2013.07.020.

Setchell, J., Costa, N., Ferreira, M., Makovey, J., Nielsen, M., & Hodges, P. W. (2017). Individuals' explanations for their persistent or recurrent low back pain: A cross-sectional survey. *BMC musculoskeletal disorders, 18*(1), 466. https://doi.org/10.1186/s12891-017-1831-7.

Sheahan, P. J., Nelson-Wong, E. J., & Fischer, S. L. (2015). A review of culturally adapted versions of the oswestry disability index: The adaptation process, construct validity, test-retest reliability and internal consistency. *Disability and rehabilitation, 37*(25), 2367–2374. https://doi.org/10.3109/09638288.2015.1019647.

Shinohara, Y., Wakaizumi, K., Ishikawa, A., Ito, M., Hoshino, R., Tanaka, C., Takaoka, S., Kawakami, M., Tsuji, O., Fujisawa, D., Fujiwara, T., Tsuji, T., Morisaki, H., & Kosugi, S. (2022). Improvement in disability mediates the effect of self-efficacy on pain relief in chronic low back pain patients with exercise therapy. *Pain research & management, 2022,* 4203138. https://doi.org/10.1155/2022/4203138.

Slade, S. C., Molloy, E., & Keating, J. L. (2009). 'Listen to me, tell me': A qualitative study of partnership in care for people with non-specific chronic low back pain. *Clinical rehabilitation, 23*(3), 270–280. https://doi.org/10.1177/0269215508100468.

Slater, D., Korakakis, V., O'Sullivan, P., Nolan, D., & O'Sullivan, K. (2019). "Sit Up Straight": Time to re-evaluate. *The Journal of orthopaedic and sports physical therapy, 49*(8), 562–564. https://doi.org/10.2519/jospt.2019.0610.

Sluka, K. A., Frey-Law, L., & Hoeger Bement, M. (2018). Exercise-induced pain and analgesia? Underlying mechanisms and clinical translation. *Pain, 159 Suppl 1*(Suppl 1), S91–S97. https://doi.org/10.1097/j.pain.0000000000001235.

Smallwood, R. F., Potter, J. S., & Robin, D. A. (2016). Neurophysiological mechanisms in acceptance and commitment therapy in opioid-addicted patients with chronic pain. *Psychiatry research. Neuroimaging, 250,* 12–14. https://doi.org/10.1016/j.pscychresns.2016.03.001.

Smeets, R. J., Vlaeyen, J. W., Kester, A. D., & Knottnerus, J. A. (2006). Reduction of pain catastrophizing mediates the outcome of both physical and cognitive-behavioral treatment in chronic low back pain. *The Journal of pain, 7*(4), 261–271. https://doi.org/10.1016/j.jpain.2005.10.011.

Soer, R., Köke, A. J., Speijer, B. L., Vroomen, P. C., Smeets, R. J., Coppes, M. H., Reneman, M. F., Gross, D. P., & Groningen Spine Study Group (2015). Reference values of the pain disability index in patients with painful musculoskeletal and spinal disorders: A cross-national study. *Spine, 40*(9), E545–E551. https://doi.org/10.1097/BRS.0000000000000827.

Song, J. S., Yamada, Y., Kataoka, R., Wong, V., Spitz, R. W., Bell, Z. W., & Loenneke, J. P. (2022). Training-induced hypoalgesia and its potential underlying mechanisms. *Neuroscience and biobehavioral reviews, 141,* 104858. https://doi.org/10.1016/j.neubiorev.2022.104858.

Soundararajan, K., Prem, V., & Kishen, T. J. (2022). The effectiveness of mindfulness-based stress reduction intervention on physical function in individuals with chronic low back pain: Systematic review and meta-analysis of randomized controlled trials. *Complementary therapies in clinical practice, 49,* 101623. https://doi.org/10.1016/j.ctcp.2022.101623.

Synnott, A., O'Keeffe, M., Bunzli, S., Dankaerts, W., O'Sullivan, P., & O'Sullivan, K. (2015). Physiotherapists may stigmatise or feel unprepared to treat people with low back pain and psychosocial factors that influence recovery: A systematic review. *Journal of physiotherapy, 61*(2), 68–76. https://doi.org/10.1016/j.jphys.2015.02.016.

Syroyid Syroyid, I., Cavero-Redondo, I., & Syroyid Syroyid, B. (2022). Effects of resistance training on pain control and physical function in older adults with low back pain: A systematic review with meta-analysis. *Journal of geriatric physical therapy (2001), 46*(3), E113–E126. https://doi.org/10.1519/JPT.0000000000000374.

Tan, H. S., Sultana, R., Han, N. R., Tan, C. W., Sia, A., & Sng, B. L. (2020). The association between preoperative pain catastrophizing and chronic pain after hysterectomy—Secondary analysis of a prospective cohort study. *Journal of pain research, 13,* 2151–2162. https://doi.org/10.2147/JPR.S255336.

Tashani, O. A., & Johnson, M. I. (2010). Avicenna's concept of pain. *The Libyan Journal of medicine, 5,* https://doi.org/10.3402/ljm.v5i0.5253. https://doi.org/10.3402/ljm.v5i0.5253.

Tang, Y. Y., Hölzel, B. K., & Posner, M. I. (2015). The neuroscience of mindfulness meditation. *Nature reviews. Neuroscience, 16*(4), 213–225. https://doi.org/10.1038/nrn3916.

Urits, I., Hubble, A., Peterson, E., Orhurhu, V., Ernst, C. A., Kaye, A. D., & Viswanath, O. (2019). An update on cognitive therapy for the management of chronic pain: A comprehensive review. *Current pain and headache reports, 23*(8), 57. https://doi.org/10.1007/s11916-019-0794-9.

Vadivelu, N., Mitra, S., Hines, R., Elia, M., & Rosenquist, R. W. (2012). Acute pain in undergraduate medical education: An unfinished chapter! *Pain practice: The official Journal of World Institute of Pain, 12*(8), 663–671. https://doi.org/10.1111/j.1533-2500.2012.00580.x.

Van Oosterwijck, J., Meeus, M., Paul, L., De Schryver, M., Pascal, A., Lambrecht, L., & Nijs, J. (2013). Pain physiology education improves health status and endogenous pain inhibition in fibromyalgia: A double-blind randomized controlled trial. *The clinical Journal of pain, 29*(10), 873–882. https://doi.org/10.1097/AJP.0b013e31827c7a7d.

van Tulder, M., Becker, A., Bekkering, T., Breen, A., del Real, M. T., Hutchinson, A., Koes, B., Laerum, E., Malmivaara, A., & COST B13 Working Group on Guidelines for the Management of Acute Low Back Pain in Primary Care (2006). Chapter 3. European guidelines for the management of acute nonspecific low back pain in primary care. *European spine Journal: Official publication of the European Spine Society, the European Spinal Deformity Society, and the European Section of the Cervical Spine Research Society, 15 Suppl 2*(Suppl 2), S169–S191. https://doi.org/10.1007/s00586-006-1071-2.

Veehof, M. M., Trompetter, H. R., Bohlmeijer, E. T., & Schreurs, K. M. (2016). Acceptance- and mindfulness-based interventions for the treatment of chronic pain: A meta-analytic review. *Cognitive behaviour therapy, 45*(1), 5–31. https://doi.org/10.1080/16506073.2015.1098724.

Velly, A. M., Look, J. O., Carlson, C., Lenton, P. A., Kang, W., Holcroft, C. A., & Fricton, J. R. (2011). The effect of catastrophizing and depression on chronic pain–a prospective cohort study of temporomandibular muscle and joint pain disorders. *Pain, 152*(10), 2377–2383. https://doi.org/10.1016/j.pain.2011.07.004.

Verbrugghe, J., Agten, A., Stevens, S., Hansen, D., Demoulin, C., O Eijnde, B., Vandenabeele, F., & Timmermans, A. (2019). Exercise intensity matters in chronic nonspecific low back pain rehabilitation. *Medicine and science in sports and exercise, 51*(12), 2434–2442. https://doi.org/10.1249/MSS.0000000000002078.

Verghese, A., & Horwitz, R. I. (2009). In praise of the physical examination. *BMJ (Clinical research ed.), 339*, b5448. https://doi.org/10.1136/bmj.b5448.

Vincent, H. K., George, S. Z., Seay, A. N., Vincent, K. R., & Hurley, R. W. (2014). Resistance exercise, disability, and pain catastrophizing in obese adults with back pain. *Medicine and science in sports and exercise, 46*(9), 1693–1701. https://doi.org/10.1249/MSS.0000000000000294.

Vlaeyen, J. W., Haazen, I. W., Schuerman, J. A., Kole-Snijders, A. M., & van Eek, H. (1995). Behavioural rehabilitation of chronic low back pain: Comparison of an operant treatment, an operant-cognitive treatment and an operant-respondent treatment. *The British Journal of clinical psychology, 34*(1), 95–118. https://doi.org/10.1111/j.2044-8260.1995.tb01443.x.

Vlaeyen, J. W. S., & Linton, S. J. (2000). Fear-avoidance and its consequences in chronic musculoskeletal pain: A state of the art. *Pain, 85*(3), 317–332. https://doi.org/10.1016/S0304-3959(99)00242-0.

Vowles, K. E., Sowden, G., & Ashworth, J. (2014). A comprehensive examination of the model underlying acceptance and commitment therapy for chronic pain. *Behavior therapy, 45*(3), 390–401. https://doi.org/10.1016/j.beth.2013.12.009.

Walker, H. K., Hall, W. D., & Hurst, J. W. (Hrsg.). (1990). *Clinical methods: The history, physical, and laboratory examinations* (3. Aufl.). Butterworths.

Wälti, P., Kool, J., & Luomajoki, H. (2015). Short-term effect on pain and function of neurophysiological education and sensorimotor retraining compared to usual physiotherapy in patients with chronic or recurrent non-specific low back pain, a pilot randomized controlled trial. *BMC musculoskeletal disorders, 16*, 83. https://doi.org/10.1186/s12891-015-0533-2.

Wand, B. M., & O'Connell, N. E. (2008). Chronic non-specific low back pain—Subgroups or a single mechanism? *BMC musculoskeletal disorders, 9*, 11. https://doi.org/10.1186/1471-2474-9-11.

Wand, B. M., O'Connell, N. E., Di Pietro, F., & Bulsara, M. (2011). Managing chronic nonspecific low back pain with a sensorimotor retraining approach: Exploratory multiple-baseline study of 3 participants. *Physical therapy, 91*(4), 535–546. https://doi.org/10.2522/ptj.20100150.

Wand, B. M., Tulloch, V. M., George, P. J., Smith, A. J., Goucke, R., O'Connell, N. E., & Moseley, G. L. (2012). Seeing it helps: Movement-related back pain is reduced by visualization of the back during movement. *The clinical Journal of pain, 28*(7), 602–608. https://doi.org/10.1097/AJP.0b013e31823d480c.

Wassinger, C. A., Williams, D. A., Milosavljevic, S., & Hegedus, E. J. (2015). Clinical reliability and diagnostic accuracy of visual scapulohumeral movement evaluation in detecting patients with shoulder impairment. *International Journal of sports physical therapy, 10*(4), 456–463.

Watson, J. A., Ryan, C. G., Cooper, L., Ellington, D., Whittle, R., Lavender, M., Dixon, J., Atkinson, G., Cooper, K., & Martin, D. J. (2019). Pain Neuroscience education for adults with chronic musculoskeletal pain: A mixed-methods systematic review and meta-analysis. *The Journal of pain, 20*(10), 1140.e1–1140.e22. https://doi.org/10.1016/j.jpain.2019.02.011.

Wertli, M. M., Rasmussen-Barr, E., Weiser, S., Bachmann, L. M., & Brunner, F. (2014). The role of fear avoidance beliefs as a prognostic factor for outcome in patients with nonspecific low back pain: A systematic review. *The spine Journal: Official Journal of the North American Spine Society, 14*(5), 816–36.e4. https://doi.org/10.1016/j.spinee.2013.09.036.

Westcott, W. L. (2012). Resistance training is medicine: Effects of strength training on health. *Current sports medicine reports, 11*(4), 209–216. https://doi.org/10.1249/JSR.0b013e31825dabb8.

Wetherell, J. L., Afari, N., Rutledge, T., Sorrell, J. T., Stoddard, J. A., Petkus, A. J., Solomon, B. C., Lehman, D. H., Liu, L., Lang, A. J., & Atkinson, H. J. (2011). A randomized, controlled trial of acceptance and commitment therapy and cognitive-behavioral therapy for chronic pain. *Pain, 152*(9), 2098–2107. https://doi.org/10.1016/j.pain.2011.05.016.

Wewege, M. A., Booth, J., & Parmenter, B. J. (2018). Aerobic vs. resistance exercise for chronic non-specific low back pain: A systematic review and meta-analysis. *Journal of back and musculoskeletal rehabilitation, 31*(5), 889–899. https://doi.org/10.3233/BMR-170920.

Whale, K., & Gooberman-Hill, R. (2022). The importance of sleep for people with chronic pain: Current insights and evidence. *JBMR plus, 6*(7), e10658. https://doi.org/10.1002/jbm4.10658.

Wielgosz, J., Kral, T. R. A., Perlman, D. M., Mumford, J. A., Wager, T. D., Lutz, A., & Davidson, R. J. (2022). Neural signatures of pain modulation in short-term and long-term mindfulness training: A randomized active-control trial. *The American Journal of psychiatry, 179*(10), 758–767. https://doi.org/10.1176/appi.ajp.21020145.

Wood, L., & Hendrick, P. A. (2019). A systematic review and meta-analysis of pain neuroscience education for chronic low back pain: Short-and long-term outcomes of pain and disability. *European Journal of pain (London, England), 23*(2), 234–249. https://doi.org/10.1002/ejp.1314.

Yang, S., & Chang, M. C. (2019). Chronic pain: Structural and functional changes in brain structures and associated negative affective states. *International Journal of molecular sciences, 20*(13), 3130. https://doi.org/10.3390/ijms20133130.

Zeidan, F., Martucci, K. T., Kraft, R. A., Gordon, N. S., McHaffie, J. G., & Coghill, R. C. (2011). Brain mechanisms supporting the modulation of pain by mindfulness meditation. *The Journal of neuroscience: The official Journal of the Society for Neuroscience, 31*(14), 5540–5548. https://doi.org/10.1523/JNEUROSCI.5791-10.2011.

Zheng, Y. N., Zheng, Y. L., Wang, X. Q., & Chen, P. J. (2024). Role of exercise on inflammation cytokines of neuropathic pain in animal models. *Molecular neurobiology*. https://doi.org/10.1007/s12035-024-04214-4.Advanceonlinepublication.doi:10.1007/s12035-024-04214-4.

Zimney, K., Van Bogaert, W., & Louw, A. (2023). The biology of chronic pain and its implications for pain neuroscience education: State of the art. *Journal of clinical medicine, 12*(13), 4199. https://doi.org/10.3390/jcm12134199.

Zou, J., & Hao, S. (2024). Exercise-induced neuroplasticity: A new perspective on rehabilitation for chronic low back pain. *Frontiers in molecular neuroscience, 17*, 1407445. https://doi.org/10.3389/fnmol.2024.1407445.

Exercise Planning in Pain Therapy

6

> **Abstract**
>
> Exercise and training play a central role in the therapy of acute and chronic pain. Various effective forms of exercise and training have been developed, which have proven to be beneficial for pain relief. The goals are, on the one hand, pain relief and, on the other hand, the restoration of function in the affected body areas. Painful or problematic movements can, however, also be modified independently of a specific form of training and adjusted to the patient's condition through progression and regression. Thus, progressive movement patterns and individualized exercise plans tailored to the patient can be established, which gradually increase activity and prevent avoidance and excessive protection.

The implementation of movement as a central pillar in multidimensional pain therapy has proven to be essential over the past few decades (Sullivan et al., 2012; Geneen et al., 2017; Mittinty et al., 2018; Cashin et al., 2022; Kechichian et al., 2022). However, restoring specific movements can be particularly challenging in chronic pain therapy, as they do not necessarily follow the laws of classical training theory due to psycho-social and neuroplastic drivers. Patients have often already changed movement patterns over months and years, which need to be reworked.

6.1 A Progressive Approach

Pain-related changes in movement do not always occur consciously. Pain serves as a protective mechanism that can cause changes in movement. These changes may initially be appropriate, but if they are maintained, they can impair recovery, prolong disabilities, and reduce quality of life. Pain influences movement and can cause both advantageous and disadvantageous changes that are individually different and must be considered in the assessment and planning of rehabilitation (Butera et al., 2016). There can be different reasons why the body changes movements pain-induced. On the one hand, maintaining *normal* movement patterns, for example after a knee distortion, is suboptimal for the regeneration of the injured structures, on the other hand, there is the risk of potentially re-damaging movements, which is why old movement patterns that led to pain are avoided (Merkle et al., 2020).

In pain therapy, three coping strategies can be identified when patients are confronted with painful movements.

1. Acceptance
2. Modification
3. Elimination

The acceptance strategy is based on the concept of pain tolerance and resistance and involves the conscious continuation of movement despite pain. This approach aims to break maladaptive behaviors, minimize worries, and increase the patient's self-efficacy. For this, exclusion of red flags, adequate education and conviction of the patient, and systematic recording of potential reactions are useful.

The modification strategy can be described as a gentle avoidance. It includes the targeted adjustment of specific movement parameters to reduce pain intensity without completely eliminating the movement. This strategy is in line with the principle of gradual exposure and promotes the neuroplastic reorganization of pain-associated cortical networks. The modification strategy will be deepened in the further course of the chapter.

The elimination strategy represents a form of strong avoidance and implies the complete exclusion of painful movement patterns. While this strategy can lead to short-term pain reduction and is temporarily useful and physiological in acute injuries, it carries the risk of promoting kinesiophobia and musculoskeletal deconditioning in chronic pain patients through negative reinforcement.

The selection of the appropriate strategy should be based on a multifactorial evaluation that takes into account both biomechanical and psycho-social factors. The pain intensity, the functional relevance of the movement, and the individual coping resources of the patient play a central role in this.

6.1.1 Movement Modification

The question that therapists and patients alike ask is about the appropriate way of performing movement and its patient-specific adaptation. This chapter places a special focus on the systematic modification of movement parameters. The aim is to provide a solid understanding of the design and implementation of individualized movement plans in pain therapy and to prevent the elimination strategy as much as possible (Vlaeyen & Linton, 2012).

The modern understanding of the necessity for movement modification is based on the preservation and enhancement of functional capacities. This view implies that while the load must be adapted to the individual patient's capacity, this does not necessarily require the complete elimination of potentially painful movement patterns. Instead, a gradual approach is recommended, in which the patient is encouraged to act within his current abilities, but also to work on expanding his limits and systematically improving those areas that currently still pose difficulties. The load modification follows the principle *As much as necessary, as little as possible*. This is based on the realization that an excessive reduction of range of motion and intensity leads to a reduction of physical capacities. Specifically, this manifests in a decrease in resilience and basic motor skills. This development results in a prolonged and more difficult rehabilitation phase, as new load stimuli must be implemented more cautiously to ensure a balance between acute new loads and the reduced resilience. A too rapid change in condition could otherwise lead to relapses and overloads. Remembering Avicenna's theories: He disagreed with Galen and saw the cause of pain not in tissue damage, but in its change in condition. If a change in condition occurs rapidly, pain would arise, if it occurs slowly, the body adapts and pain would not occur. This theory states that a rapid change in tissue condition increases the risk of pain, while a gradual change allows the body to adapt and thus does not induce pain. These considerations can be interpreted as an early conceptualization of the principle of progressive overload. This approach aims to gradually increase the patient's load tolerance without exerting excessive stress on the neuromuscular system. This should be particularly considered in patients with chronically reduced resilience.

On the micro level, exercise planning focuses on the specific adaptation possibilities of individually problematic movements. A central principle here is on the one hand the preservation of functions and activities. This strategy not only serves to maintain the mechanical-physical tissue resilience, but also fulfills an important psychological function: It prevents the development of cognitive downward spirals, minimizes avoidance behavior and reduces the risk of a progressing kinesiophobia (Nijs et al., 2015). In addition to maintenance training, on the other hand, improving the patient's existing abilities is a goal of movement therapy. To effectively implement this approach, a detailed and systematic examination of the patient is essential. The aim of this examination is the precise definition of the individual comfort and discomfort zones (Fig. 6.1). These can manifest in various parameters that lead to pain, such as a specific duration when jogging, a certain

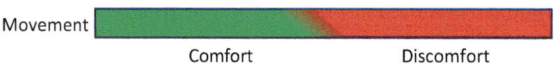

Fig. 6.1 Comfort and discomfort zone, own production

weight when bench pressing, or a specific angle in shoulder movements. The analysis of these zones is of high importance to prevent an inadequate and complete avoidance of certain movement patterns.

In addition to maintaining non-painful, or tolerable and non-pain-exacerbating movement patterns, an attempt should be made to systematically reduce the discomfort zone. The gradual expansion of the comfort zone while simultaneously reducing the discomfort zone requires a systematic progression in the exercise plan. Although there is no universally applicable formula for this progression in the practice of chronic pain therapy, there are various modification parameters that can be individually adjusted and gradually expanded.

The following modification parameters can be identified for a movement:

1. Load/Weight
2. Range of Motion (ROM)
3. Support surface
4. Closed/open chain
5. Speed
6. Reactivity/Perturbation

Even marginal modifications of a movement can often lead to a significant reduction in pain perception. When reducing parameters such as load or ROM, the principle *As much as necessary, as little as possible* applies again to avoid deconditioning.

For a training that includes multiple movements or exercises, the following overarching parameters can be modified:

1. Number of sets
2. Number of repetitions
3. Number of exercises
4. Rest duration between sets/exercises
5. Frequency of training per week

In practical application, it is advisable to first evaluate whether minimal adjustments, such as extending the breaks between sets or a moderate reduction in the number of repetitions, can already have a significant and satisfactory influence on pain perception for the patient. If this is the case, it is often possible to avoid completely eliminating painful exercises—a practice that was often applied too hastily in the past.

In conclusion, it can be summarized that on the one hand, the preservation of the comfort zone and on the other hand, its expansion or the reduction of the discomfort zone should be aimed for in movement therapy. The successful implementation of an individualized and progressive movement therapy for pain patients requires a high degree of expertise and tact. The continuous re-evaluation and adjustment of the training parameters, taking into account both physical and psychological factors, forms the basis for sustainable therapeutic success.

By specifically applying the discussed modification strategies, an optimal balance between stress and regeneration can be achieved, which can ultimately lead to an increase in resilience, a reduction in pain perception and avoidance strategies, and an improvement in the patient's quality of life.

6.1.2 Are Pains Allowed During Exercises?

When creating training recommendations in the context of physiotherapy and rehabilitation, the question often arises whether pain during exercises is acceptable. This question requires a differentiated consideration that takes into account both scientific findings and individual patient factors.

Firstly, it is important to note that training completely without pain is not possible in many cases, especially in patients with chronic pain conditions who have continuous resting pain. Moreover, logically, a higher training dose is possible if the load progression does not only occur in the absence of pain. Another significant advantage of training with controlled pain lies in the desensitization and re-evaluation of pain perceptions. Patients often automatically associate pain with damage/injury or the risk of such, which can lead to fear and avoidance behavior. Through targeted education using Pain Neuroscience Education (PNE), the therapist can clarify that pain can also arise without acute tissue damage through neurobiological processes and is not necessarily a sign of injury risk. This education is crucial to improve the patient's understanding of their pain and to promote active participation in the rehabilitation process. Paradoxically, many therapists still adopt a pain-avoiding attitude by modifying or stopping exercises when patients express pain. However, this practice contradicts newer findings in pain research and can be counterproductive to the healing process.

Controlled training into pain can help to dissolve the association *pain = damage* and reduce the avoidance of supposedly dangerous movements (Nijs et al., 2015). This approach is based on the concept of Graded Exposure (GE), in which patients are gradually introduced to feared movements. This can help them learn that these movements, despite short-term pain intensification, can be safe and even healing in the long term. Several studies underline the effectiveness of painful exercises in the rehabilitation process. Smith and colleagues (2017) showed that painful exercises can cause greater pain relief in the short term compared to pain-free exercises. This may initially seem contrary, but can be explained by various neurobiological mechanisms (see below). Particularly interesting is the observation that even a short-term symptom worsening due to intensive training can lead to a greater long-term pain reduction of about 25% compared to non-painful training (Sandal et al., 2016). This underlines the need to prepare patients for possible temporary pain intensifications and to emphasize the long-term benefits.

A neurobiological explanation for the pain-relieving effect of painful exercises lies in the activation of the descending inhibitory system, known as Conditioned Pain Modulation (CPM) (Smith et al., 2019). This system is based on the concept of Diffuse Noxious Inhibitory Control (DNIC), which explains pain inhibition through competing pain stimuli (Yarnitsky, 2010). In CPM, a painful stimulus leads to the activation of descending pain-inhibiting pathways in the central nervous system, which can reduce pain perception in other regions of the body. This mechanism could explain why painful exercises can paradoxically lead to an overall reduction in pain perception. Furthermore, exercises in the pain area can lead to improved pain management. They train pain acceptance, a concept from Acceptance and Commitment Therapy (ACT), which has proven effective in the treatment of chronic pain. Through controlled confrontation with pain, patients learn that they can function and improve their quality of life despite pain. This can help to break up often deeply rooted avoidance behavior and increase the patient's self-efficacy expectation (Smith et al., 2019). Training with controlled pain can strengthen this belief by giving patients direct experiences of success.

Despite these encouraging findings, the question arises as to the tolerable pain intensity. Some scientific recommendations are based on the numerical scale of the NRPS and consider values of 3–5 as acceptable (Ageberg et al., 2010; Sandal et al., 2016), while higher values should be avoided. However, it is important to note that these numbers should be interpreted individually and not understood as rigid limits. The subjective perception and significance of a pain value can vary greatly from patient to patient and is influenced by various factors, such as previous pain experiences, cultural background, expectations, and psychosocial factors. Therefore, it is crucial not only to pay attention to the numerical pain indication but also to consider the patient's non-verbal communication. Facial expressions, body posture, and the way pain is expressed can provide valuable clues about the patient's actual burden. Supplementary questions about the tolerability of pain and the subjective assessment of danger can provide additional information. For example, one patient might find a pain value of 3 disturbing and show fear of worsening, while another might classify a value of 6 as normal and harmless. This individual variability underscores the need for a personalized approach in pain therapy. The therapist should build a trusting relationship with the patient to openly discuss pain experiences and expectations. Situational consultations during training allow the patient's pain tolerance to be continuously evaluated and the exercise intensity to be adjusted accordingly.

In addition, it is important to distinguish between different pain qualities. While a dull muscle pain or a slight pull in the joints are often harmless, sharp, stabbing, or radiating pains should be examined more closely. The therapist must perform a careful differential diagnosis here to rule out potential contraindications for painful exercises.

Another important aspect is the temporal dynamics of pain. It should be observed how the pain develops during and after the exercise. Pain that occurs during the exercise but quickly subsides is often less concerning than pain that lasts for hours or days. The use of pain diaries can be helpful here to recognize patterns and adjust the training planning.

An action plan for pain monitoring (Fig. 6.2) could – depending on the patient and individual factors – look as follows:

6.2 Specific Exercise Recommendations

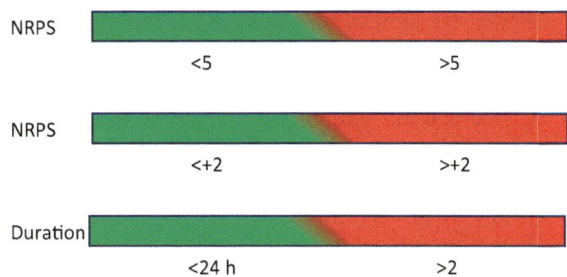

Fig. 6.2 Pain monitoring, own production. Action plan for 1. Pain intensity, 2. -increase and 3. -duration

Continue if: 🟢

- Pain is tolerable (Example: less than or equal to NRPS 5)
- Pain is constant during or after activity or increases by up to two points
- New symptoms or increases in pain subside within 24 hours

Adjust if: 🔴

- Pain is too severe (for example, more than NRPS 5)
- Pain increases by more than 2 points on the NRPS
- This lasts more than 24 hours
- New symptoms occur such as signs of inflammation or significant reduction of ROM or strength

In summary, it can be said that pain during training does not necessarily have to be avoided and can even have positive effects. However, the dosage should be individually adjusted, with human interaction and communication with the patient being of crucial importance. A well-trained therapist can use pain as a tool to optimize rehabilitation and help the patient improve pain management. Ultimately, the goal should be to enable the patient to manage their pain independently and to lead an active and fulfilled life despite occasional pain. This requires continuous education, encouragement, and support from the therapist, as well as the patient's willingness to question old thought patterns and allow new experiences.

6.2 Specific Exercise Recommendations

This chapter presents various examples of movement-induced pain problems, based on which a hypothetical exercise planning and adjustment is made. In all presented cases, there is no trauma, and radiations, neurological abnormalities, and other red flags are clinically excluded. The focus is exclusively on movement-specific pain indications.

For each example, both domains of movement modification are explained:

1. Activity maintenance: Here it is shown how in the specific case an adjustment of the activity within the comfort zone can take place to continue to enable movement. This also includes training peripheral, non-painful muscle groups.
2. Expansion of movement capacities: This aspect includes the gradual approach to the discomfort zone through targeted progressions, with the painful region being directly addressed. Through movement adjustment, movements learned by the brain or classified as threatening and thus painful can be bypassed and unlearned.

In the following case examples, the inclusion of structural information and specific pathologies is deliberately omitted. This approach is based on the consideration of nociplastic mechanisms. In nociplastic pain patients, it has been shown that function-related intervention strategies are often more effective than structure-related approaches. The focus is on an analysis of the individual patient situation, including a careful evaluation of comfort and discomfort zones. Based on these findings, realistic goals are formulated together with the patient. The interventions focus on the modification of movement patterns and their gradual increase, always taking into account the individual load capacity and pain tolerance. It should be emphasized that alternative intervention possibilities—such as movement patterns in opposite directions of the problematic movement, stretching exercises or other movement measures—should by no means be considered less significant or relevant. The focus of this chapter and the exercise examples contained therein is rather on the initiation of movement towards the specific problematic movement of the patient.

6.2.1 Chronic Lower Back Pain

Example 1

A patient reports having had pain in the lower lumbar region for a year, which occurs centrally when bending and lifting. The complaints began with a classic lumbago. The patient now tries to lift more from the legs to relieve the back. Nevertheless, the pain persists with stronger back strain, such as normal bending, lifting light objects, or deadlifting, even with a neutral lumbar spine position without curvature. ◄

Problematic Movement: Trunk/Lumbar spine flexion from standing

Pain Reports:

- Deadlift: Painful from 50 kg and a depth of approx. 80° hip flexion, NRPS 6 (Fig. 6.3)
- Weight-free bending: Painful (NRPS 4) from a finger-floor distance of 60 cm (Fig. 6.4)

6.2 Specific Exercise Recommendations

Fig. 6.3 painful deadlift

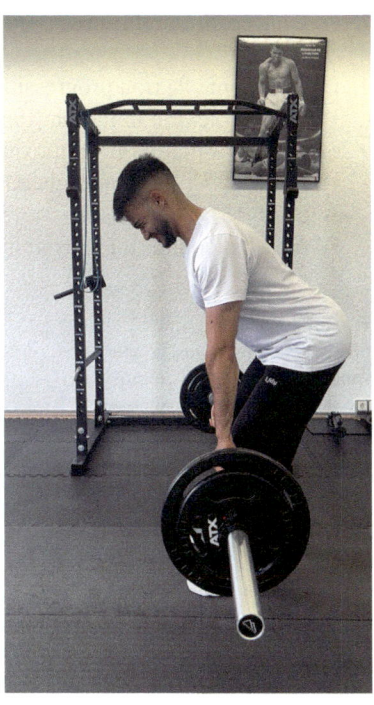

Fig. 6.4 painful bending

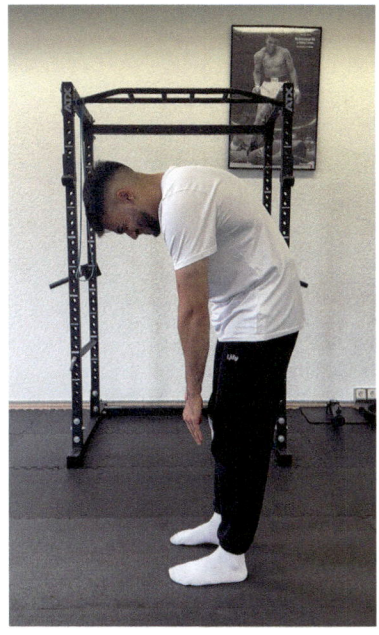

Exercise Recommendations:

1. Lumbar spine flexion progression from alternative less painful positions:
    - Indirect flexion initiation (Fig. 6.5, 6.6 und 6.7):
    - Flexion initiation from the quadruped position (see Fig. 6.8, 6.9 und 6.10):
    - Direct flexion initiation bending forward with rounded back (Fig. 6.11, 6.12 und 6.13):
    - Assisted counterforce exercises (see Fig. 6.14, 6.15, 6.16 und 6.17):

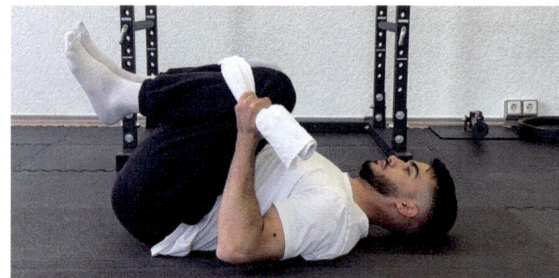

Fig. 6.5 Knees to chest bilaterally. Continuing lumbar spine flexion over maximum hip flexion with emphasis through a towel

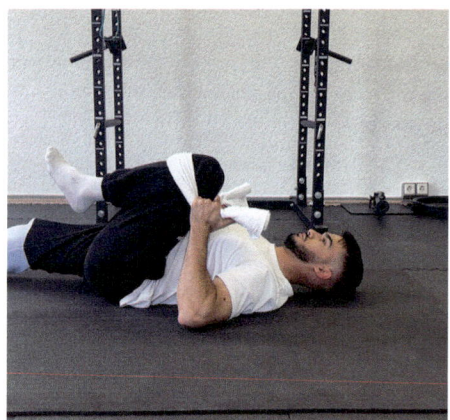

Fig. 6.6 Knee to chest unilaterally. Regression to 6.5, less continuing lumbar spine flexion due to contralateral hip extension

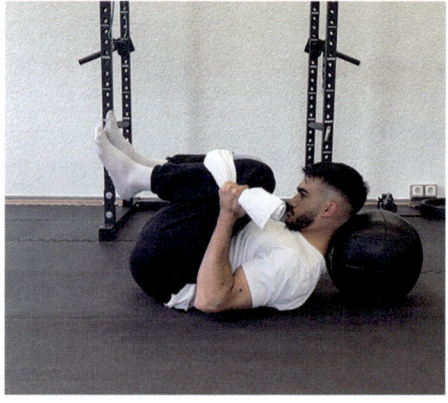

Fig. 6.7 Knees to chest bilaterally with head elevation. Progression to 6.5. More flexion pre-setting from cranial and more continuing lumbar spine flexion

6.2 Specific Exercise Recommendations

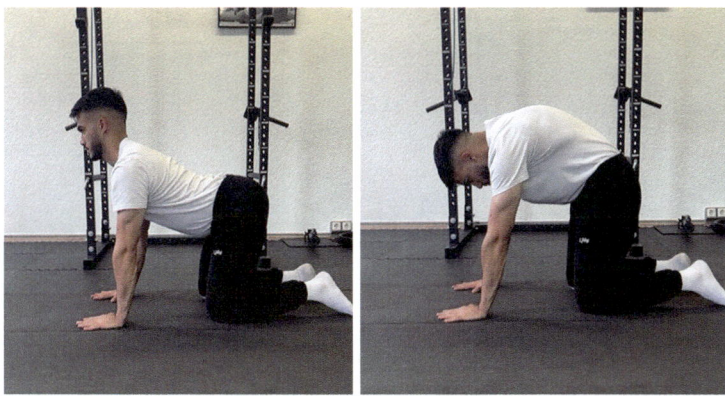

Fig. 6.8 Lumbar spine flexion from standing position. Closer to the problematic movements than a flexion from the supine position

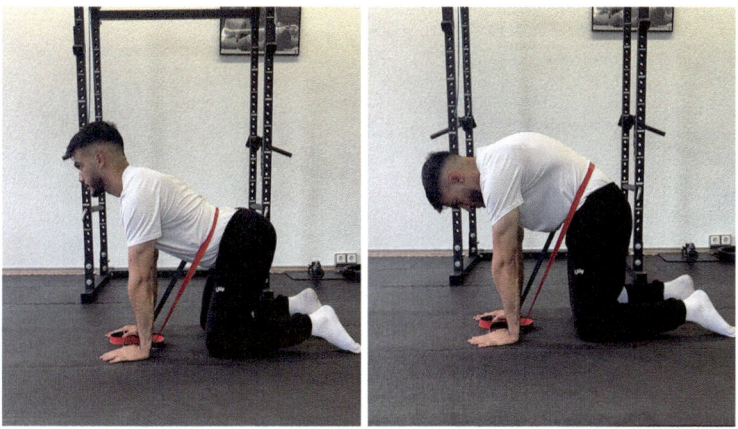

Fig. 6.9 Lumbar spine flexion from standing position with band. Progression of intensity compared to 6.8

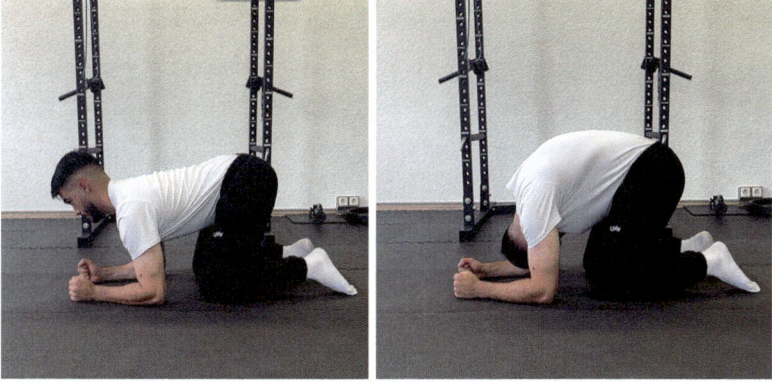

Fig. 6.10 Lumbar spine flexion from standing position with elbow support. Progression of kinematics compared to 6.8. The elbow support provides more upper body inclination and more hip flexion, thus more deep lumbar spine flexion

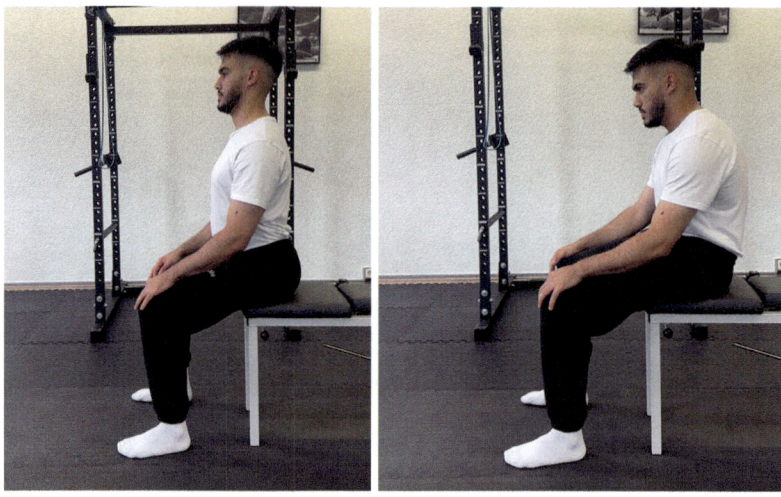

Fig. 6.11 Lumbar spine flexion from sitting position

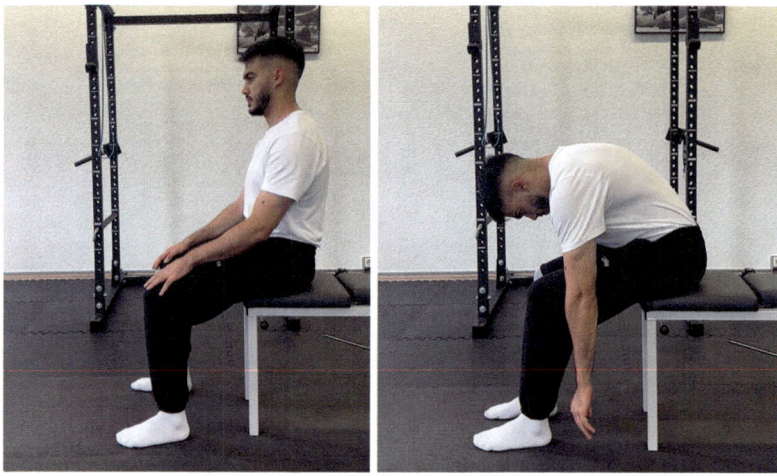

Fig. 6.12 Lumbar spine flexion with upper body inclination from sitting position

6.2 Specific Exercise Recommendations

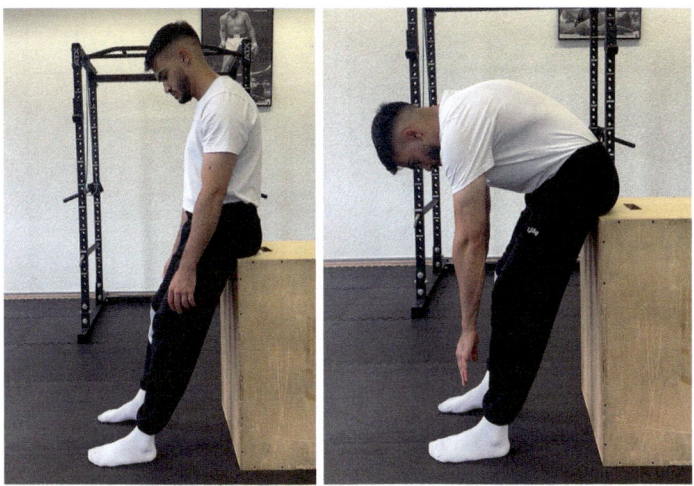

Fig. 6.13 Lumbar spine flexion from assisted standing position

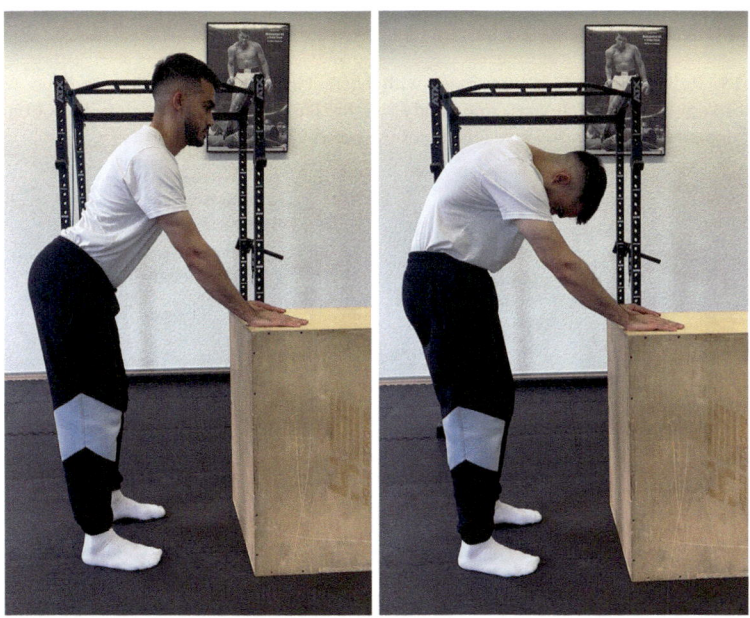

Fig. 6.14 Lumbar spine flexion from standing position with support. By transferring weight through the hands, the patient can be given a sense of security and the load can be reduced. In addition, the upper body inclination is initiated with a neutral lumbar spine and the lumbar spine flexion is added later. From a cognitive perspective, this is not the bending movement that the patient has stored as painful

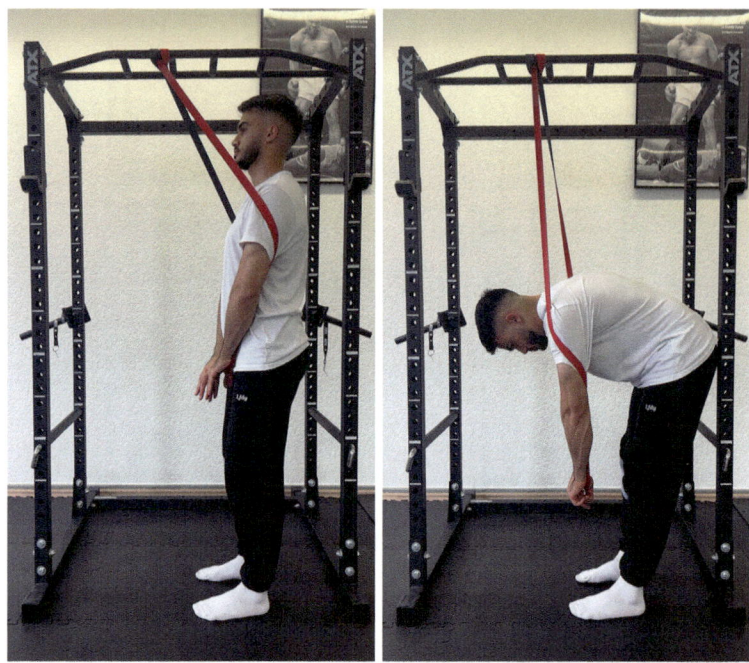

Fig. 6.15 Relieving bending movement with band. Grasp a sufficiently firm band with the palms of your hands, which takes some body weight. This allows a more relaxed position for the patient and possibly less protective tension of the posterior muscle chain

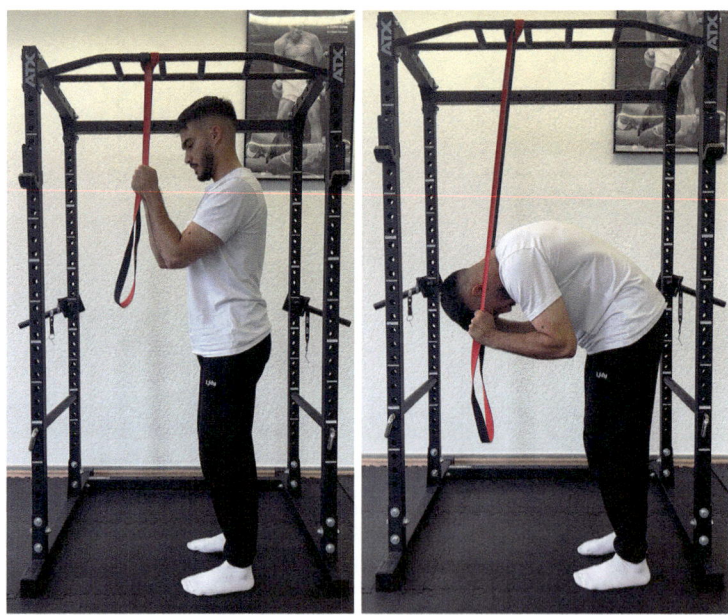

Fig. 6.16 Bending with antagonistic resistance. By working the anterior muscle chain against the band, the focus may be shifted away from the painful work of the posterior muscle chain

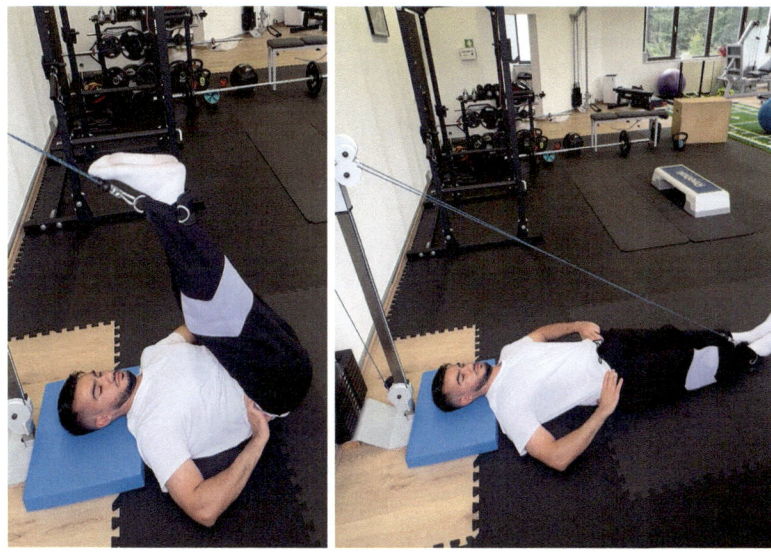

Fig. 6.17 Indirect lumbar spine flexion on the cable pull. This exercise can indirectly train the lumbar spine. The hip flexion makes the posterior muscle chain and the lumbar spine biomechanically more resilient to flexion, however, this exercise does not imply lumbar spine flexion and the patient may see less risk in this than in direct bending movements. By reversing the Punctum Fixum and Punctum Mobile, a detour is often possible for movements coded as painful

2. Maintenance training of the deadlift:
   - Perform warm-up sets (under 50 kg) with full range of motion
   - 2–3 training sets (from 50 kg, depending on individual load capacity) with adjusted range of motion up to approx. 70° hip flexion
   - Progression: Slow increase of the weight and/or the range of motion over several weeks
   - Variation of grip techniques (e.g., sumo style, conventional style) to determine the best tolerated form
3. Jefferson Curls with moderate weight:
   - Range of motion up to a finger floor distance of 50–70 cm (Fig. 6.18), depending on tolerable pain and reaction in the following hours
   - Start with very light weight and gradual increase

Fig. 6.18 Jefferson Curl hip and lumbar spine dominant

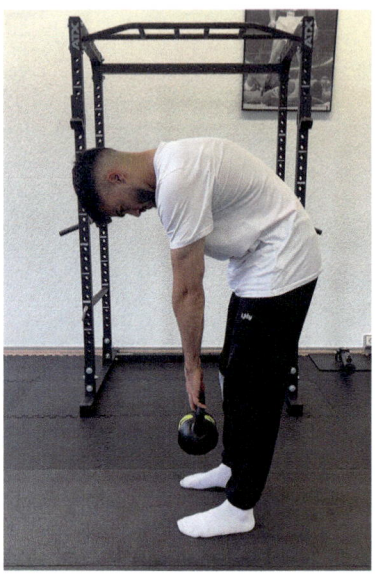

Fig. 6.19 Jefferson Curl thoracic spine dominant. Regression to 6.18 through less leverage (biomechanically) and less similar movement to the patient's problematic movement (cognitively), which is hip and lumbar spine dominant. Sometimes it is worth educating the patient to clarify that performing a new movement, such as this one, is a movement modification and not the same movement that usually causes problems. This may make the patient more likely to engage

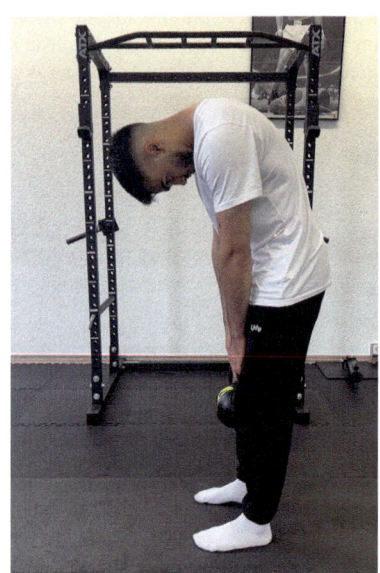

- Focus on controlled movement execution and conscious perception of back flexion
- Alternative regressions: Change of levers and support surfaces (see Fig. 6.19, 6.20, 6.21 und 6.22):
4. Building up the load capacity of surrounding structures:
    - Hip Thrusts

6.2 Specific Exercise Recommendations

Fig. 6.20 Jefferson Curl from assisted standing. Regression to 6.18

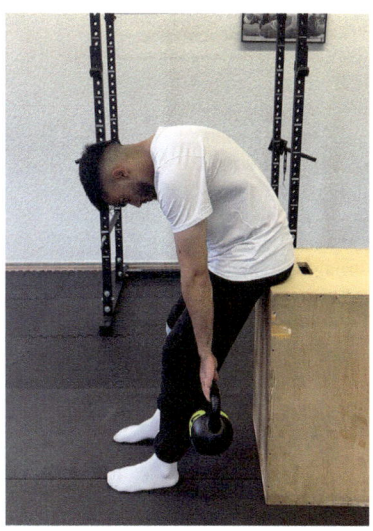

Fig. 6.21 Lumbar spine flexion with ball from assisted standing. Biomechanical regression to 6.20 through closer weight guidance and less leverage

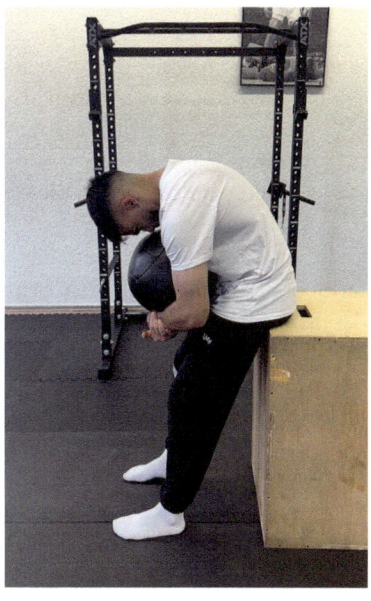

Fig. 6.22 Jefferson Curl from sitting. Regression to 6.20 through a more distant position to the patient's problematic bending movement from standing (cognitively), possibly however kinematically seen a progression due to the stronger hip and thus lumbar spine flexion

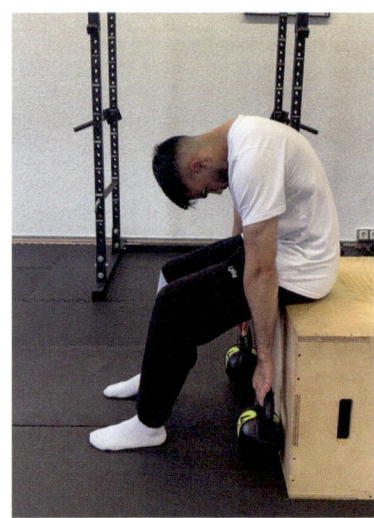

- Squats
- Core exercises:
  - static holding exercises like planks in various variations
  - Integration of controlled anti-rotation exercises (e.g., Pallof Press)
  - Introduction of dynamic movements with small amplitude (e.g., Dead Bugs, Bird Dogs)
  - Increase of complexity by combination of movements and increase of instability

These exercises aim to indirectly strengthen and mobilize the surrounding structures of the lumbar spine. Controlled execution and gradual increase promote desensitization of the affected area. At the same time, the general resilience of the musculoskeletal system is improved, which can contribute to a long-term reduction of back pain. It is important to always perform the exercises adapted to pain and to adjust the intensity and range of motion individually to the patient's tolerance. Often, it is not important what exactly is done, but that something is done and moments of conscious improvement are generated through progressions.

6.2.2 Chronic high cervical pain

Example 2

A patient has been suffering from pain in the upper cervical spine area for several months. She has difficulties with everyday rotational movements, such as looking over her shoulder while driving. As compensation, she turns more from the trunk and tries to relieve the cervical spine and rotate little. Out of concern for her intervertebral discs, she has given up her hobby, playing volleyball, as she fears that the increasingly extended high cervical posture during jumps and the landings in general could be harmful to the intervertebral discs. After playing volleyball, she always had temporarily increased complaints, especially after longer playing phases. The training frequency also correlated with the intensity of the complaints on the weekend. To avoid taking painkillers on the weekend, she now completely refrains from playing volleyball. ◄

Problematic movement: Cervical spine rotation

Pain reports:

- Resting pain: Constant feeling of tension in the entire cervical spine, NRPS 2 (Fig. 6.23)
- Rotation: Painful from 20° on both sides, NRPS 8 (Fig. 6.24)
- After volleyball: Increased feeling of tension for 2–3 h (NRPS 5)

Fig. 6.23 tense cervical spine

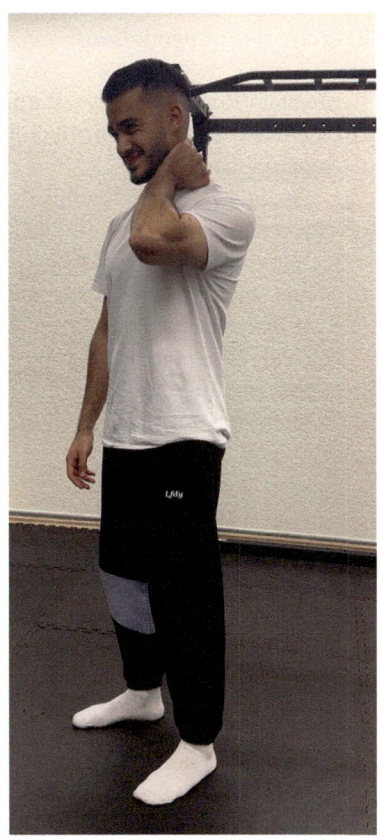

Fig. 6.24 painful cervical spine rotation

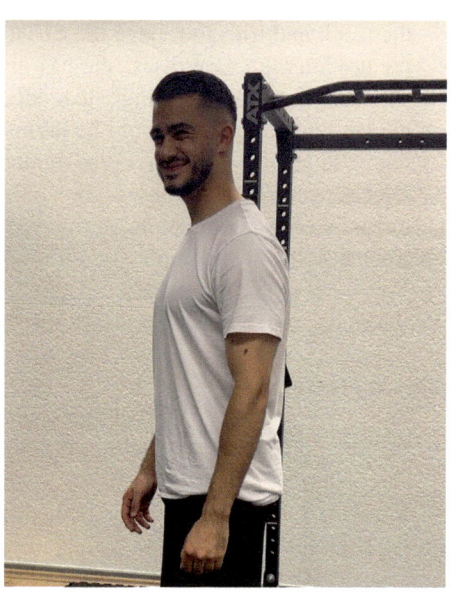

Exercise recommendations:

1. Maintain/Resume volleyball training
   - Education about pain monitoring and the usefulness of physical activity/participation
   - Gradual re-entry: Initially 1–2 times weekly volleyball training in the comfort zone for 4–6 weeks, then gradual expansion possible
   - Introduction of a warm-up program focusing on cervical spine mobilization and stabilization before training
   - If discomfort persists despite several weeks of adapted volleyball training, changes in playing position or technique or implementation of breaks during training for self-perception and relaxation of the cervical spine are possible, in order not to completely eliminate participation

6.2 Specific Exercise Recommendations

2. Rotation exercises from alternative less painful positions
   - Rotation of the head with less muscle activity (Fig. 6.25 und 6.26):
   - Indirect cervical spine rotation (Fig. 6.27 und 6.28):
3. Progressive strength training
   - Isometric exercises for cervical muscle groups (Fig. 6.29, 6.30, 6.31, 6.32, 6.33 und 6.34):
   - Dynamic exercises (Fig. 6.35, 6.36, 6.37, 6.38, 6.39 und 6.40):

Perform all exercises with adjusted ROM and intensity with tolerable pain and increase difficulty in the absence of negative reactions to increase load capacity and improve mobility.

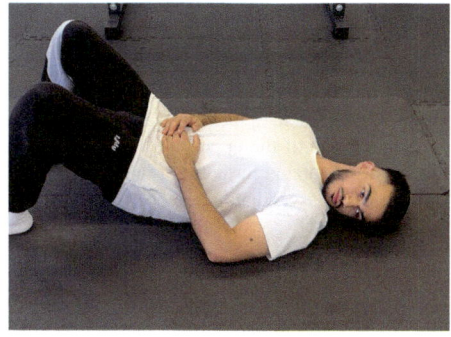

Fig. 6.25 Cervical spine rotation from supine position. The weight transfer to the ground usually allows for a safer execution and greater range of motion for the patient

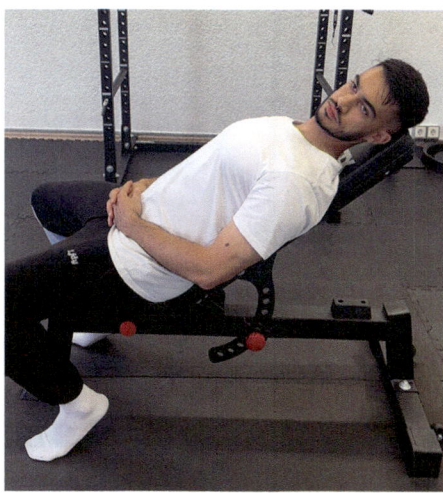

Fig. 6.26 Cervical spine rotation from elevated supine position. Progression to 6.25

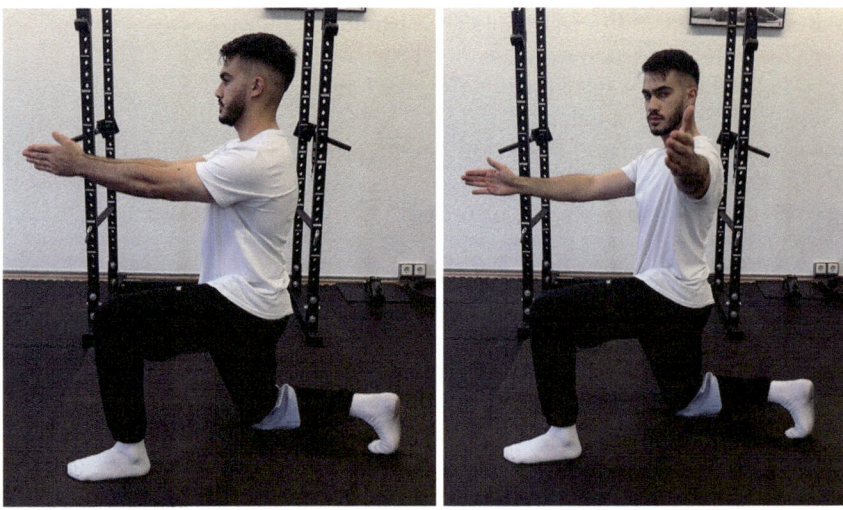

Fig. 6.27 Thoracic spine-dominant rotation. Through the visual fixation of the moving palms and the rotation of the upper body with horizontal shoulder adduction, the cervical spine is biomechanically rotated further, but the movement is not an implicit cervical spine rotation exercise and may serve as a cognitive opener

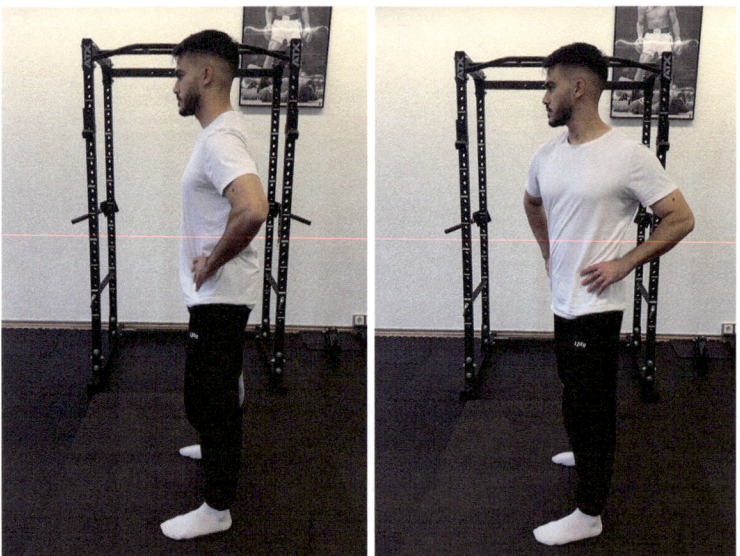

Fig. 6.28 Thoracic spine rotation without head rotation. Through the visual fixation of a point and a thoracic spine rotation without head rotation, an indirect counter-rotating cervical spine rotation is created. In the following example, there is a reversal of Punctum Fixum and Mobile, with the thoracic spine rotating to the left and the cervical spine indirectly rotating to the right

6.2 Specific Exercise Recommendations

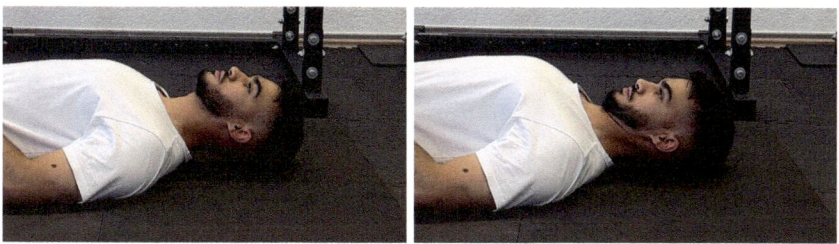

Fig. 6.29 Chin-in from supine position. Isometric activation of the high cervical flexors and deep cervical extensors

Fig. 6.30 Isometric cervical extension

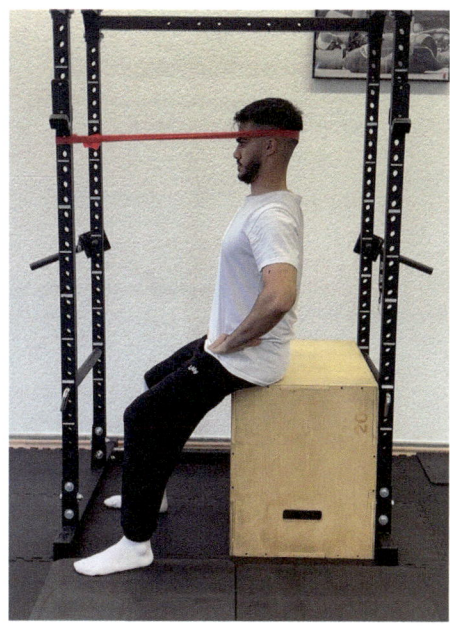

Fig. 6.31 Isometric cervical flexion

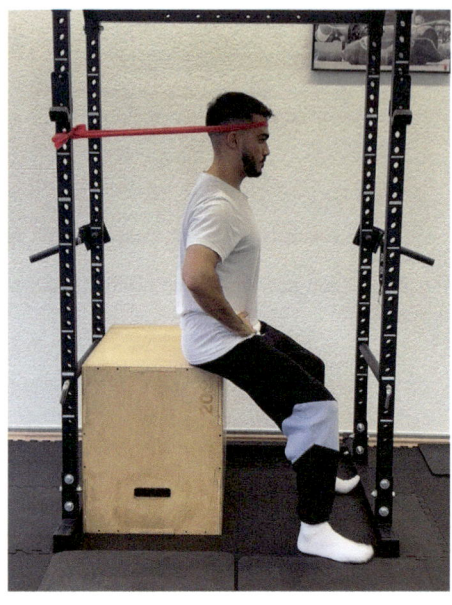

Fig. 6.32 Isometric cervical lateral flexion to the left

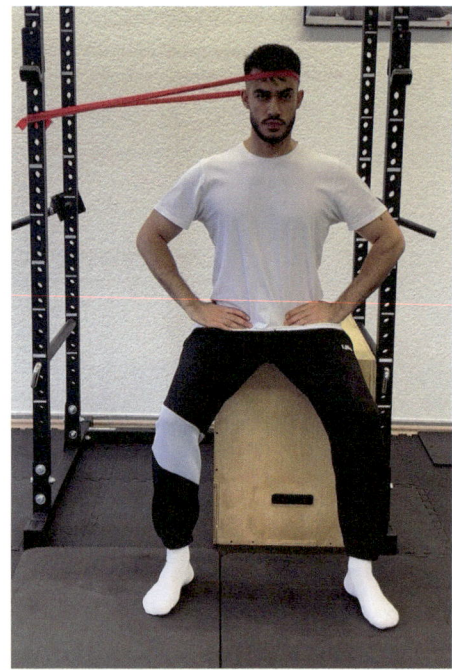

6.2 Specific Exercise Recommendations

Fig. 6.33 Isometric cervical rotation to the left. It is difficult to create a torque into the rotation with a band. It helps to sit further forward so that the pull goes dorsolaterally

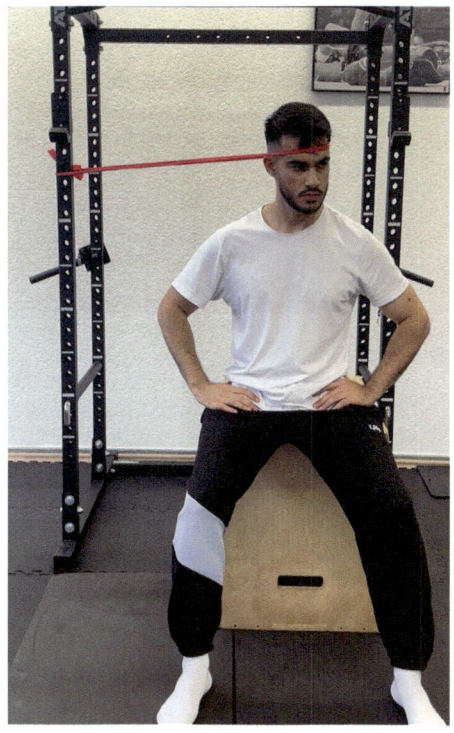

Fig. 6.34 Isometric cervical rotation to the left with the hand. With the hand, a better anti-rotation activity can be triggered by a pressure on the lateral forehead towards the medial

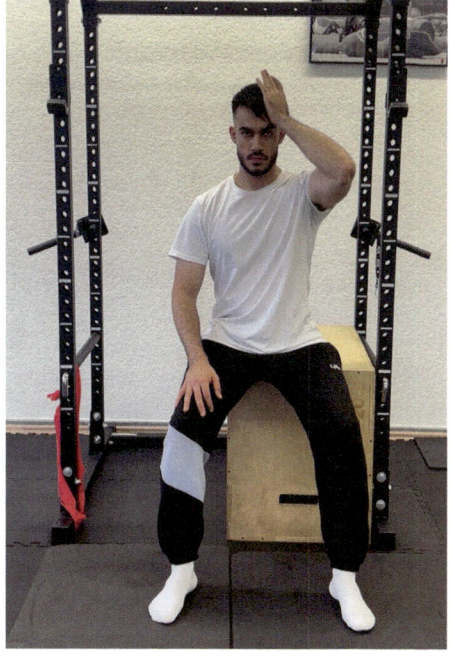

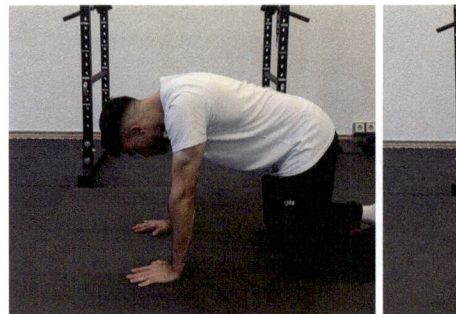
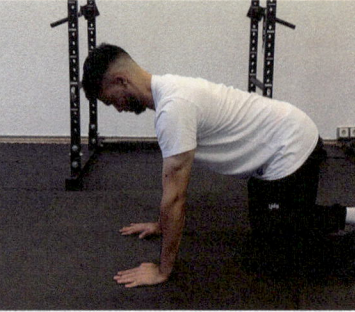

Fig. 6.35 Deep cervical mobilization. The nose always points towards the ground. This achieves movement of deep cervical and high thoracic segments

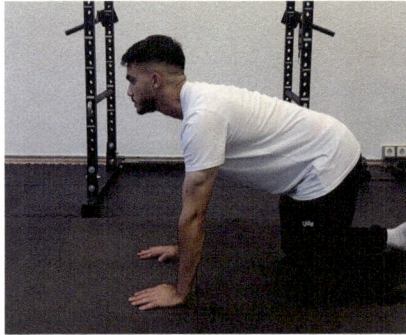
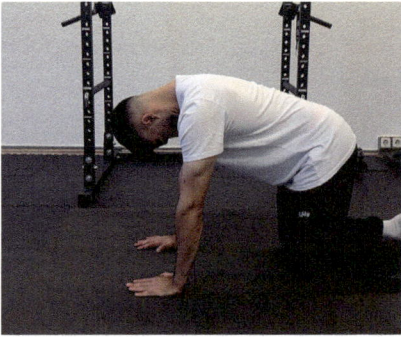

Fig. 6.36 High cervical mobilization. Nose and head swing along, look forward and down at the back. Progression to 6.35 in individual patient cases, who particularly have problems in high cervical regions

Fig. 6.37 Dynamic strengthening of cervical flexion. Example for cervical flexion. Extension from prone position

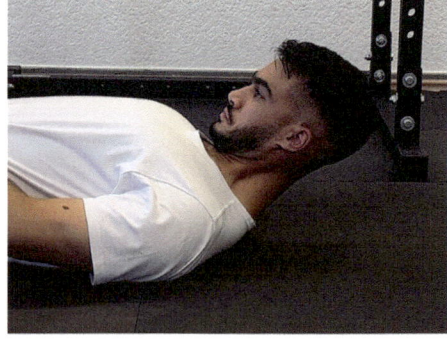

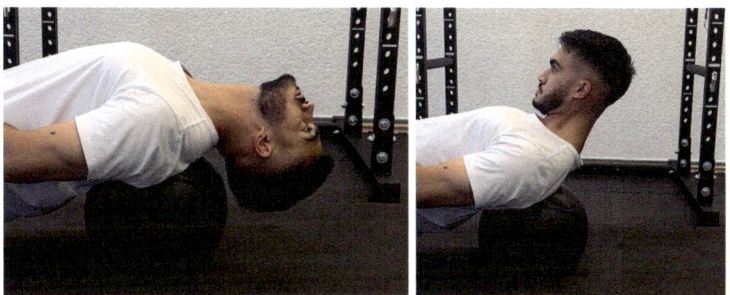

Fig. 6.38 Dynamic strengthening of cervical flexion from overhang. Progression to 6.37 due to larger range of motion

Fig. 6.39 Dynamic strengthening of cervical flexion with band

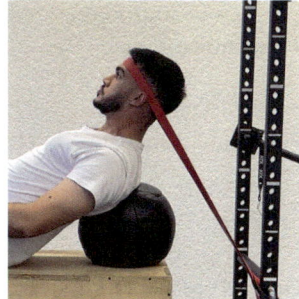

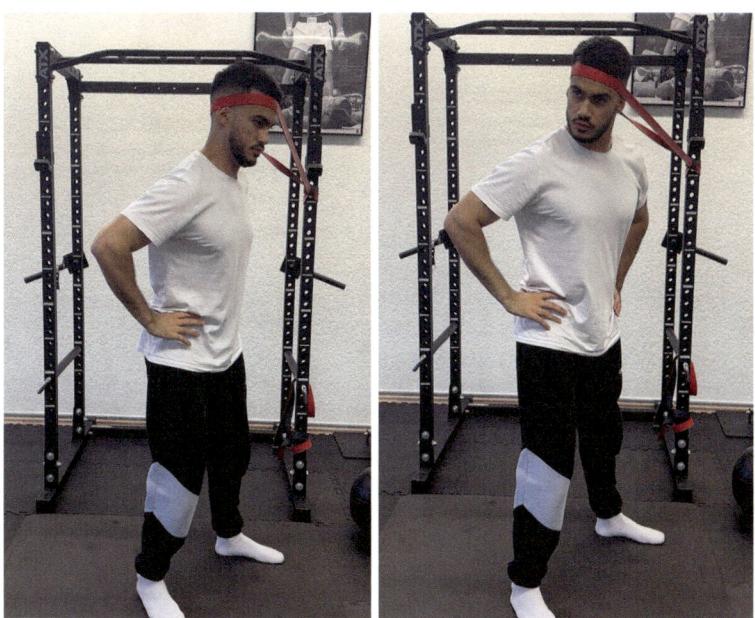

Fig. 6.40 Dynamic strengthening of cervical rotation with band

6.2.3 Chronic Neck Pain

Example 3

An office worker has been plagued by persistent neck pain and tension for several months. Ergonomic workplace and posture settings have not yet had the desired effect. She experiences neck pain after sitting for a long time, which then leads to concentration problems, which is why she tries to sit as straight and upright as possible to delay the onset of increased pain. However, she is not successful in this. In addition, shoulder abduction is very painful for the neck, which is why she avoids this movement to prevent further tension. The shoulder has therefore become somewhat stiffer according to her perception. ◄

Problematic Movement: prolonged sitting, shoulder abduction

Pain Indications:

- persistent neck pain NRPS 2, after 2–3 h sitting NRPS 7 (Fig. 6.41)
- Shoulder abduction NRPS 6 from 80° (Fig. 6.42)

Fig. 6.41 painful neck

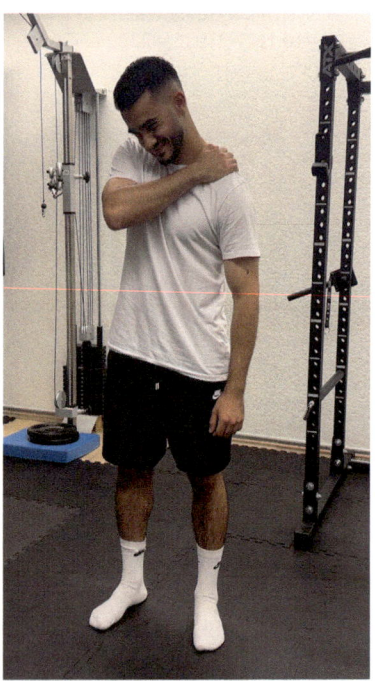

Fig. 6.42 painful shoulder abduction

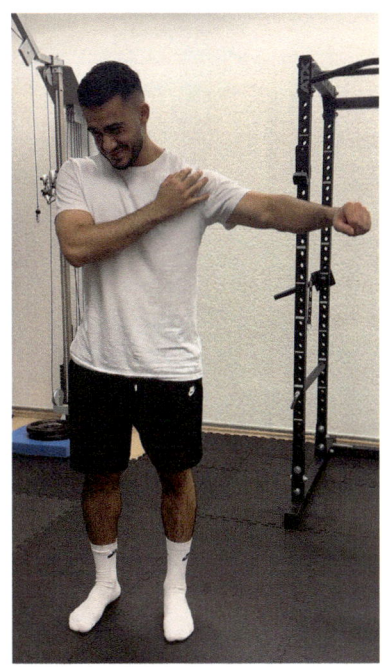

Exercise Recommendations:

1. Starting a movement routine at work:
   - Education about the necessity of posture variation
   - Education about the necessity of movement, even of those that feel stiff or painful, which subsequently bring positive results
   - General movements of the arms, shoulders, and spine
2. Shoulder mobility exercises (Fig. 6.43, 6.44 and 6.45):
3. Building up the load capacity of the neck muscles (Fig. 6.46, 6.47, 6.48, 6.49 and 6.50):
   - Progression of the exercise plan with additional pull and push exercises

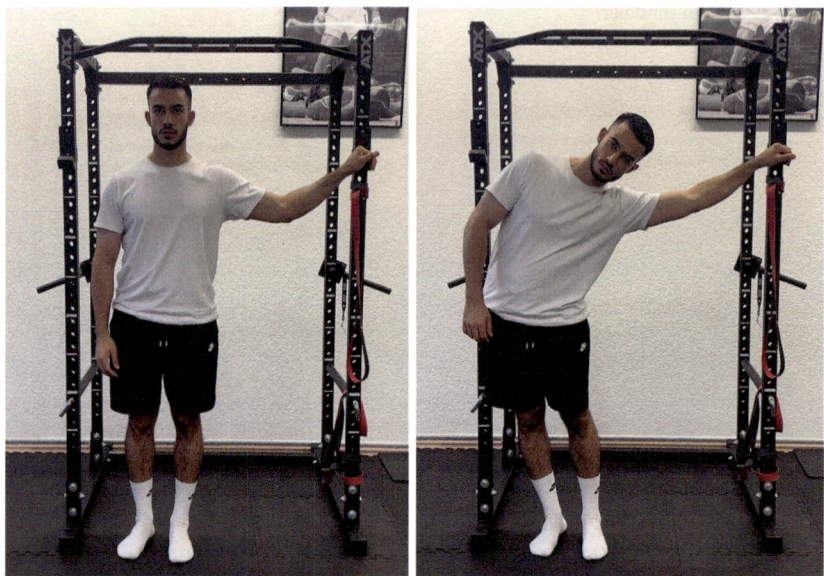

Fig. 6.43 Passive shoulder abduction with fulcrum. By swapping Punctum Fixum and Mobile, the abducting muscles are less activated and indirectly a greater abduction is achieved than would be the case actively against gravity

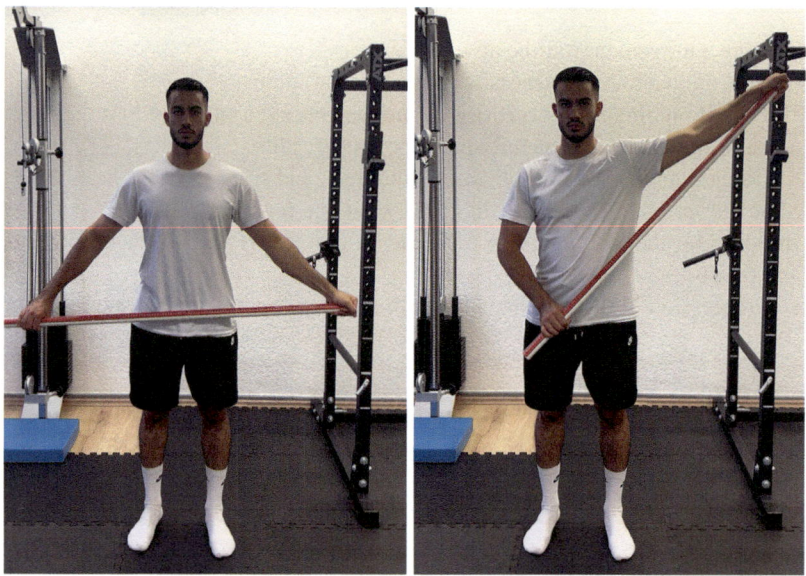

Fig. 6.44 Assistive shoulder abduction with rod. Progression to 6.43 through more active work of the abducting muscles. The push of the right hand relieves the left shoulder compared to abduction without a rod

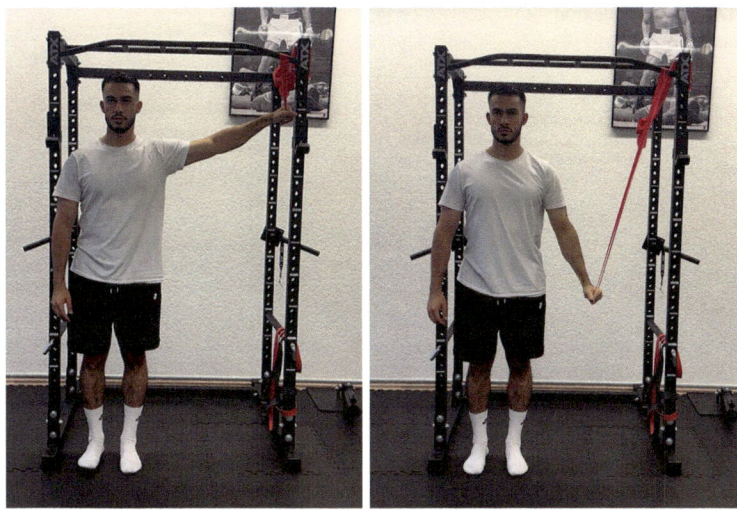

Fig. 6.45 Shoulder abduction with antagonistic resistance. The adducting muscles are eccentrically active during abduction and can relieve the abducting muscles and facilitate abduction. The movement task is an adduction, which can also be a cognitive approach to the abduction coded as painful

Fig. 6.46 Shoulder abduction with resistance

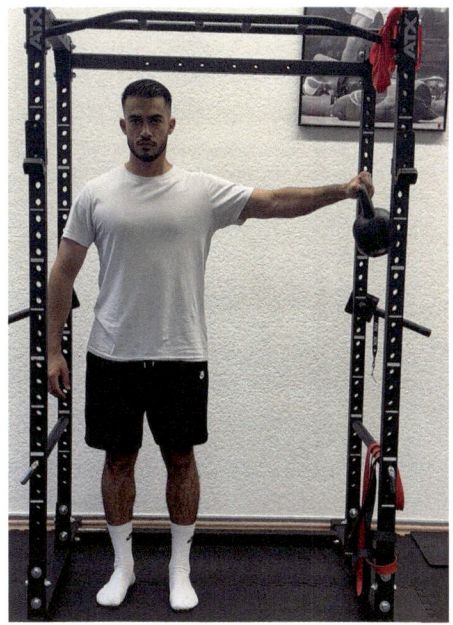

Fig. 6.47 Shoulder flexion with resistance

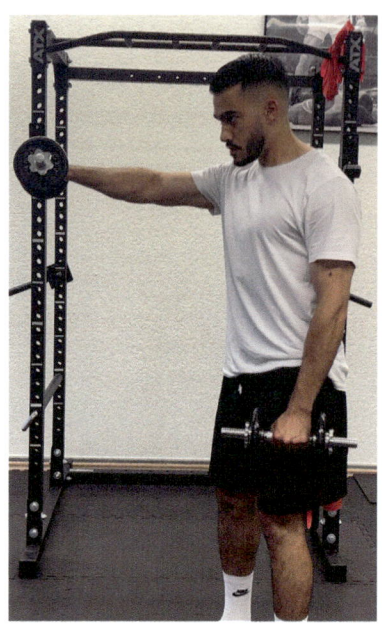

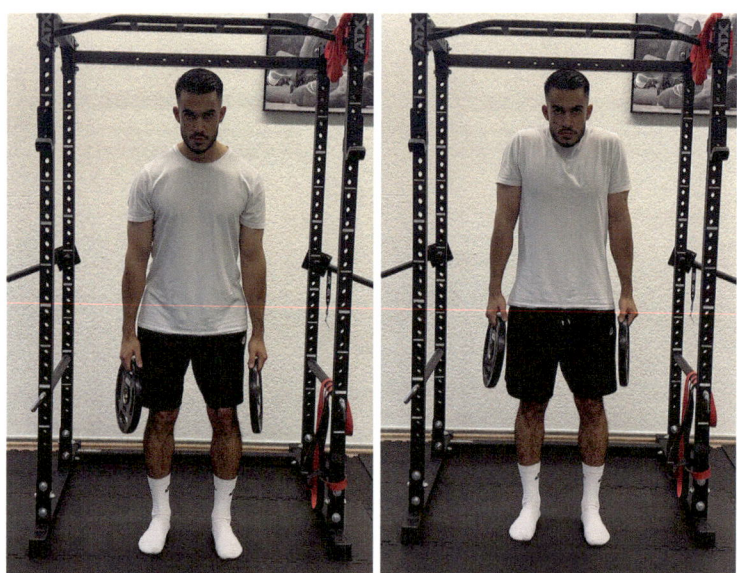

Fig. 6.48 Shrugs with resistance

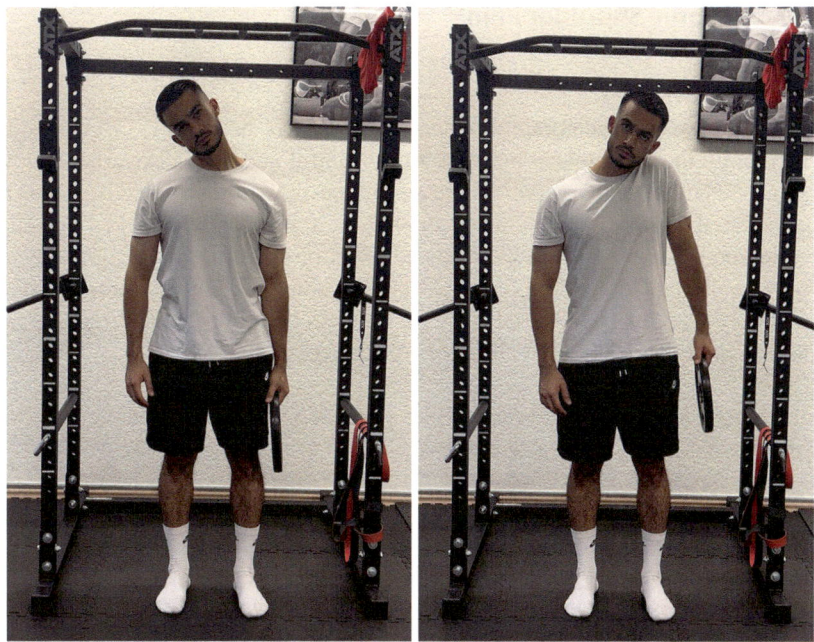

Fig. 6.49 Unilateral shrugs. Progression to 6.48 through ipsilateral cervical spine lateral flexion in the concentric phase and contralateral cervical spine lateral flexion in the eccentric phase

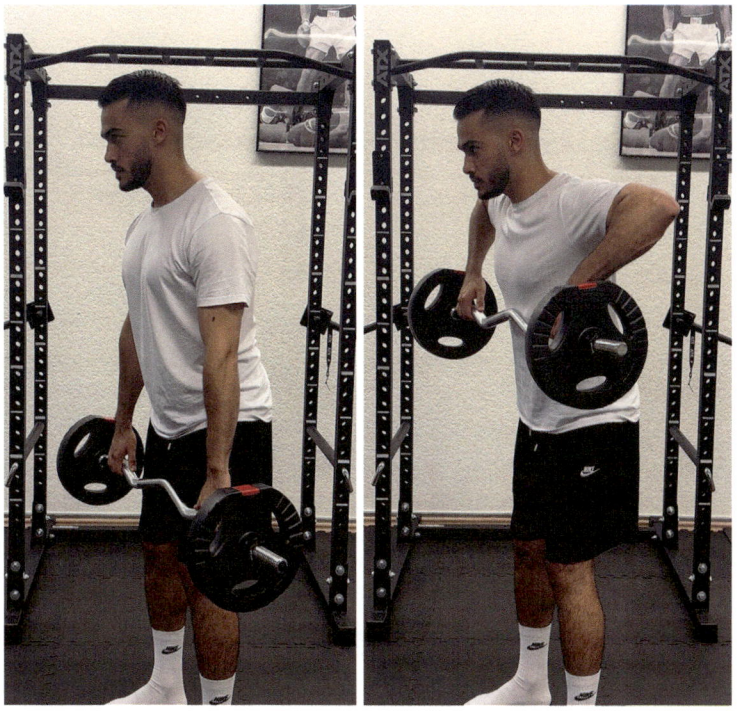

Fig. 6.50 Upright Rowing

6.2.4 Chronic Shoulder Pain

Example 4

A patient has long-standing persistent postoperative pain in the right shoulder. Especially the arm elevation above 90° is painful and thus all overhead movements like the tennis serve or pressure-intensive strength exercises like the overhead press. He has minimized strength exercises for the shoulder and eliminated pressure exercises like overhead press or even the (non-painful) bench press or lat pull-down to avoid stressing the shoulder. He used to play tennis regularly with his friends, but since he wants to be a full-fledged training partner, he prefers not to play tennis so as not to lower the level. ◄

Problematic Movement: Shoulder elevation and pressure-intensive overhead movements.

Pain Indications:

- Shoulder flexion NRPS 2 from 90° and end-stage NRPS 5 (Fig. 6.51)
- Overhead press from 100° NRPS 3, even with light weight (Fig. 6.52)
- Tennis serve NRPS 6
- Feeling of stiffness from 120° shoulder elevation

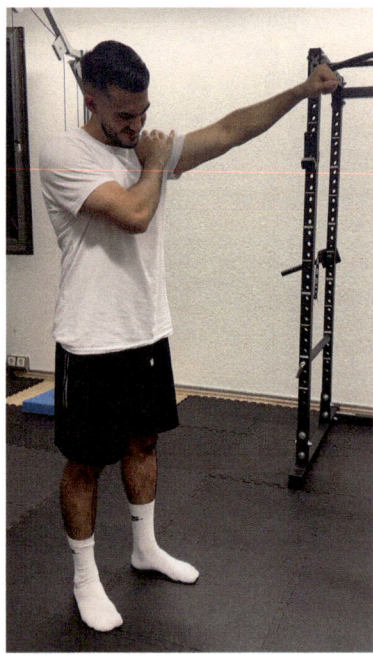

Fig. 6.51 Painful shoulder flexion

Fig. 6.52 Painful overhead press

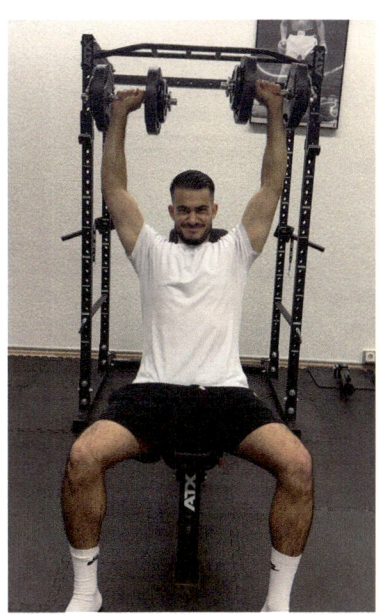

Exercise Recommendations:

1. Maintaining/Resuming tennis and strength training
   - Open communication with training partners about limitations
   - Playing tennis without serving
   - Resume non-painful pressure exercises, such as bench press
   - Resume non-painful pulling exercises, including those over 90° arm elevation, such as lat pull-down
2. Mobilization exercises from alternative less painful positions (Fig. 6.53 and 6.54)
3. Adjustment of painful overhead movements (Fig. 6.55, 6.56 and 6.57)
   - Incline Press for load capacity building over 90° (Fig. 6.55):
   - Gradual increase of overhead pressure exercises by adjusting the ROM in the Overheadpress to a tolerable angle (Fig. 6.56):
   - Front raises to a tolerable angle (Fig. 6.57):
4. Training surrounding structures at the border to the painful area:
   - Lateral Raises
   - Open lateral rowing
   - Cable pullovers

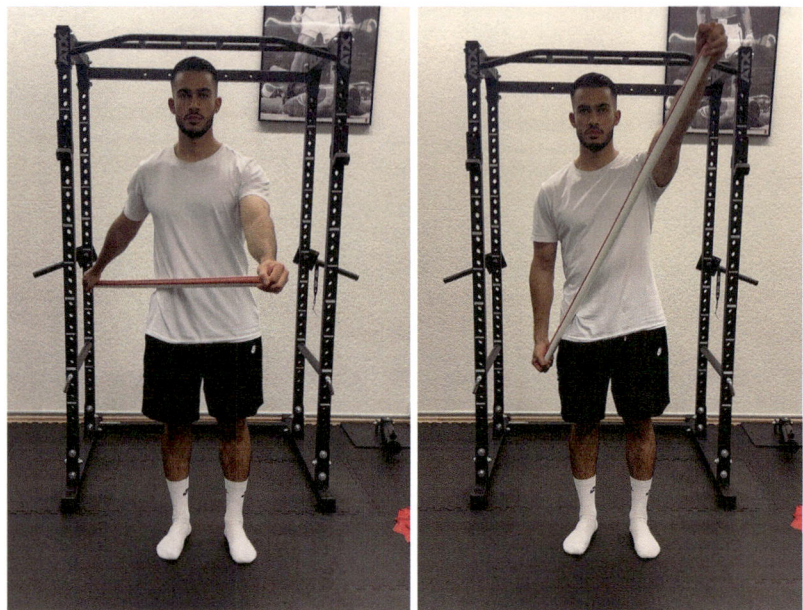

Fig. 6.53 Assistive shoulder flexion with rod

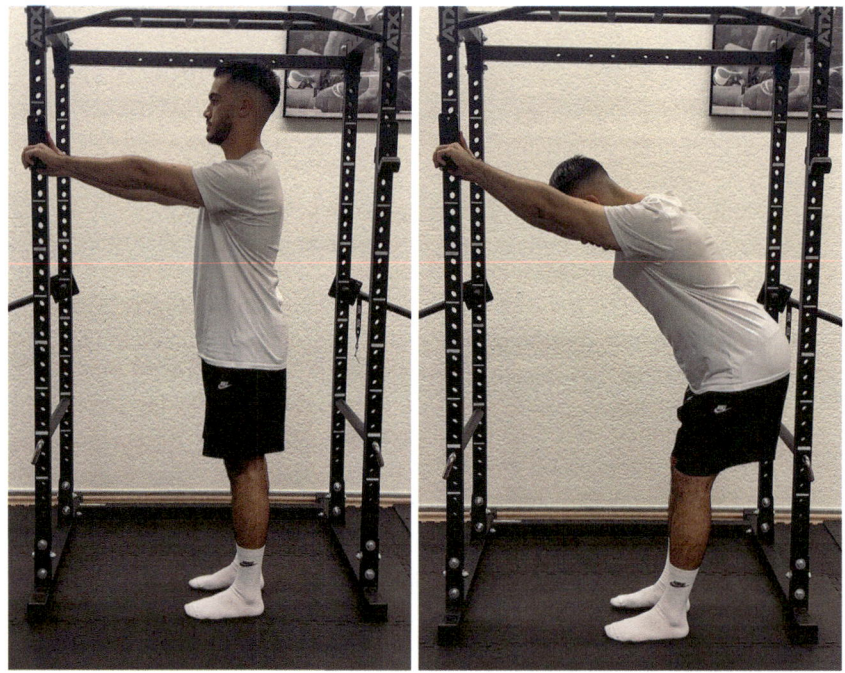

Fig. 6.54 Shoulder flexion with abutment on the wall

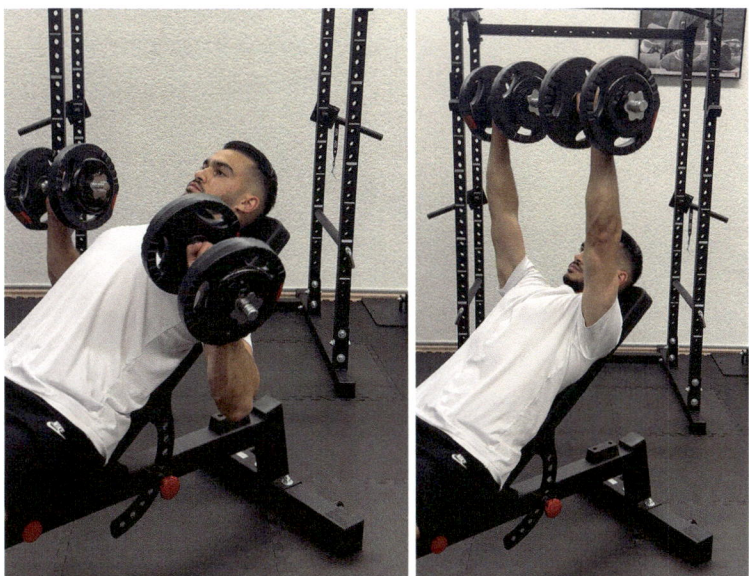

Fig. 6.55 Incline Dumbbell Bench Press

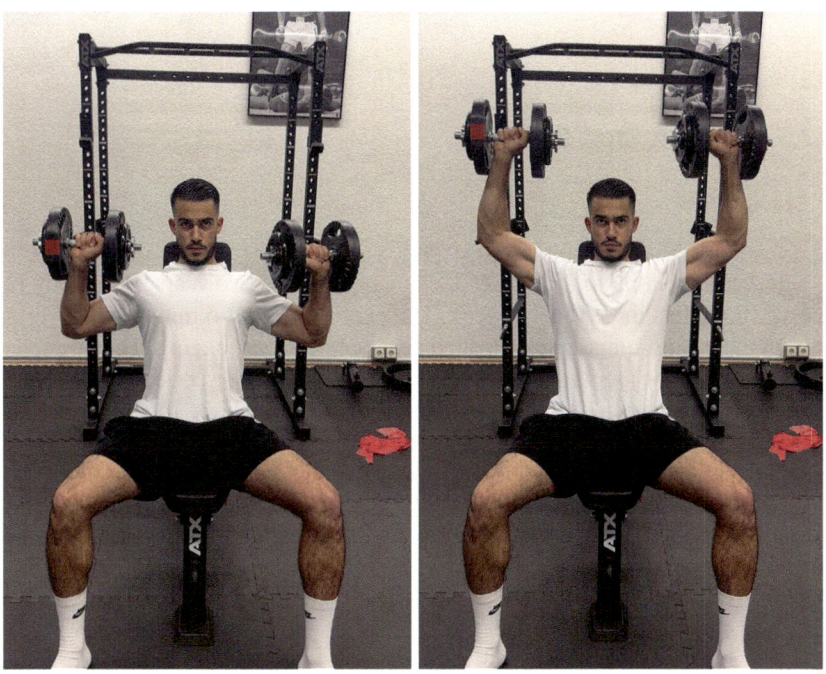

Fig. 6.56 Adjusted Overhead Press. Another possible regression is the Overhead Press in the closed chain with a barbell or in a guided device

Fig. 6.57 Front Raise

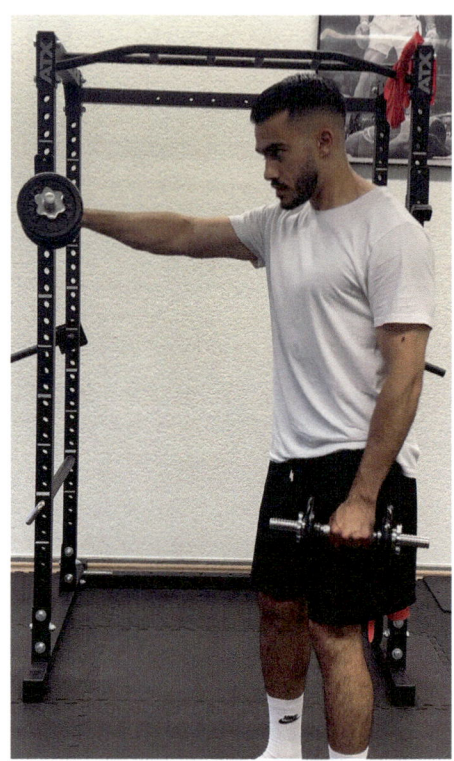

6.2.5 Chronic Knee Pain

> **Example 5**
>
> An ambitious runner has been experiencing persistent knee pain on the left side, caudo-ventral to the kneecap, while jogging for two years. He usually runs 5–7 kilometers three times a week. The pain starts after 5 minutes and worsens with increasing running time, which also persists after jogging. Therefore, he is considering not jogging at all. In strength training, he experiences pain during knee-dominant exercises such as squats or lunges, which is why he was recommended a general multi-week break from strength training. In addition, he reports increasing knee stiffness, especially in the deep squat. ◄

Problematic Movement: Running, knee-dominant strength exercises, and end-range knee flexion.

Pain Reports:

- Running from minute 5 NRPS 6, increasing from minute 15 NRPS 8, pain after running up to 24 hours at NRPS 4

6.2 Specific Exercise Recommendations

- Squats with 40 kg from 60° knee flexion painful, NRPS 3 (Fig. 6.58)
- Lunges painful in the front leg already from 50° without additional weight NRPS 6 (Fig. 6.59)
- Deep squat stiffness feeling in the knee (Fig. 6.60)

Exercise Recommendations:

1. Maintenance/Adjustment of Running Training
   - Reduction of weekly running volume: A sensible strategy could be to reduce the weekly running volume from about 15 km to, for example, approximately 10 km. This could be achieved through two units of 5 km or three units of 3.3 km. This adjustment aims to reduce the load on the knee joint without having to completely abandon running training.
   - Adjustment of running mechanics such as reducing stride length and increasing cadence. This technique optimization could make it possible to maintain or even cautiously increase the previous running volume without increasing the intensity of pain.
   - Combined adjustment: Volume reduction and running technique optimization. Here, the running volume would initially be temporarily reduced to create a basic relief. At the same time, the running mechanics are adjusted. With increasing adaptation and pain relief, the running volume could then be gradually increased again.

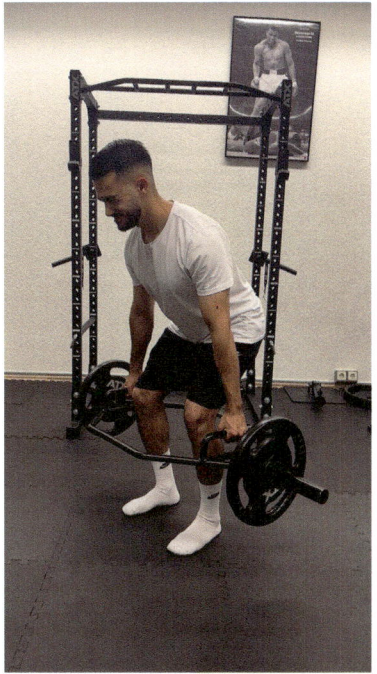

Fig. 6.58 painful squat

Fig. 6.59 painful lunge

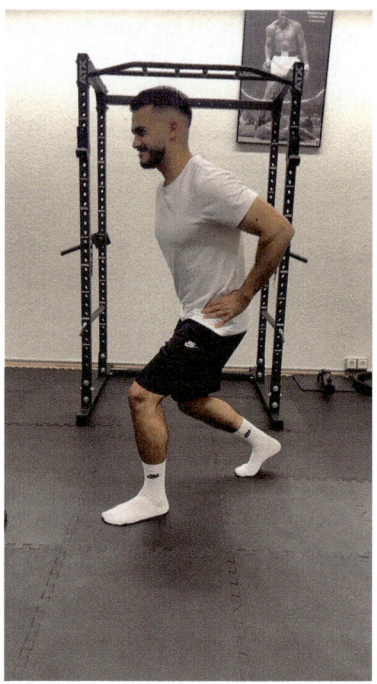

Fig. 6.60 stiff deep squat

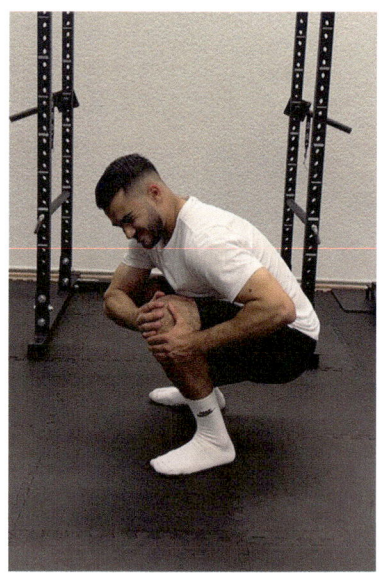

6.2 Specific Exercise Recommendations

To reliably assess the effectiveness of an adjustment, it is advisable to implement it consistently over a period of several weeks. Only in this way can possible changes in symptoms be accurately observed and evaluated. It is important to note that an adjustment should not be prematurely classified as ineffective if no noticeable improvements have occurred after just one week. Often, the body needs more time to respond to changes and show positive effects, especially with nociplastic pain.

2. Maintaining/Adjusting Strength Training
   - No general break from strength sports
   - Continue or even intensify pain-free hip-dominant exercises (examples: deadlifts, ab-/adductor on the machine, hip thrusts)
   - Continue to train low-pain knee-dominant exercises such as leg extensions or curls
   - Adjust painful squats:
     – Continue to work in full range of motion with under 40 kg.
     – From 40kg, reduce ROM to up to 50° knee flexion for a low-pain comfort zone, for example on the hex bar
     – B-Stance variant, painful knee forward and load more on the rear foot. This reduces knee flexion and load on the front knee (Fig. 6.61)
     – Lift hip-dominantly and minimize knee flexion (Fig. 6.62)
     – Isometric strength exercises (Fig. 6.63, 6.64 and 6.65):

Fig. 6.61 B-Stance Squat

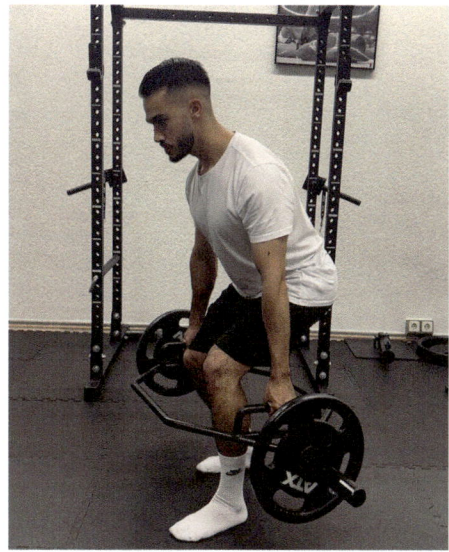

Fig. 6.62 Hip-dominant squat. Similar to deadlift

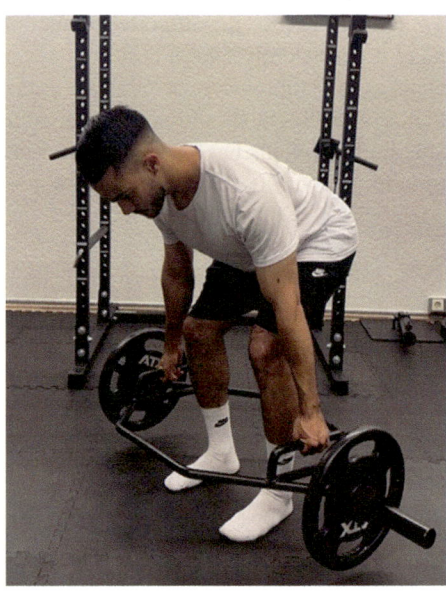

Fig. 6.63 Bilateral wall sit

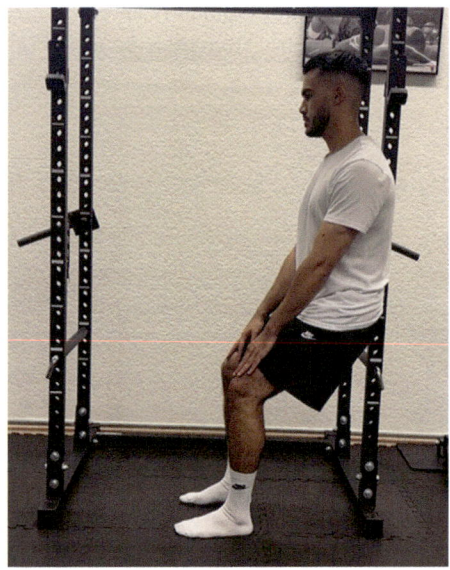

Fig. 6.64 Unilateral wall sit. Progression to 6.63

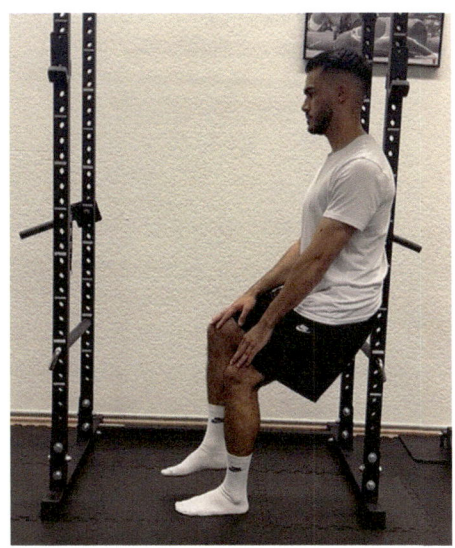

Fig. 6.65 Isometric flexed single-leg stand. Regression to 6.63, due to the upper body tilt more involvement of posterior muscle groups

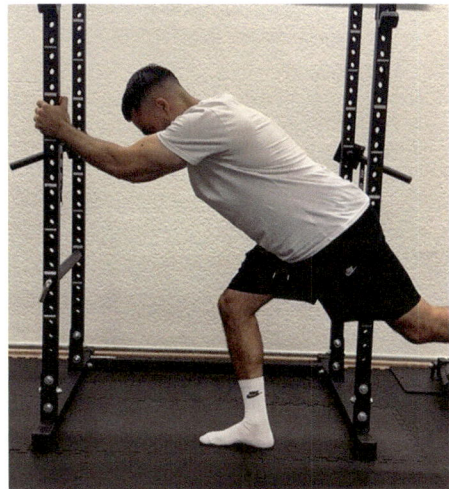

- Adjust painful lunges:
  - Narrower step and adjusted depth.
  - Step-Downs below the painful knee flexion from 50° in small amplitude (Fig. 6.66 and 6.67)
3. Plyometric Initiation
    - Since running is a movement consisting of cyclic unilateral jumps, plyometric exercises should be used to improve knee resilience. Especially after a running break, to progressively reintroduce running. Depending on whether the eccentric phase or concentric phase causes more problems (if at all

Fig. 6.66 Step-Down foot lateral down

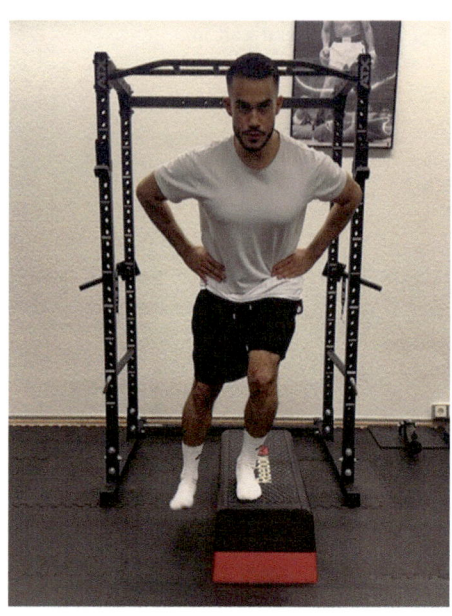

Fig. 6.67 Stepdown foot ventral down. Regression to 6.66 due to the upper body tilt more knee flexion

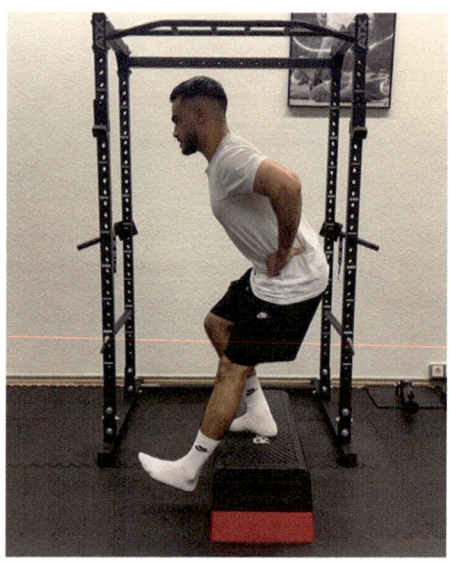

identifiable from pain history), the less painful movement form can continue to be trained and the more problematic movement can be slowly worked on. An exemplary progression for the eccentric phase (Figs. 6.68 6.69, 6.70, 6.71, 6.72 and 6.73):

6.2 Specific Exercise Recommendations

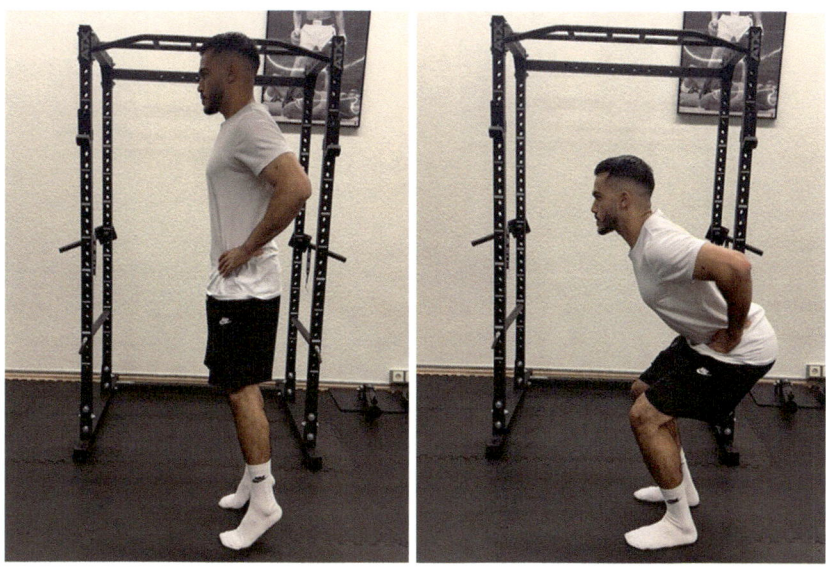

Fig. 6.68 Bilateral landing from a standstill. This movement is not a jump. (Only a fall occurs from the toe stand, without jumping upwards)

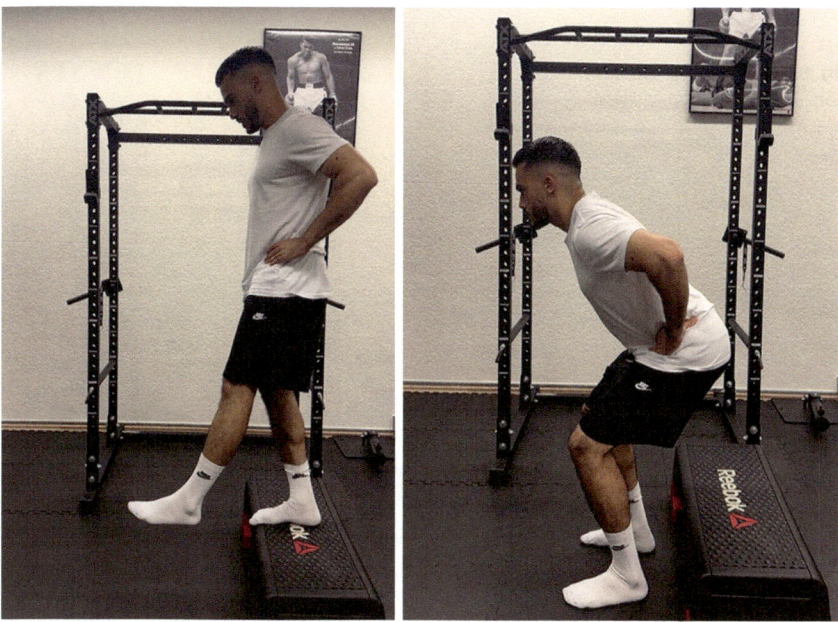

Fig. 6.69 Bilateral landing from an elevation

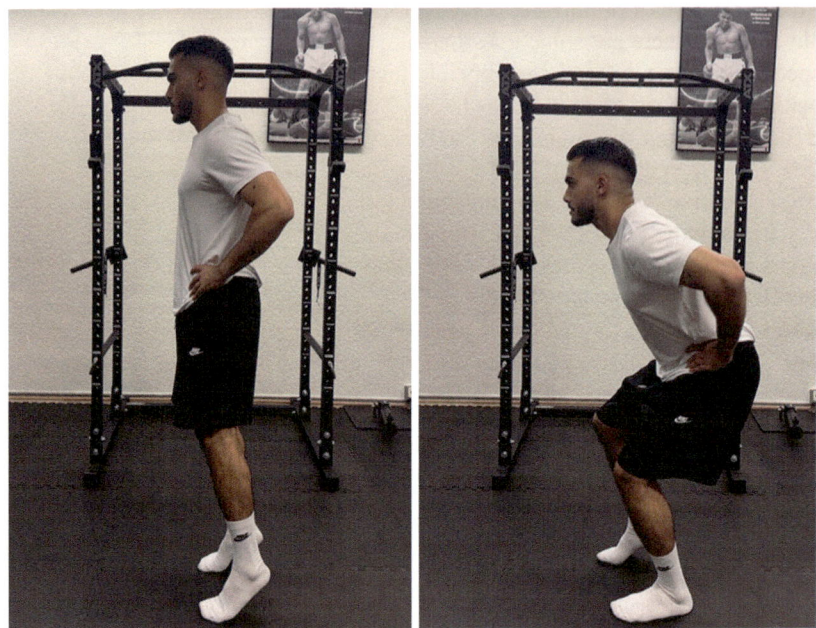

Fig. 6.70 Shifted landing from a standstill. Preparation for unilateral landings. The right foot here serves as a light support for weight reduction and for more stability

Fig. 6.71 Unilateral landing from a standstill. Progression to 6.70

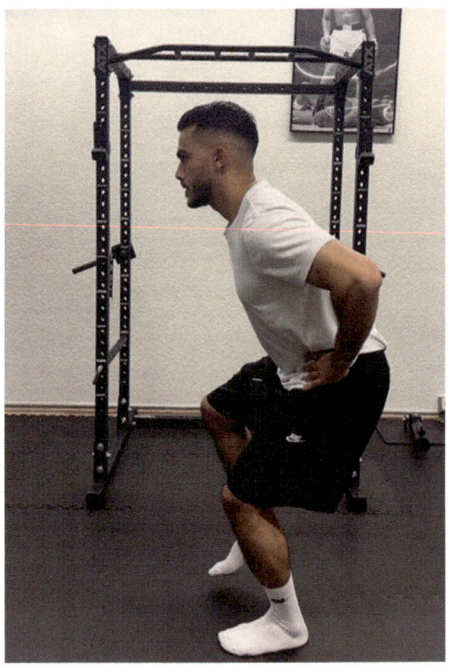

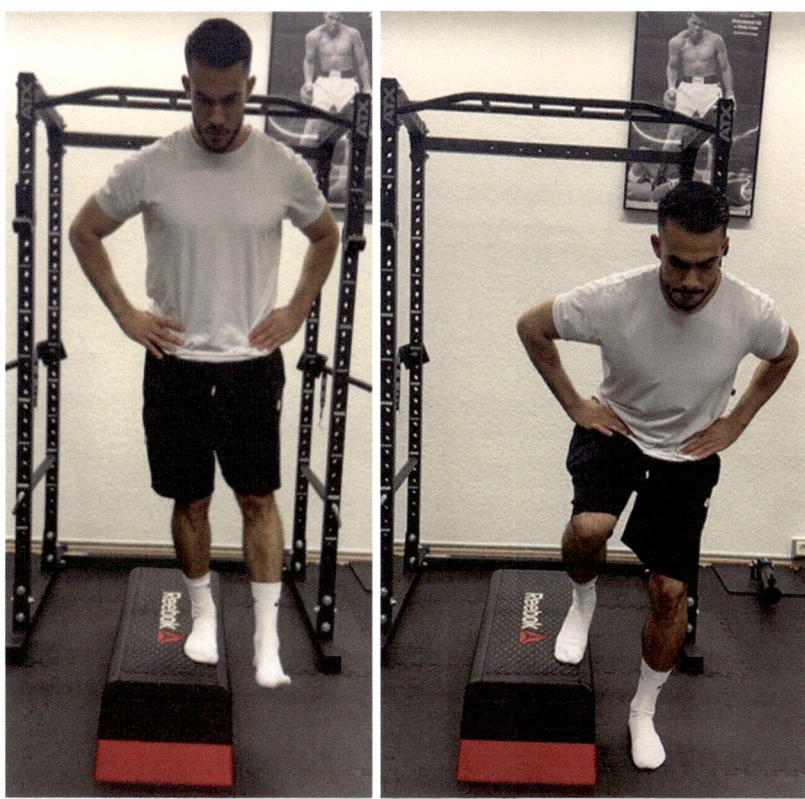

Fig. 6.72 Shifted landing from an elevation. Preparation for unilateral landing from an elevation. The right foot here serves as a light support for weight reduction and for more stability

Fig. 6.73 Unilateral landing from an elevation

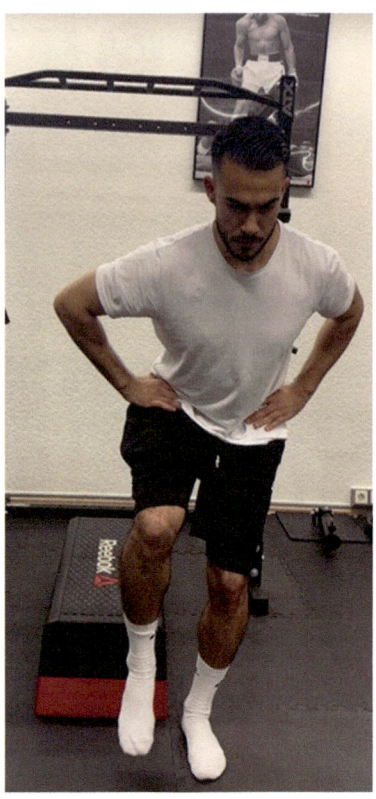

4. End-range knee flexion mobility training
   - Improvement of knee flexion (Fig. 6.74, 6.75, 6.76 and 6.77):

6.2 Specific Exercise Recommendations

Fig. 6.74 Deep squat with holding

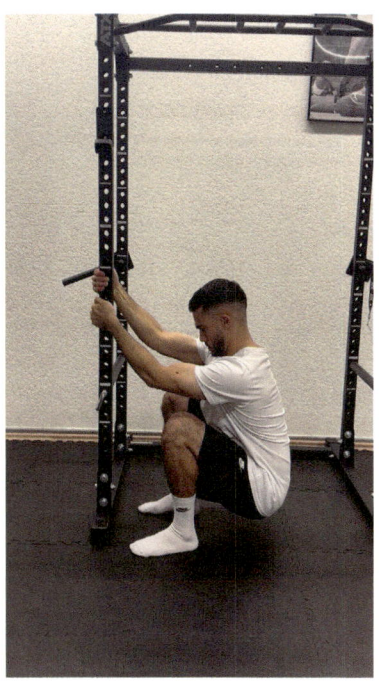

Fig. 6.75 Heel sit variant 1. The near-knee support position allows for better dosing of tolerable pressure on the knee joint

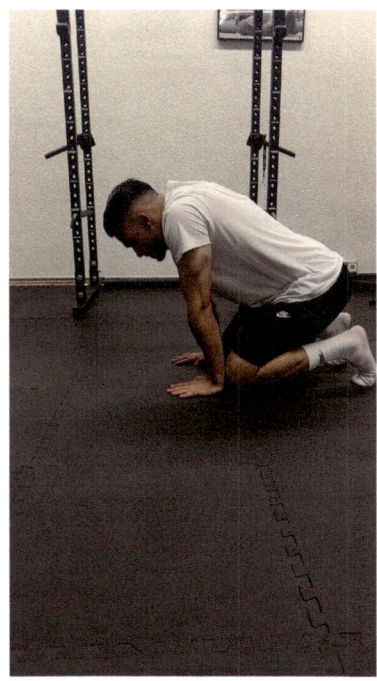

Fig. 6.76 Heel-sit Variant 2

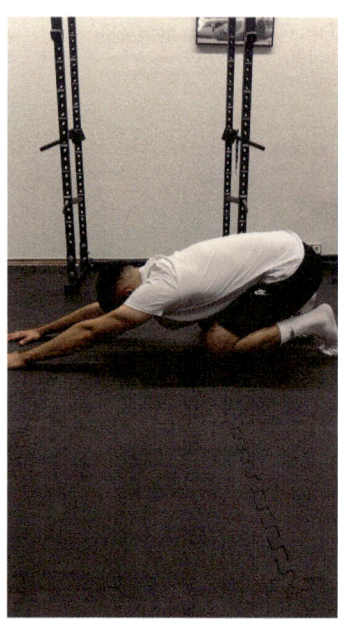

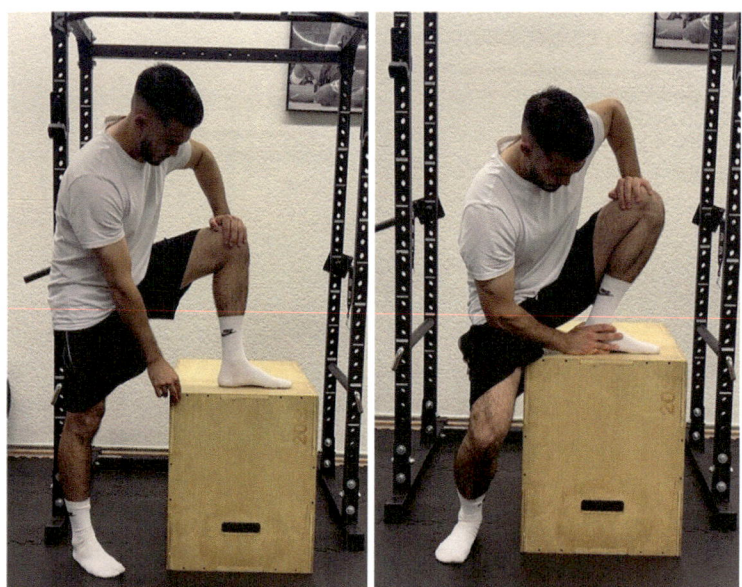

Fig. 6.77 Unilateral Knee Mobilization on an Elevation

6.2 Specific Exercise Recommendations

The exercise recommendations in these five examples contain progressive-dynamic movement approaches, without giving the impression of a specific exercise plan. It is intended as a stimulus for creative movement modifications and pro- and regressions. However, this should not question the possibility, if not even individual necessity, of other pain-relieving strategies such as relaxation techniques, stretching exercises or other forms of movement, such as walking, swimming or other activities. The goal was to provide insight into possible movement modifications while maintaining the highest possible activity level and gradual approach to the problematic/pain-avoided action, which is particularly relevant in physio- and sports therapeutic practice. This chapter deliberately avoided presenting specific formulas, standardized training or periodization models, as well as rigid content and time sequences. Instead, the importance of pronounced clinical expertise in situation-dependent adaptability and the sensible progression or regression of movement interventions is emphasized. This ability for individualized therapy design allows the therapist to flexibly respond to the changing needs and capacities of the patient.

In the therapy of chronic pain, it is crucial to understand that no linear improvement is to be expected. Rather, the healing process is often characterized by fluctuations that can include both progress and temporary setbacks. This non-linearity requires a high degree of flexibility from the therapist and the ability to continuously adapt the therapy concept. The perception of pain in chronic conditions is influenced by a multitude of factors that go far beyond purely biomechanical aspects. Accordingly, exercise therapy, whose effectiveness is often attributed exclusively to biomechanical changes, should also be adapted to contextual, mental and cognitive factors and increased gradually. The regressions modified from the problematic movements form the progression towards the old, problematic movements in the course of rehabilitation. Whether the gradual increase initially takes place through the expansion of the range of motion or the increase in training volume or intensity should be decided situationally and adapted to individual factors. It is important to consider not only physical aspects but also psycho-social factors, as proposed by O'Sullivan and colleagues (2018) in the context of CFT. The goal should still be to get closer to the problematic movement, both from a biomechanical and cognitive perspective. This includes not only the kinematic approach to the problematic movement but also addressing movement fears and negative beliefs about pain. Vlaeyen and Linton (2012) emphasize in their fear-avoidance model the importance of gradually counteracting feared or perceived dangerous movements to break the vicious circle of fear and avoidance behavior.

The flexibility in therapy design requires a profound understanding of pain physiology, movement biomechanics, and psycho-social influencing factors from the therapist. Only in this way can truly patient-centered therapy be designed that is oriented towards the individual needs, goals, and reactions of the patient. This may seem more complex at first glance than standardized protocols, but in the long term, it leads to more sustainable results and higher patient satisfaction, as studies on personalized pain therapy show (Foster et al., 2018).

The key to success lies in the ability to keep patients moving as much as possible and to gradually expand this, without negligently provoking overloads or negative experiences. In the event of relapse events, such as significant pain increase or functional restrictions, it is essential to promote the patient's resilience, avoid maladaptive cognitions and the progression of kinesiophobia, and reactivate motivation through education and modified therapeutic approaches. The focus should be on strengthening self-efficacy and implementing adaptive coping strategies to ensure sustainable rehabilitation. Setbacks are normal and should not be dramatized. This approach not only promotes physical functionality but also supports the development of self-efficacy and a positive understanding of movement in chronic pain patients.

Pain. A symptom—countless measures to alleviate it. Therapists should adhere to scientific guidelines, whose authors, contrary to popular belief, are not just professors or laboratory researchers without patient contact. Finally, based on current research results, some do's and don'ts can be formulated, which should represent core strategies of chronic pain therapy:

Do's:

1. Maintaining activity: Continuous physical activity promotes functionality and reduces the risk of secondary complications (Geneen et al., 2017).
2. Maintaining functional behaviors: Continuing adaptive routines strengthens self-efficacy and supports everyday coping (Foster et al., 2018).
3. Hedonistic activities: The integration of joyful activities promotes positive affects and can modulate pain perception (Flink et al., 2015). Interventions should be fun.
4. Education on pain physiology: Sound knowledge about pain mechanisms can reduce catastrophizing thoughts and improve self-management (Moseley & Butler, 2015).
5. Focus on quality of life: Instead of a pure pain reduction of the affected body part, the expansion of the quality of life of the affected person should be prioritized (Kamper et al., 2015).
6. Maintaining social relationships: Social interaction and support are essential for mental well-being and pain adaptation (Karayannis et al., 2019).

Don'ts:

1. Uncritical information intake. Solution: Selective evaluation of information sources to avoid maladaptive beliefs.
2. Overvaluation of imaging diagnostics. Solution: Consideration of the limited correlation between structural findings and pain experience (Brinjikji et al., 2015).
3. Pathologizing physiological phenomena. Solution: Differentiation between normal variations and clinically relevant red-flag findings.
4. Equating pain with tissue damage. Solution: Conveying the complex bio-psycho-social pain model (Moseley & Butler, 2015).

5. Maladaptive pain reactions such as protection and avoidance. Solution: Promotion of adaptive coping strategies to avoid hypervigilance and catastrophizing.
6. Antagonistic handling of pain. Solution: Implementation of acceptance-based interventions as a basis for behavioral changes (McCracken & Vowles, 2014).

Your patients are waiting for you. And they look forward to a therapist who is empathetic, can respond to the patient's needs, incorporates current scientific findings into his therapies, restores movement, joy and activity, demands active participation through positive communication and motivation, avoids nocebos, increases the patient's self-efficacy expectation, increases physical resilience, reduces worries and fears, and thus sustainably improves quality of life.

References

Ageberg, E., Link, A., & Roos, E. M. (2010). Feasibility of neuromuscular training in patients with severe hip or knee OA: The individualized goal-based NEMEX-TJR training program. *BMC musculoskeletal disorders, 11*, 126. https://doi.org/10.1186/1471-2474-11-126

Brinjikji, W., Luetmer, P. H., Comstock, B., Bresnahan, B. W., Chen, L. E., Deyo, R. A., Halabi, S., Turner, J. A., Avins, A. L., James, K., Wald, J. T., Kallmes, D. F., & Jarvik, J. G. (2015). Systematic literature review of imaging features of spinal degeneration in asymptomatic populations. *AJNR. American journal of neuroradiology, 36*(4), 811–816. https://doi.org/10.3174/ajnr.A4173

Butera, K. A., Fox, E. J., & George, S. Z. (2016). Toward a Transformed Understanding: From Pain and Movement to Pain With Movement. *Physical therapy, 96*(10), 1503–1507. https://doi.org/10.2522/ptj.20160211

Cashin, A. G., Booth, J., McAuley, J. H., Jones, M. D., Hübscher, M., Traeger, A. C., Fried, K., & Moseley, G. L. (2022). Making exercise count: Considerations for the role of exercise in back pain treatment. *Musculoskeletal Care, 20*(2), 259–270. https://doi.org/10.1002/msc.1597

Flink, I. K., Smeets, E., Bergboma, S., & Peters, M. L. (2015). Happy despite pain: Pilot study of a positive psychology intervention for patients with chronic pain. *Scandinavian journal of pain, 7*(1), 71–79. https://doi.org/10.1016/j.sjpain.2015.01.005

Foster, N. E., Anema, J. R., Cherkin, D., Chou, R., Cohen, S. P., Gross, D. P., Ferreira, P. H., Fritz, J. M., Koes, B. W., Peul, W., Turner, J. A., Maher, C. G., & Lancet Low Back Pain Series Working Group (2018). Prevention and treatment of low back pain: Evidence, challenges, and promising directions. *Lancet (London, England), 391*(10137), 2368–2383. https://doi.org/10.1016/S0140-6736(18)30489-6

Geneen, L. J., Moore, R. A., Clarke, C., Martin, D., Colvin, L. A., & Smith, B. H. (2017). Physical activity and exercise for chronic pain in adults: An overview of Cochrane Reviews. *The Cochrane database of systematic reviews, 4*(4), CD011279. https://doi.org/10.1002/14651858.CD011279.pub3

Kamper, S. J., Apeldoorn, A. T., Chiarotto, A., Smeets, R. J., Ostelo, R. W., Guzman, J., & van Tulder, M. W. (2015). Multidisciplinary biopsychosocial rehabilitation for chronic low back pain: Cochrane systematic review and meta-analysis. *BMJ (Clinical research ed.), 350*, h444. https://doi.org/10.1136/bmj.h444

Karayannis, N. V., Baumann, I., Sturgeon, J. A., Melloh, M., & Mackey, S. C. (2019). The Impact of Social Isolation on Pain Interference: A Longitudinal Study. *Annals of behavioral medicine : A Publication of the Society of Behavioral Medicine, 53*(1), 65–74. https://doi.org/10.1093/abm/kay017

Kechichian, A., Lafrance, S., Matifat, E., Dubé, F., Lussier, D., Benhaim, P., Perreault, K., Filiatrault, J., Rainville, P., Higgins, J., Rousseau, J., Masse, J., & Desmeules, F. (2022). Multimodal Interventions Including Rehabilitation Exercise for Older Adults With Chronic Musculoskeletal Pain: A Systematic Review and Meta-analyses of Randomized Controlled Trials. *Journal of geriatric physical therapy (2001)*, *45*(1), 34–49. https://doi.org/10.1519/JPT.0000000000000279

McCracken, L. M., & Vowles, K. E. (2014). Acceptance and commitment therapy and mindfulness for chronic pain: Model, process, and progress. *The American psychologist*, *69*(2), 178–187. https://doi.org/10.1037/a0035623

Merkle, S. L., Sluka, K. A., & Frey-Law, L. A. (2020). The interaction between pain and movement. *Journal of Hand Therapy : Official Journal of the American Society of Hand Therapists*, *33*(1), 60–66. https://doi.org/10.1016/j.jht.2018.05.001

Mittinty, M. M., Vanlint, S., Stocks, N., Mittinty, M. N., & Moseley, G. L. (2018). Exploring effect of pain education on chronic pain patients' expectation of recovery and pain intensity. *Scandinavian Journal of Pain*, *18*(2), 211–219. https://doi.org/10.1515/sjpain-2018-0023

Moseley, G. L., & Butler, D. S. (2015). Fifteen Years of Explaining Pain: The Past, Present, and Future. *The Journal of Pain*, *16*(9), 807–813. https://doi.org/10.1016/j.jpain.2015.05.005

Nijs, J., Lluch Girbés, E., Lundberg, M., Malfliet, A., & Sterling, M. (2015). Exercise therapy for chronic musculoskeletal pain: Innovation by altering pain memories. *Manual Therapy*, *20*(1), 216–220. https://doi.org/10.1016/j.math.2014.07.004

O'Sullivan, P. B., Caneiro, J. P., O'Keeffe, M., Smith, A., Dankaerts, W., Fersum, K., & O'Sullivan, K. (2018). Cognitive Functional Therapy: An Integrated Behavioral Approach for the Targeted Management of Disabling Low Back Pain. *Physical Therapy*, *98*(5), 408–423. https://doi.org/10.1093/ptj/pzy022

Sandal, L. F., Roos, E. M., Bøgesvang, S. J., & Thorlund, J. B. (2016). Pain trajectory and exercise-induced pain flares during 8 weeks of neuromuscular exercise in individuals with knee and hip pain. *Osteoarthritis and Cartilage*, *24*(4), 589–592. https://doi.org/10.1016/j.joca.2015.11.002

Smith, B. E., Hendrick, P., Smith, T. O., Bateman, M., Moffatt, F., Rathleff, M. S., Selfe, J., & Logan, P. (2017). Should exercises be painful in the management of chronic musculoskeletal pain? A systematic review and meta-analysis. *British Journal of Sports Medicine*, *51*(23), 1679–1687. https://doi.org/10.1136/bjsports-2016-097383

Smith, B. E., Hendrick, P., Bateman, M., Holden, S., Littlewood, C., Smith, T. O., & Logan, P. (2019). Musculoskeletal pain and exercise-challenging existing paradigms and introducing new. *British Journal of Sports Medicine*, *53*(14), 907–912. https://doi.org/10.1136/bjsports-2017-098983

Sullivan, A. B., Scheman, J., Venesy, D., & Davin, S. (2012). The role of exercise and types of exercise in the rehabilitation of chronic pain: Specific or nonspecific benefits. *Current Pain and Headache Reports*, *16*(2), 153–161. https://doi.org/10.1007/s11916-012-0245-3

Vlaeyen, J. W. S., & Linton, S. J. (2012). Fear-avoidance model of chronic musculoskeletal pain: 12 years on. *Pain*, *153*(6), 1144–1147. https://doi.org/10.1016/j.pain.2011.12.009

Yarnitsky, D. (2010). Conditioned pain modulation (the diffuse noxious inhibitory control-like effect): Its relevance for acute and chronic pain states. *Current Opinion in Anaesthesiology*, *23*(5), 611–615. https://doi.org/10.1097/ACO.0b013e32833c348b

GPSR Compliance

The European Union's (EU) General Product Safety Regulation (GPSR) is a set of rules that requires consumer products to be safe and our obligations to ensure this.

If you have any concerns about our products, you can contact us on ProductSafety@springernature.com

In case Publisher is established outside the EU, the EU authorized representative is:

Springer Nature Customer Service Center GmbH
Europaplatz 3
69115 Heidelberg, Germany

Batch number: 08998957

Printed by Printforce, the Netherlands